Animal Health and Nutrition

Animal Health and Nutrition

Edited by **Shawn Kiser**

SYRAWOOD
PUBLISHING HOUSE

New York

Published by Syrawood Publishing House,
750 Third Avenue, 9th Floor,
New York, NY 10017, USA
www.syrawoodpublishinghouse.com

Animal Health and Nutrition
Edited by Shawn Kiser

International Standard Book Number: 978-1-68286-145-5 (Hardback)

The publisher's policy is to use permanent paper from mills that operate a sustainable forestry policy. Furthermore, the publisher ensures that the text paper and cover boards used have met acceptable environmental accreditation standards.

Trademark Notice: Registered trademark of products or corporate names are used only for explanation and identification without intent to infringe.

Printed in the United States of America.

Contents

Permissions

List of Contributors

Preface

The main aim of this book is to educate learners and enhance their research focus by presenting diverse topics covering this vast field. This is an advanced book which compiles significant studies by distinguished experts. This book addresses successive solutions to the challenges arising in the area of application, along with it; the book provides scope for future developments.

The discipline of animal health and nutrition focuses mainly on the dietary habits and nutritional requirements of animals. This book discusses the fundamentals as well as modern approaches of animal nutrition. Latest researches on pathogens, host and microbe interactions, infectious diseases, development of vaccines, etc. are included in this book. It consists of contributions made by international experts. It will also provide a number of innovative topics for research which interested readers can take up. This book is meant for students who are looking for an elaborate reference text on animal health and nutrition.

It was a great honour to edit this book, though there were challenges, as it involved a lot of communication and networking between me and the editorial team. However, the end result was this all-inclusive book covering diverse themes in the field.

Finally, it is important to acknowledge the efforts of the contributors for their excellent chapters, through which a wide variety of issues have been addressed. I would also like to thank my colleagues for their valuable feedback during the making of this book.

Editor

Brucellosis, genital campylobacteriosis and other factors affecting calving rate of cattle in three states of Northern Nigeria

Hassan M Mai[1,2*], Peter C Irons[1] and Peter N Thompson[1]

Abstract

Background: Reproductive diseases limit the productivity of cattle worldwide and represent an important obstacle to profitable cattle enterprise. In this study, herd brucellosis and bovine genital campylobacteriosis (BGC) status, and demographic and management variables were determined and related to predicted calving rate (PrCR) of cattle herds in Adamawa, Kaduna and Kano states, Nigeria. Serum samples, preputial scrapings, questionnaire data, trans-rectal palpation and farm records were used from 271 herds. The Rose-Bengal plate test and competitive enzyme-linked immunosorbent assay were used for *Brucella* serology and culture and identification from preputial samples for BGC. A herd was classified as positive if one or more animals tested positive. The PrCR was determined as the number of calvings expected during the previous 6 and next 6 months as a percentage of the number of postpubertal heifers and cows in the herd. A multilevel linear regression model was used to estimate the herd-level effect of *Brucella abortus* seropositivity, *Campylobacter fetus* infection and other factors on calculated PrCR.

Results: The reproductive performance of the cattle herds was generally poor: Only 6.5% of the nursing cows were pregnant and 51.1% were non-pregnant and acyclic; the mean annual PrCR was 51.4%. *Brucella abortus* and *C. fetus* infection of herds were independently associated with absolute reduction in PrCR of 14.9% and 8.4%, respectively. There was also a strong negative association between within-herd *Brucella* seroprevalence and PrCR. Presence of small ruminants, animal introduction without quarantine and the presence of handling facilities were associated with lower PrCR, whereas larger herd size, supplementary feeding, routine mineral supplementation and care during parturition were associated with higher PrCR.

Conclusions: Brucellosis and BGC may be largely responsible for the poor reproductive performance of indigenous Nigerian cattle. Farmer education and measures to improve the fertility of cattle herds are suggested.

Keywords: Bovine genital campylobacteriosis, Brucellosis, Calving rate, Reproductive efficiency

Background

Cattle are the largest livestock enterprise in the agricultural sector in Nigeria, with a national herd of about 15.3 million [1]. However, the productivity and reproductive efficiency of indigenous Nigerian cattle are low [2,3]. About 95% of all food animal populations in Nigeria are in the hands of nomadic and semi-nomadic traditional farmers, who utilise relatively inefficient production systems [4]. Therefore, the causes of poor productivity need to be identified and addressed [5].

Reproductive indices reported in nomadic cattle herds in Nigeria include age at first calving of 60 months, calving interval of 17 to 24 months, annual calf crop of 40% and total lifetime number of calves produced by a cow of 2.5 [6]. Other reported indices include age at puberty of 40.2 months [7], calving to first conception of 7.8 months [8] and first service conception rate of 46.7% [9]. These indices are affected by several factors such as poor genetic material [2,3], adverse environmental factors [10], inadequate veterinary services [3], age and parity of the dam [5], inadequate nutrition [11], suckling [8], inadequate

* Correspondence: hassanmai@hotmail.com
[1]Department of Production Animal Studies, Faculty of Veterinary Science, University of Pretoria, Private Bag X04, Onderstepoort 0110, South Africa
[2]Animal Production Programme, School of Agriculture and Agricultural Technology, Abubakar Tafawa Balewa University, P. M. B. 0248, Bauchi, Nigeria

oestrus detection [12] and widespread infectious and parasitic diseases [3,13,14].

Measurement of annual calving percentage is a good measure of herd reproductive performance; however, it involves visiting the farm at least monthly for a period of one year to monitor and record calvings as they occur, and even then it depends on the farmer's records, which are often poor and inadequate, or their recall. Predicted annual calving rate (PrCR), on the other hand, is a robust indicator of breeding performance and herd fertility, taking into account the number of pregnant animals and estimated ages of foetuses based on trans-rectal palpation, as well as estimated ages of calves in the herd at a single time point [5,15,16]. It is also independent of the season in which the data are collected, which can be a confounder when other indices are used in herds with seasonal calving patterns [17]. However, single-day examination of a herd and prediction of calving rate may be prone to bias in that it cannot account for future cases of abortion and is dependent on accurate aging of pregnancies.

Brucellosis, caused by *Brucella abortus*, and bovine genital campylobacteriosis, commonly caused by *Campylobacter fetus venerealis* [18], are known to be prevalent in Nigeria and have been implicated in infertility [13,14]. They result in huge economic losses due to abortion, repeat breeding, decrease in number of calves, culling and replacing affected animals and decreased milk production due to clinical mastitis [3,13,19-22]. In contrast, studies of trichomonosis in Nigeria have revealed a low or zero prevalence [23-25]. These venereal diseases are transmitted by communal bulls in management systems commonly found in various locations across Africa [26]; however, their influence on reproductive performance has not been well studied on a herd basis in communal farming systems [27,28].

The purpose of this study was firstly to estimate the reproductive efficiency of cattle herds in Northern Nigeria, as reflected by PrCR, and secondly to investigate the effect of brucellosis, BGC, and other managemental and environmental factors, on PrCR.

Methods

This study was performed in conjunction with a survey to determine prevalence of and risk factors for brucellosis, BGC and trichomonosis in cattle herds of Northern Nigeria [23,29,30]. The research protocol was approved by the Animal Use and Care Committee and the Research Committee of the University of Pretoria (Protocol no. V073-08).

Study areas and study design

Three states, namely Adamawa, Kaduna and Kano, were selected from the 19 Northern states of Nigeria. Adamawa state is situated at 8-11°N and 11.5-13.5°E, Kaduna state at 9-11.3°N and 10.3-9.6°E, and Kano state is at 12°N and 9°E (Figure 1). All three states have Sudan or sub-Sudan savannah in the north and tropical grasslands of Guinea savannah in the south.

The study design was previously described [29]. Briefly, a cross sectional study was conducted using multistage cluster sampling. Sample size was calculated to estimate a 40% herd prevalence of brucellosis with 10% absolute precision and using a design effect of 2.8 to account for the multistage sampling design. Each of the three selected states was divided into three administrative geographical zones, and two local government areas (LGA's) were randomly selected from each zone, giving a total of six LGA's from each state, using as sampling frame a list of all LGA's in each zone. Approximately 50% of wards were randomly selected from a list of all wards in each selected LGA (Figure 1). Since no sampling frames were available for selection of herds within wards, herds were selected by visiting the farms and enrolling them as they consented to participation. An average of three herds was selected per ward, giving an average of 15 herds selected per LGA. A total of 271 herds was sampled.

Animal and herd classification

Selected herds were visited once each between July 2008 and June 2009. Herd and individual animal data collection, and animal sampling were done during this visit.

All the postpubertal bulls, postpubertal heifers, breeding bulls and cows were sampled in each selected herd. A postpubertal bull was defined as a bull that had been successfully mounting other cows or heifers by achieving intromission. A postpubertal heifer was a female that had been observed exhibiting oestrus or standing to be mounted by a bull or on trans-rectal examination had either of the functional structures, i.e. corpus luteum or follicle, on their ovaries.

Four management systems were encountered during the study. The pastoral management system was characterized by cattle grazing on fallow land close to the place of settlement of the owners during the rainy season but covering long distances, some even migrating, during the critical period of the dry season in search of natural pasture. Agro-pastoral management was characterized by cattle grazing locally and supplementation with mostly crop residues particularly during the dry and pre-rainy seasons. Commercial management systems were organized farms that were usually fenced with paddocked, improved pastures and concentrate provided as supplementary feeds. Zero-grazing systems were farms in which the cattle were confined or even tethered with restricted movement and feed was provided.

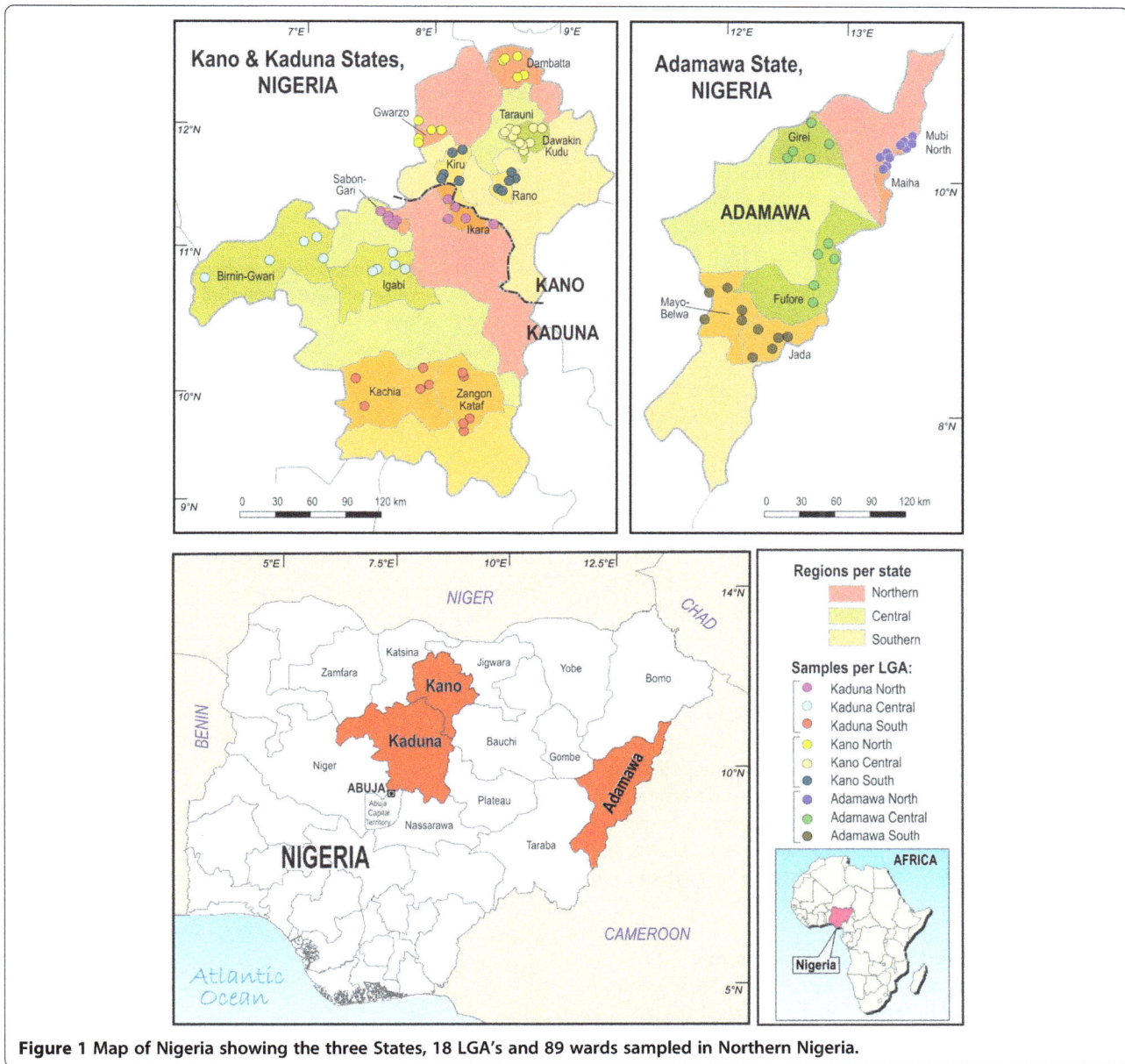

Figure 1 Map of Nigeria showing the three States, 18 LGA's and 89 wards sampled in Northern Nigeria.

Sample collection and testing for *Brucella abortus*

Animals selected for blood sampling for brucellosis were first calf heifers which had calved at least six weeks previously, cows and postpubertal heifers and bulls. About 10 ml of blood was collected from the jugular, coccygeal or saphenous veins into Vacutainer® tubes, and placed into an ice bath and transported to the laboratory for centrifugation, serum separation and storage at -20°C until ready for analysis. The Rose-Bengal plate agglutination test (RBPT) for brucellosis using RBP antigen (VLA, Weybridge, UK) and confirmation of RBPT-positive samples with competitive enzyme-linked immunosorbent assay (c-ELISA) (VLA, Weybridge, UK) were carried out

as recommended by OIE [31]. Sampling and testing methods are discussed in detail in Mai *et al.* [29], where the estimated animal-level sensitivity and specificity of the applied test system were calculated to be 87.9% and 99.8%, respectively.

Sample collection and isolation of *Campylobacter fetus* from bulls

Preputial scrapings were collected from all breeding bulls and other postpubertal bulls in the herds as described by Irons *et al.* [32] and used to isolate *C. fetus* as described by OIE [31]. At 72 h, a representative of a dew-drop colony that was Gram-negative, vibroid in shape and oxidase- and catalase-positive was transferred to a blood agar base (Oxoid, CM0055), streaked for purity and incubated under microaerophilic conditions for 72 h. Each culture and incubation was verified by using control strains of *C. f. fetus* and *C. f. venerealis* (ATCC 33247 and 19438 respectively). These isolates obtained were subjected to biochemical testing for H_2S production using TSI agar (Oxoid, CM0277B), aerobic growth, growth at 25°C and 42°C and in the presence of 1% glycine, 3.5% NaCl and sensitivity to cephalothin and nalidixic acid.

Additional data collection
Interview-based, structured questionnaires were administered to the livestock owners on each farm at the time of sample collection, in order to gather information on potential animal-level and herd-level factors affecting PrCR. As far as possible, the herdsmen were interviewed in the presence of the owner or farm manager for about 30 to 45 minutes. Interview questions were focused on events on the farm over the past 12 to 24 months. Management, herd structure, location and environmental variables with a potential impact on PrCR were recorded. The reproductive status of each animal, such as suckling/non-suckling, age and parity, as well as method of breeding, feeding, breed, etc. were obtained.

Age was estimated using farm records, dentition and, in some cases, cornual rings. Body condition score (BCS) was obtained as described by Pullan [33] and assigned by the same veterinarian for all animals. Pregnancy diagnosis, including age of foetus, and cyclicity were determined in all mature females using trans-rectal palpation as described by Arthur *et al.* [34]. All data were stored in a Microsoft Excel spreadsheet (Microsoft Corp., Redmond, WA, U.S.A.).

Determination of predicted annual calving rate
For the calculation of PrCR in each herd, the formula of Voh Jr and Otchere [5] and Stonaker *et al.* [15] was used to determine the number of animals likely to calve during a 12-month period (the previous 6 months and the next 6 months), as follows:

$$PrCR = \text{Number of calvings due in one year}$$
$$/\text{No. of postpubertal heifers and cows}$$
$$= (b + e + g + 2h + i)$$
$$/(a + b + c + d + e + f + g + h + i)$$

where:

a is the number of open, dry cows
b is the number of open cows nursing a calf under 6 months of age
c is the number of open cows nursing a calf 6 months of age and over

d is the number of pregnant dry cows under 2 months of gestation
e is the number of pregnant cows under 2 months of gestation and nursing a calf under 6 months of age
f is the number of pregnant cows under 2 months of gestation and nursing a calf 6 months of age and over
g is the number of pregnant dry cows at 2 months of gestation and over

Table 1 Herd structure, breed, management system and reproductive status of cattle sampled from three states of Northern Nigeria

Variables and categories	Total	Proportion of group (%)
Herd structure		
Bulls	602	6.0
Heifers	1,134	11.3
Cows	3,068	30.4
Bull calves and growers	1,285	12.8
Young bulls	1,038	10.3
Heifer calves and growers	1,276	12.7
Young heifers	1,663	16.5
Total[a]	10,066	
Breed		
Bunaji	3,097	64.4
Gudali	870	18.1
Other *Bos indicus*	448	9.3
Bos taurus	120	2.5
B. taurus x *B. indicus*	272	5.7
Total[b]	4,807	
Management system		
Pastoral	1,263	26.3
Agro-pastoral	2,793	58.1
Commercial	650	13.5
Zero-grazing	101	2.1
Total[b]	4,807	
Reproductive status		
Suckling	1,818	43.3
Non-pregnant	1,545	36.8
Cyclic	609	14.5
Non-cyclic	936	22.3
Pregnant	273	6.5
Non-Suckling	2,384	56.7
Non-pregnant	1,290	30.7
Pregnant	1,094	26.0
Total[c]	4,202	

[a]Total number of animals in the sampled herds.
[b]Number of mature animals.
[c]Number of mature females.

Table 2 Reproductive status of heifers sampled from the three states of Northern Nigeria

Age (years)	Cyclic	Acyclic or reproductive problem	Pregnant	Total
< 2	2	5	0	7
2	21 (21.2)	65 (65.7)	13 (13.1)	99
3	208 (54.6)	92 (23.1)	81 (21.3)	381
4	212 (44.2)	54 (11.3)	214 (44.6)	480
5	54 (36.2)	10 (6.7)	85 (57.0)	149
6	1	10	2	13
7	0	5	0	5
Total	498	241	395	1134

h is the number of pregnant cows at 2 months of gestation and over and nursing a calf under 6 months of age

i is the number of pregnant cows at 2 months of gestation and over and nursing a calf 6 months of age and over.

The numerator for calculating annual PrCR therefore includes calves of 6 months of age or less (*b*, *e* and *h*) and all females which were pregnant on trans-rectal palpation, i.e. were more than 2 months in calf (*g*, *h* and *i*). This was considered the best period to choose as the pregnancy diagnosis results were accurate (carried out by an experienced veterinary surgeon and theriogenologist)

and most farmers/herdsmen could remember calves of less than 6 months old [5,15,16]. The '*h*' group was likely to produce two calves in one year and was therefore counted twice.

Statistical analysis

The unit of analysis was the herd and the outcome variable was the PrCR. Each independent variable (brucellosis, BGC and the management and environmental variables) was tested for bivariable association with the outcome using Student's *t*-test or ANOVA. Variables associated with the outcome at $P < 0.2$ were selected for the multivariable model. A multilevel, mixed-effects linear regression model with state as a fixed effect and nested random effects for LGA and ward was then constructed. Backward elimination was applied until all remaining variables were significant ($P < 0.05$), after which all other predictor variables were tested by adding them back into the model and retained if significant. Significance of the random effects for LGA and ward was assessed by comparing models with and without random effects using a likelihood ratio test. Fit of the final model was evaluated using a plot of residuals versus fitted values and a normal probability plot of residuals. The association between within-herd *Brucella* seroprevalence and PrCR was also determined. All statistical analyses were done using STATA 12 (Stata Corporation, College Station, TX, USA) and a significance level of $\alpha = 0.05$ was used.

Table 3 Age and parity of cattle sampled from three states of Northern Nigeria

Age (years)	Parity 0	1	2	3	4	5	6	7	8	9	10	Total
<2	7	0	0	0	0	0	0	0	0	0	0	7
2	99	4	0	0	0	0	0	0	0	0	0	103
3	381	46	0	0	0	0	0	0	0	0	0	427
4	480	241	21	0	0	0	0	0	0	0	0	742
5	149	581	131	40	2	0	0	0	0	0	0	903
6	13	284	285	65	21	0	0	0	0	0	0	668
7	5	50	204	107	25	6	0	0	0	0	0	397
8	0	6	91	143	57	10	2	0	0	0	0	309
9	0	2	6	78	50	22	5	1	0	0	0	164
10	0	0	6	33	50	36	7	1	0	0	0	133
11	0	0	1	8	14	13	8	6	1	0	0	51
12	0	0	0	6	7	15	9	10	6	1	0	54
13	0	0	0	0	0	2	3	3	1	1	0	10
14	0	0	0	0	1	0	0	0	0	0	1	2
15	0	0	0	0	0	0	0	0	1	3	4
Total	1134	1214	745	480	227	104	34	21	8	3	4	3974
% of total	28.5	30.5	18.7	12.1	5.7	2.6	0.9	0.5	0.2	0.1	0.1	

Table 4 Bivariable analysis of categorical predictors for predicted calving rate in herds in three states of Northern Nigeria

Predictor and level	No. tested	Calving rate (%) Mean	SD	P-value
Brucella infection[a]				<0.001
No	59	76.8	9.2	
Yes	192	43.6	21.8	
Campylobacter fetus infection[a]				<0.001
No	166	57.3	22.2	
Yes	66	33.1	18.0	
State[a]				0.033
Adamawa	87	46.1	23.5	
Kaduna	98	55.2	22.8	
Kano	66	52.7	25.8	
Method of breeding[a]				0.026
AI and natural mating	44	52.5	24.0	
AI only	11	70.1	25.0	
Natural mating only	196	50.1	23.8	
Use of AI[a]				0.11
No	196	50.1	23.8	
Yes	55	56.0	25.0	
Management system[a]				<0.001
Zero-grazing	3	76.2	12.3	
Commercial	26	66.2	25.4	
Agro-pastoral	146	58.1	21.3	
Pastoral	76	32.6	17.3	
Supplementary feeding[a]				<0.001
None	25	21.9	7.6	
Fodder/bran	105	46.3	22.1	
Concentrate	121	62.0	21.5	
Mineral supplementation[a]				<0.001
No	69	32.2	17.6	
Yes	182	58.7	22.2	
Pasture establishment[a]				0.122
No	187	50.0	23.8	
Yes	64	55.5	24.9	
Water source[a]				<0.001
Piped	69	63.2	21.2	
Natural flowing	112	46.6	22.5	
Natural static	70	47.6	25.8	
Housing[a]				<0.001
Open barbed wire	153	46.4	23.3	
Open half way and roofed	66	63.1	24.6	
Open solid enclosure	32	51.5	18.9	

Table 4 Bivariable analysis of categorical predictors for predicted calving rate in herds in three states of Northern Nigeria *(Continued)*

Hygiene/floor type[a]				<0.001
Floored	63	63.1	23.0	
Unfloored/natural bear earth	188	47.5	23.3	
Isolation and observation of the cow during parturition and removal of afterbirth[a]				<0.001
No	94	35.1	19.1	
Yes	154	61.4	21.4	
Regular herd prophylactic measures[a]				<0.001
No	97	40.0	22.1	
Yes	154	58.6	22.5	
Borrow/share bull[a]				<0.001
No	166	60.4	21.8	
Yes	85	33.9	18.2	
Presence of small ruminants[a]				<0.001
No	97	65.6	19.5	
Yes	154	42.5	22.5	
Presence of dogs[a]				0.036
No	227	52.9	24.5	
Yes	24	37.5	13.7	
Presence of chickens[a]				0.0002
No	161	55.7	23.3	
Yes	90	43.8	23.9	
Multiple herds[a]				0.013
No	166	54.1	23.6	
Yes	85	46.1	25.3	
Purpose of keeping animals[a]				0.0002
Small scale local dairy	187	52.5	24.1	
Dairy and Beef	29	61.3	23.2	
Beef	35	37.5	18.9	
Initial purchase of stock from a market[a]				<0.001
Inherited	118	55.1	24.0	
Other farms	14	71.5	21.2	
Market	119	45.4	27.7	
Buying-in new animals and quarantine[a]				<0.001
Buy <3 + quarantine	30	68.4	11.8	
Buy >3 or no quarantine	147	38.3	20.2	
Close herd	74	70.6	15.9	
Socio-economic status of farmer[a]				0.031
Full-time	176	53.6	23.7	
Part-time	75	46.4	24.9	
Specialist attending to animals[a]				<0.001
No	48	32.6	17.9	

Table 4 Bivariable analysis of categorical predictors for predicted calving rate in herds in three states of Northern Nigeria *(Continued)*

Yes	203	55.9	23.3	
Presence of crush/local chute or other means of handling/restrain at the farm[a]				0.061
No	187	49.8	23.9	
Yes	64	56.3	24.9	

[a]Variable significant (P < 0.20) for calving rate and therefore considered in the multivariable model.

Results

Herd structure

The structure of the 271 herds sampled is shown in Table 1. The average bull: female ratio was one mature male to eight mature females. The herd size ranged between 7 and 119 animals (median: 34; interquartile range (IQR): 25, 43).

Reproductive parameters

Because a few herds had no postpubertal heifers or cows, PrCR could be calculated for only 251 herds. The mean annual PrCR was 51.4%, ranging between 0% and 100%, while the pregnancy rate, defined as the proportion of cows and postpubertal heifers that were pregnant, was 32.5%.

Reproductive status and BCS

A total of 4,202 females consisting of 1,134 heifers and 3,068 cows were studied. The proportion suckling, and pregnancy and cyclicity status are shown in Table 1. The BCS ranged from 2 to 5 (median: 3; IQR: 3, 4). Using two categories of BCS (≤ 3 and ≥ 3.5), there was a significant difference in the BCS between cyclic and non-cyclic cows ($P < 0.0001$) and between suckling and non-suckling cows ($P < 0.0001$) (data not shown).

Reproductive status of heifers and parity of cows and heifers

The reproductive performance records of heifers indicated that at <2 years some heifers started cycling; peak cyclicity (55%) and pregnancy (57%) were attained at 3 and 5 years respectively. The median age at puberty was between 2 and 3 years (Table 2). Table 3 shows the distribution of parity by age. The median age at first calving was between 4 and 5 years.

Number of calves per cow lifetime in the herd and productive life of the cows

A total of 2,840 cows were examined for which we had complete information about their ages (Table 3). The cows had produced a total of 6,054 calves, i.e. 2.1 calves produced/cow. Furthermore, Table 3 shows that very few animals were kept beyond 10 years.

Factors associated with PrCR

The distribution of the various environmental and managemental factors and their bivariable association with PrCR at the herd level are shown in Table 4. The crude absolute difference in PrCR between *Brucella* positive and *Brucella* negative herds was 33.2%, while that between *C. fetus* positive and *C. fetus* negative herds was 24.2%. All of the 59 herds that were *Brucella* negative had a PrCR of over 50%, while 124/192 (65%) of the *Brucella* positive herds had a PrCR of <50% (Figure 2). The mean PrCR for *Brucella* positive, *Brucella* negative, *C. fetus* positive and *C. fetus* negative herds were 43.6%, 76.8%, 33.1% and 57.3% respectively. In addition, there was a strong negative association between within-herd *Brucella* seroprevalence and PrCR ($P < 0.001$) (Figure 3).

The final regression model of factors associated with PrCR is shown in Table 5. The random effects for LGA and ward were not significant and therefore the normal multiple regression model without random effects was used. The residuals were normally distributed and the residual vs. fitted plot showed no evidence of non-linearity or heteroscedasticity. After adjustment for confounding by the other variables in the model, *Brucella* herd infection was associated with an absolute reduction in PrCR of 14.9%. In addition to this, *C. fetus* herd infection was associated with a further reduction in PrCR of 8.4%.

Herds that gave fodder and bran were associated with 6.5% higher PrCR ($P = 0.044$) and herds that gave concentrate with 7.9% higher PrCR ($P = 0.037$) than herds that did not. In addition, mineral supplementation and isolation and observation of cows during parturition and removal of afterbirth were associated with higher PrCR than herds in which these practices were absent. Furthermore, the presence of small ruminants, the presence of a handling facility and the introduction of new animals, particularly the introduction of >3 animals without quarantine, were significantly associated with lower PrCR in such herds (Table 5). Herd size was initially not significant in the bivariable analysis but after adding it to the final model and adjusting for other variables there was a significant positive association with PrCR.

Discussion

Reproductive indices are vital in the determination and management of herd fertility. It is apparent from this study that several factors are responsible for poor reproductive efficiency of cattle in Northern Nigeria. Previous studies on the reproductive performance of cattle in traditional herds in Northern Nigeria are more than two decades old [5] and there is a lack of data quantifying the impact of infectious causes of infertility [13,14]. This report provides current information on reproductive efficiency and factors affecting calving rates in cattle in

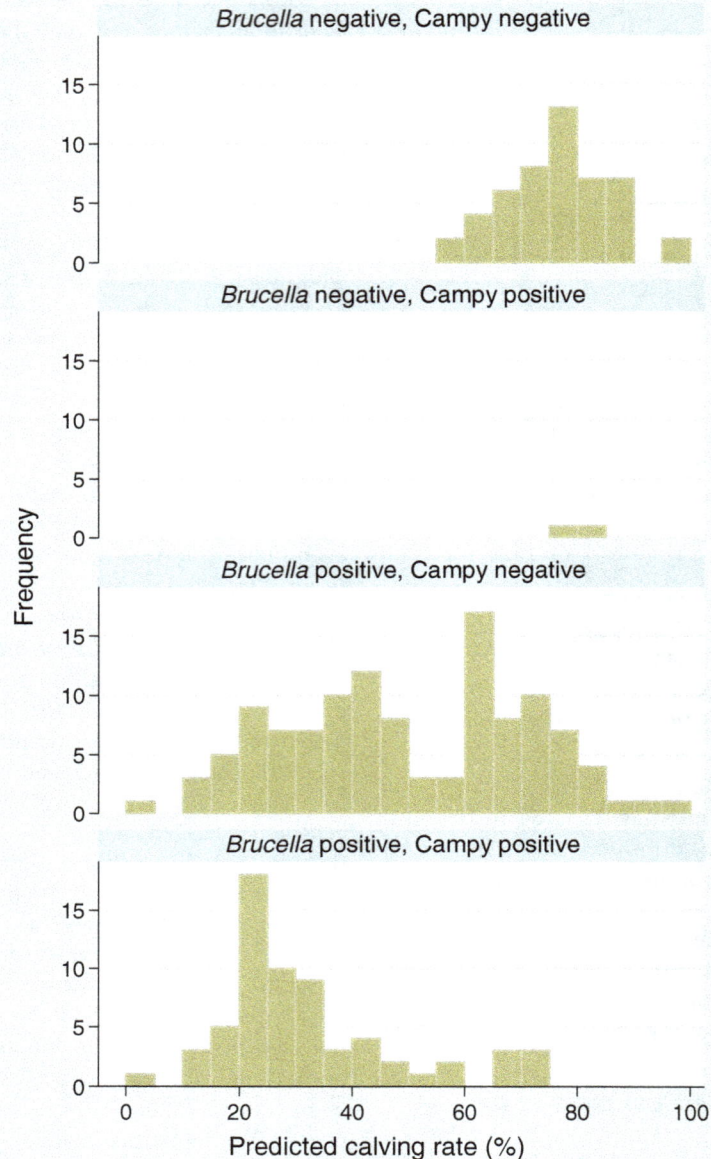

Figure 2 Predicted calving rate in *Brucella abortus* positive and negative herds, and *Campylobacter fetus* positive and negative herds in three states of Northern Nigeria.

Nigeria. It is the only report that considers various management systems in one study.

The average herd size of 37 in agro-pastoral production systems obtained in this study is similar to 38.3 reported by Voh Jr and Otchere [5] in agro-pastoral herds; but the herd size of 34.1 in pastoral herds (data not shown) is lower than 45.9 reported by Otchere [35] in the same management system.

From the global perspective, the previous few decades have witnessed a steady rise in bovine infertility [36]. The overall calving rate of 51.4% found in this study is similar to the 52 to 55% calving rate reported in Colombia [15] and the 55% observed by Voh Jr and Otchere [5] in the traditional agro-pastoral system in Nigeria. The pregnancy rate of 32.5% in this study is lower than the 42% reported by Voh Jr and Otchere [5]. Nevertheless, our study does not provide conclusive evidence to support a decline in fertility of the study population in Northern Nigeria.

It is apparent from this study that brucellosis and BGC have a significant impact on PrCR, and that there

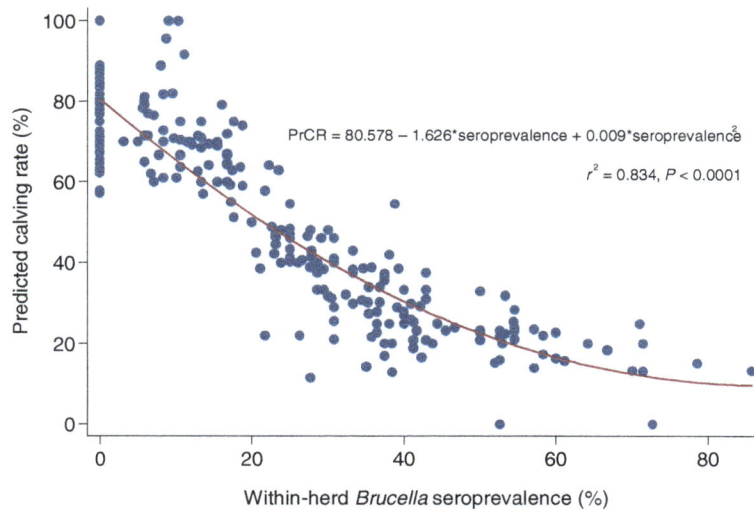

Figure 3 Scatter plot of predicted calving rate (PrCR) vs. within-herd *Brucella* seroprevalence, with least squares quadratic fit, in cattle sampled from three states of Northern Nigeria.

is a clear negative relationship between within-herd *Brucella* seroprevalence and PrCR. The outcome of brucellosis such as abortion, retained afterbirth, stillbirth and birth of weak calves or calf mortality affect the overall calving rate of infected herds. This tends to agree with reports by Aguair *et al.* [37] and Degefa *et al.* [38]. It is also consistent with the report that a 10% decrease in the number of calves was observed in *Brucella* positive cows [19]. Bovine genital campylobacteriosis causes similar clinical signs and therefore may be associated with infertility thereby lowering calving rate and other reproductive indices [39,40]. Due to the fact that almost all *C. fetus* positive herds were also positive for *Brucella*, it was not possible to accurately quantify the impact of BGC alone. However, a combination of brucellosis and BGC was associated with poorer PrCR in this study than brucellosis alone (Figure 2), which would suggest that BGC has an additional negative effect. Despite this, our data confirm that it is possible to maintain good calving rate with only brucellosis or BGC infections, and even with both infections present a PrCR in excess of 70% is possible, provided that the within-herd seroprevalence of brucellosis is below about 20% (Figure 3). The fact that females often abort once and following that they reproduce normally in the case of brucellosis, and the acquired immunity conferred by *C. fetus* challenge, may explain the acceptable PrCR observed in some infected herds.

Although management system was not significant in the multivariable analysis of PrCR, the model showed that the observed difference in PrCR between the management systems was partially accounted for by the other variables in the multivariable model. In the bivariable analysis, the PrCR differed significantly between the

various management systems ($P < 0.001$). The crude PrCR being lowest in the pastoral system may be as a result of the movement of the pastoral Fulani herdsmen and interaction of their cattle with other Fulani herdsmen particularly at watering points during the dry season which may expose them to infection thereby lowering the PrCR. In previously published data from the same study we showed that the presence of brucellosis was positively associated with the pastoral management system [29].

It was shown from this study that providing supplementary feeding and mineral supplementation were associated with higher PrCR, as were the isolation and observation of cows during parturition and removal of the afterbirth, and the presence of a handling facility were associated with lower PrCR. Such effects may be by proxy, in that the education level of the herd owner, availability of other sources of income, focus on other activities may all have impact on the general level of management, condition and health of the herd. Likewise, larger herd size is likely to be associated with increased animal movements, with the associated increased risk of contact with infectious agents. Indeed, farmers that introduced > 3 animals without quarantine were found to have 15% lower PrCR than farmers that did not. In the initial crude analysis, the association with herd size was obscured due to confounding; in the multivariable analysis PrCR was significantly associated with herd size, with larger herds having higher PrCR. The reason for this is not clear. The commercial and zero-grazing herds showed higher PrCR but had smaller herd sizes.

It was observed that over 61% of the multiple herd owners introduced >3 animals without quarantine in their herds. This is a risky practice due to the potential for

Table 5 Factors associated with predicted calving rate in cattle herds in Northern Nigeria: results of a multiple linear regression model

Risk factor and level	Coefficient	95% CI	P- value
Brucella infection			
No	1	-	-
Yes	-14.9	-20.01, -9.62	<0.001
Campylobacter fetus infection			
No			
Yes	-8.41	-12.93, -3.88	<0.001
State			
Adamawa	1	-	-
Kaduna	1.76	-2.84, 6.35	0.452
Kano	-0.24	-5.40, 4.92	0.928
Supplementary feeding			
None	1	-	-
Fodder and bran	6.54	0.46, 12.63	0.044
Concentrate	7.86	0.46, 15.30	0.037
Mineral supplementation			
No	1		
Yes	6.45	1.71, 11.20	0.008
Isolation and observation of cow during parturition and removal of afterbirth			
No	1		
Yes	7.54	3.09, 11.98	0.001
Small ruminants			
No	1	-	-
Yes	-7.81	-12.41, -3.22	0.001
Buy in new animals			
Closed herd	1	-	-
Buy <3 + quarantine	-6.44	-12.53, -0.38	0.038
Buy >3 or no quarantine	-15.23	-20.31, -10.16	<0.001
Presence of crush, chute or other form of restraint on the farm			
No	1	-	-
Yes	-9.97	-16.08, -3.76	0.002
Herd size			
≤ 15	1	-	
> 15	4.98	1.17, 8.80	0.011

introducing infections that may lower the calving rate. Reports indicate that ownership of multiple herds potentially increases the risk of a herd being infected with brucellosis [41], which may also affect the calving rate.

Herds that had small ruminants had significantly lower PrCR. Cross infection of infectious reproductive diseases may be possible between species thereby lowering the PrCR. This tends to agree with findings by Megersa *et al.* [19] regarding mixed herds/flocks. The association between presence of a handling facility and lower PrCR may be due to the fact that such farmers may be likely to share their facilities with other farmers, leading to increased contact with other herds.

The median age at puberty observed in this study (2 to 3 years) is shorter than reports by Mukasa-Mugerwa [3] who showed average age at puberty of *Bos indicus* as 40 months. However, the median age at first calving agreed with estimates of 4 to 5 years reported by Voh Jr and Otchere [5] and 5 years by Zemjanis [6]. In addition, the reported age at first calving in indigenous tropical cattle of between 3 and 5 years, between 4 and 7 years for the second time and between 5 and 8 years for the third [42] are consistent with our findings. This study also revealed that age at first calving in cattle in Northern Nigeria can also be as low as 2 to 3 years, meaning that some animals attained puberty and conceived at about 1 to 2 years old. Oyedipe *et al.* [11] indicated that under improved management where seasonal nutritional stress is reduced, it is possible to achieve average age at first calving a little over 3 years.

The previously reported reproductive lifespan of cattle in Northern Nigeria of up to 10 years [5] is consistent with our findings. Almost all of the cows had been culled by the age of 10 years. We can therefore conclude from this finding that the productive life of cattle in this study area is up to 10 years. The low lifetime number of calves per cow may be attributed to late age at first calving, long calving intervals and early culling age. It is an underestimation of true lifetime production in that it includes animals which are still in the productive state. Suckling and nutrition are in a large part responsible for this reproductive inefficiency [5].

Body condition score is a management tool that has proved useful in the assessment of the nutritional status of dairy and beef cows [43,44]. Poor BCS of cows, mainly caused by poor management, was also considered to play a major role in reducing pregnancy rates [45]; their results further suggest that an abrupt loss of nutritional status postpartum can impair uterine involution, and cause pregnancy failure in the early foetal development period when the placentomes develop. In addition, a one unit reduction in BCS from previous partum to 30 days postpartum resulted in a 2.4-fold increase in pregnancy loss [45]. Highly significant associations between BCS and pregnancy status ($P < 0.0001$) and BCS and cyclicity status ($P < 0.0001$) were observed in this study.

The limitations to this study were that the determination of age at puberty and age at first calving relied on observations of the farmers and herdsmen who are mostly uneducated, and on the herd size, the management system, etc. These may introduce some bias to the study.

Conclusion

The reproductive performance of the cattle herds studied in Northern Nigeria was generally poor. *Brucella abortus* and *C. fetus* infections were associated with reduced PrCR. In addition, presence of small ruminants, lack of quarantine and presence of handling facility were also associated with lower PrCR. Suckling and nutrition contributed to the high prevalence of anoestrus. However, improved feeding, attention during parturition and herd size improved the PrCR. Herd health management programmes, proper feeding and care during parturition should be encouraged while failure to quarantine, sharing handling facilities and mixing herds with small ruminants should be avoided.

Abbreviations

BCS: Body condition score; BGC: Bovine genital campylobacteriosis; c-ELISA: Competitive enzyme-linked immunosorbent assay; IQR: Interquartile range; LGA: Local government area; RBPT: Rose-Bengal plate agglutination test; PrCR: Predicted calving rate.

Competing interests

The authors declare that they do not have any competing interests.

Authors' contributions

HMM conceived and designed the project, conducted blood and preputial samples collection and administration of questionnaires, involved in RBPT and c-ELISA testing of the serum, culture and isolation of preputial samples, performed data analysis and write-up of the manuscript. PNT was the major supervisor and project leader; he participated in data analysis, interpretation, and editing. PCI was co-supervisor, involved in organizing the data and helped in revision of the manuscript. All the authors read and approved the final manuscript.

Authors' information

HMM has a DVM, MSc and PhD in Theriogenology, Department of Production Animal Studies, Faculty of Veterinary Science, University of Pretoria. PNT has a BVSc, MMedVet and PhD and is Professor of Veterinary Epidemiology in the Department of Production Animal Studies, Faculty of Veterinary Science, University of Pretoria. PCI has a BVSc, MMedVet and PhD, is a Diplomate of the American College of Theriogenologists and a Professor in Theriogenology, Department of Production Animal Studies, Faculty of Veterinary Science, University of Pretoria.

Acknowledgement

The authors are grateful to Drs. J Kabir, MA Qadeers and DJU Kalla for their contributions and to those that assisted in sample collection, laboratory analysis and preparation of the map. The partial funding by the Department of Production Animal Studies, University of Pretoria is appreciated.

References

1. Anon: Animal population. World Animal Health Information Database (WAHID). 2011.
2. Pullan NB. Productivity of white Fulani cattle in Jos Plateau, Nigeria. II. Nutritional factors. Trop Anim Health Prod. 1979;12:17–24.
3. Mukasa-Mugerwa E: A review of reproductive performance of female *Bos indicus* (Zebu) Cattle. ILCA Monograph No.6. 1989.
4. Rikin UM. Brucellosis of cattle in Nigeria. Proposals for a control under intensive and extensive husbandry systems. Acta Vet Scand. 1988;84 (Suppl):95–7.
5. Voh Jr AA, Otchere EO. Reproductive performance of Zebu cattle under traditional agro-pastoral management in Northern Nigeria. Anim Reprod Sci. 1989;19:191–203.
6. Zemjanis R: Veterinarians and animal production in Nigeria. A Paper presented at the Annual meeting of the Nigerian Veterinary Medical Association. Nigeria: Port-Harcourt; 25-28th September, 1974.
7. Knudson PM, Sohael AS. The Vom herd: a study of the performance of a mixed Friesian/Zebu herd in a tropical environment. Trop Agric (Trinidad). 1970;47:189–203.
8. Eduvie LO, Dawuda PM. Effect of suckling on reproductive activities of Bunaji cows during the postpartum period. J Agric Sci Cambridge. 1986;107:235–8.
9. Voh Jr AA, Buvanendran V, Oyedipe EO. Artificial insemination of indigenous Nigerian cattle following synchronization of oestrus with PGF2& 1. Preliminary fertility trial. Brit Vet J. 1987;143:136–42.
10. Mai HM. Some environmental and physiological factors affecting fertility rates in artificially inseminated cattle herds. MSc thesis. Ahmadu Bello University, Zaria, Nigeria: Veterinary Surgery and Medicine Department; 1997.
11. Oyedipe EO, Osori DIK, Akerejola O, Saror D. Effects of levels of nutrition on onset of puberty and conception rates of Zebu heifers. Theriogenology. 1982;18:525–39.
12. Mai HM, Ogwu D, Eduvie LO, Voh Jr AA. Detection of oestrus in Bunaji cows under field conditions. Trop Anim Health Prod. 2002;34:35–47.
13. Mshelia GD, Amin JD, Egwu GO, Yavari CA, Murray RD, Woldehiwet Z. Detection of antibodies specific to *Campylobacter fetus* subsp. *venerealis* in the vaginal mucous of Nigerian breeding cows. Vet Ital. 2010;46:337–44.
14. Ocholi RA, Kwaga JKP, Ajogi I, Bale JO. Phenotypic characterization of *Brucella* strains isolated from livestock in Nigeria. Vet Microbiol. 2004;103:47–53.
15. Stonaker HH, Villar J, Osorio G, Salazar J. Differences among cattle and farms as related to beef cow reproduction in the Eastern plains of Colombia. Trop Anim Health Prod. 1976;8:147–54.
16. Reed JBH, Doxey DL, Forbes AB, Finlay RS, Geering IW, Smith SD, et al. Productive performance of cattle in Botswana. Trop Anim Health Prod. 1974;6:1–21.
17. Fahey J, O'Sullivan K, Crilly J, Mee JF. The effect of feeding and management practices on calving rate in dairy herds. Anim Reprod Sci. 2002;74:133–50.
18. Schmidt T, Venter EH, Picard JA. Evaluation of PCR assays for the detection of *Campylobacter fetus* and identification of subspecies in South African. J S Afr Vet Assoc. 2010;81:87.
19. Megersa B, Biffa D, Abunna F, Regassa A, Godfroid J, Skjerve E. Seroprevalence of brucellosis and its contribution to abortion in cattle, camel, and goat kept under pastoral management in Borana, Ethiopia. Trop Anim Health Prod. 2011;43:651–6.
20. Esuruoso GO. Current status of brucellosis in Nigeria and preliminary evaluation of probable cost and benefit of proposed brucellosis control programme for the country. In: Geemwy WA, editor. Proceedings of the Second International Symposium on Veterinary Epidemiology and Economics. Canberra: Australian Government Publishing Services; 1979. p. 644–9.
21. Akhtar A, Riemann HP, Thurmond MC, Franti CE. The association between antibody titres against *Campylobacter fetus* and milk production efficiency in dairy cattle. Vet Res Commun. 1993;17:183–91.
22. Bawa EK, Adekeye JO, Oyedipe EO, Umoh JU. Prevalence of bovine campylobacteriosis in indigenous cattle of three states in Nigeria. Trop Anim Health Prod. 1991;23:157–60.
23. Mai HM, Irons PC, Kabir J, Thompson PN. Prevalence of genital campylobacteriosis and trichomonosis of bulls in Northern Nigeria. Acta Vet Scand. 2013;55:56.
24. Adeyeye AA, Ate IU, Bale JO, Lawal AI. A survey for bovine trichomoniasis in cattle at slaughter in the Sokoto metropolitan abattoir, Sokoto state, Nigeria. Sokoto J Vet Sci. 2011;8:18–21.
25. Akinboade OA. Incidence of Bovine Trichomoniasis in Nigeria. Rev Elev Med Vet Pays Trop. 1980;33(4):381–4.
26. Tekleye B, Kasali OB, Mukawa-Mugerwa E, Scholtens RG, Yigzaw T: Infertility problems of cattle in Africa. Proceedings of the 6th Tanzania Veterinary Association Scientific Conference. Arusha: Tanzania; 5th-7th December, 1988:152.
27. Njiro SM, Kidanemariam AG, Tsotetsi AM, Katsande TC, Mnisi M, Lubisi BA, et al. A study of some infectious causes of reproductive disorders in cattle owned by resource-poor farmers in Gauteng Province, South Africa. J S Afr Vet Assoc. 2011;82:213–8.

28. Mokantla E, McCrindle CME, Sebei JP, Owen R. An investigation in to the causes of low calving percentage in communally grazed cattle in Jericho, North West Province. J S Afr Vet Assoc. 2004;75:30–6.

29. Mai HM, Irons PC, Kabir J, Thompson PN. A large seroprevalence survey of brucellosis in cattle herds under diverse production systems in Northern Nigeria. BMC Vet Res. 2012;8:144.

30. Mai HM, Irons PC, Kabir J, Thompson PN. Herd-level risk factors for *Campylobacter fetus* infection, *Brucella* seropositivity and within-herd seroprevalence of brucellosis in cattle in Northern Nigeria. Prev Vet Med. 2013;111:256–67.

31. OIE. Manual of Diagnostic Tests and Vaccines for Terrestrial Animals. Paris, France: World Organization for Animal Health; 2011. http://www.oie.int/manual-of-diagnostic-tests-and-vaccines-for-terrestrial-animals/.

32. Irons PC, Schutte AP, Van Der Walt ML, Bishop GC. Genital Campylobacteriosis in cattle. In: Coetzer JAW, Thompson G, Tustin RC, editors. Infectious Diseases of Livestock. 3rd ed. South Africa: Oxford University Press; 2004. p. 1459–68.

33. Pullan NB. Condition scoring of white Fulani cattle. Trop Anim Health Prod. 1978;10:118–20.

34. Arthur GH, Noakes DE, Pearson H, Parkinson TJ. Veterinary Reproduction and Obstetrics. 7th ed. Philadelphia: W.B. Saunders; 1996.

35. Otchere EO. Traditional Cattle Production in the Subhumid Zone of Nigeria. In: von Kaufmann R, Chater S, Blench R, editors. Livestock Systems Research in Nigeria's Subhumid Zone. Addis Ababa: International Livestock Center for Africa; 1986. p. 110–40.

36. Lopez-Gatius F. Is fertility declining in dairy cattle? A retrospective study in northeastern Spain. Theriogenology. 2003;60:89–99.

37. Aguiar DM, Cavalcante GT, Labruna MB, Vasconcellos SA, Rodrigues AAR, Morais ZM, et al. Risk factors and seroprevalence of *Brucella* spp. in cattle from western Amazon, Brazil. Arq Inst Biol. 2007;74:301–5.

38. Degefa T, Duressa A, Duguma R. Brucellosis and some reproductive problems of indigenous Arsi cattle in selected Arsi zones of Oromia regional state, Ethiopia. Global Vet. 2011;7:45–53.

39. Campero CM, Anderson ML, Walker RL, Blanchard PC, BarBano L, Chiu P, et al. Immunohistochemical identification of *Campylobacter fetus* in natural cases of bovine and ovine abortions. J Vet Med B. 2005;52:138–41.

40. Jimenez DF, Perez AM, Carpenter TE, Martinez A. Factors associated with infection by *Campylobacter fetus* in beef herds in the Province of Buenos Aires, Argentina. Prev Vet Med. 2011;101:157–62.

41. Richey EJ, Harrell CD: *Brucella abortus* disease (brucellosis) in beef cattle. IFAS Extension: University of Florida; 1997:1-6. http://www.agro.uba.ar/users/catala/Informacion%20Brucelosis/brucellosis%201.pdf.

42. Wilson RT. Livestock production in central Mali: Reproductive aspects of sedentary cows. Anim Reprod Sci. 1985;9:1–9.

43. Hady PJ, Demecq JJ, Kaneene JB. Frequency and precision of body condition scoring in dairy cattle. J Dairy Sci. 1994;77:1543–7.

44. Montiel F, Ahuja C. Body condition and suckling as factors influencing the duration of postpartum anestrus in cattle: a review. Anim Reprod Sci. 2005;85:1–26.

45. Lopez-Gatius F, Santolaria P, Yaniz J, Rutllant J, Lopez-Bejar M. Factors affecting pregnancy loss from gestation day 38 to 90 in lactating dairy cows from a single herd. Theriogenology. 2002;57:1251–61.

2

Epidermolysis bullosa in Danish Hereford calves is caused by a deletion in *LAMC2* gene

Leonardo Murgiano[1], Natalie Wiedemar[1], Vidhya Jagannathan[1], Louise K Isling[2], Cord Drögemüller[1] and Jørgen S Agerholm[2,3]*

Abstract

Background: Heritable forms of epidermolysis bullosa (EB) constitute a heterogeneous group of skin disorders of genetic aetiology that are characterised by skin and mucous membrane blistering and ulceration in response to even minor trauma. Here we report the occurrence of EB in three Danish Hereford cattle from one herd.

Results: Two of the animals were necropsied and showed oral mucosal blistering, skin ulcerations and partly loss of horn on the claws. Lesions were histologically characterized by subepidermal blisters and ulcers. Analysis of the family tree indicated that inbreeding and the transmission of a single recessive mutation from a common ancestor could be causative. We performed whole genome sequencing of one affected calf and searched all coding DNA variants. Thereby, we detected a homozygous 2.4 kb deletion encompassing the first exon of the *LAMC2* gene, encoding for laminin gamma 2 protein. This loss of function mutation completely removes the start codon of this gene and is therefore predicted to be completely disruptive. The deletion co-segregates with the EB phenotype in the family and absent in normal cattle of various breeds. Verifying the homozygous private variants present in candidate genes allowed us to quickly identify the causative mutation and contribute to the final diagnosis of junctional EB in Hereford cattle.

Conclusions: Our investigation confirms the known role of laminin gamma 2 in EB aetiology and shows the importance of whole genome sequencing in the analysis of rare diseases in livestock.

Keywords: Cattle, Epidermolysis bullosa, Laminin gamma 2, Hereditary, Congenital, Skin

Background

Heritable forms of epidermolysis bullosa (EB) constitute a heterogeneous group of skin disorders of genetic aetiology that are characterised by skin and mucous membrane blistering and ulceration in response to even minor trauma. EB is classified into four major types based on the level of blister formation in the dermo-epidermal interface, i.e. within the epidermis, basement membrane zone or uppermost dermis. In EB simplex, blisters develop within the epidermis, while for junctional and dystrophic EB cleavage occurs in the lamina lucida or below the lamina densa, respectively. The fourth major type, Kindler Syndrome, is characterized by blisters in the lamina lucida and below the lamina densa. In humans, many subtypes of which some have extracutaneous lesions have been identified [1-4].

In contrast to the situation in man, where more than 1000 mutations in at least 18 genes encoding structural proteins have been associated with EB and thousands of EB patients have been thoroughly diagnosed [3,4], rather few cases have been characterized to the molecular level in domestic animals. In cattle, EB simplex was associated with a mutation in *keratin 5* [5] and dystrophic EB was associated with *COL7A1* mutations in cattle [6] and dogs [7] while junctional EB has been diagnosed in sheep (*LAMC2* mutation) [8], horses (*LAMC2* and *LAMA3* mutations) [9-11], and dogs (*LAMA3* mutation) [12]. In addition to these, genetically uncharacterized EB cases in animals have been reported [13].

In addition to genetically characterised cases in crossbred Holstein calves [5] and Rotes Höhenvieh cattle [6],

* Correspondence: jager@sund.ku.dk
[2]Department of Veterinary Disease Biology, Section for Veterinary Pathology, Faculty of Health and Medical Sciences, University of Copenhagen, Ridebanevej 3, DK-1870 Frederiksberg C, Denmark
[3]Department of Large Animal Sciences, Section for Veterinary Reproduction and Obstetrics, Faculty of Health and Medical Sciences, University of Copenhagen, Dyrlaegevej 68, DK-1870 Frederiksberg C, Denmark
Full list of author information is available at the end of the article

sporadic [14-17] and multiple genetically linked cases within single herds have been reported [18-20]. In these cases, a presumptive diagnosis of EB was based on presence of congenital blistering of the skin and mucous membranes and histopathological detection of dermoepidermal cleavage and in some cases supported by transmission electron microscopy (TEM) findings. Here we report the occurrence of EB in a Danish herd of Hereford cattle and its genetic characterization using positional cloning and whole genome sequencing.

Methods

Cases

The first case of EB, a female Hereford calf with a body weight of 30 kg, was born in March 2007 (case 1). The calf was euthanized four days old by intravenous injection of an overdose of pentobarbital sodium and submitted for necropsy. A second case of unregistered sex was stillborn in December 2007 (case 2). EB was diagnosed retrospectively based on the owner's description of lesions as the calf was destroyed. The third case was a male Hereford calf with a body weight of 48 kg that died immediately after parturition in July 2009 (case 3) and was submitted for necropsy. The herd consisted of four breeding females in 2007. None of the parents of affected calves had signs of a blistering skin disorder. The study was performed according to Danish legislation and the cases published with the consent of the owner.

Pathology

A complete necropsy was performed in both calves and specimens of skin and mucous membranes were sampled for histology. Samples were taken from within lesions, from the border between lesions and adjacent grossly normal tissue and from normal skin areas distant to lesions. Specimens were fixed in 10% neutral buffered formalin, processed by routine methods, embedded in paraffin, sectioned at 5 μm, and stained by haematoxylin and eosin. Selected sections were stained with periodic acid-Schiff (PAS).

DNA samples and genotyping

Four-generation pedigrees of the cases were obtained from the Danish Cattle Database and analysed for inbreeding loops. Tissue samples were collected from the one of the available affected calves (case 1). In addition, blood samples were gathered from both parents of case 1 and the sire of case 3. DNA was extracted using standard methods. Genotyping of these animals was performed using the BovineHD BeadChip (illumina), including 777,961 evenly distributed single nucleotide polymorphisms (SNPs) and standard protocols as recommended by the manufacturer.

Homozygosity mapping

PLINK software [21] was used to search for extended intervals of homozygosity with shared alleles as described previously [22]. Individuals and SNPs were selected using the commands --keep, and --extract while final files were generated through the --merge command. Homozygosity analysis was carried out on all cases using the commands --cow, --homozyg and --homozyg-group.

Whole genome re-sequencing and searching for variants

A fragment library with a 300 bp insert size was prepared and collected in a single lane of Illumina HiSeq2500 paired-end reads (2 × 100 bp); the fastq files were created using Casava 1.8. We obtained a total of 487,657,379 paired-end reads, which were then mapped to the cow reference genome UMD3.1/bosTau6 and aligned using Burrows-Wheeler Aligner (BWA) version 0.5.9-r16 [23] with default settings. The mapping showed that 403,122,849 reads had unique mapping positions. The SAM file generated by BWA was then converted to BAM and the reads sorted by chromosome using samtools [24]. Polymerase chain reaction (PCR) duplicates were marked using Picard tools [25]. We used the Genome Analysis Tool Kit (GATK version 2.4.9, [26]) to perform local realignment and to produce a cleaned BAM file. The genome data have been made freely available under accession no. PRJEB7527 at the European Nucleotide Archive [27].

Search for variants was then made with the unified genotyper module of GATK. The variant data for each sample was obtained in variant call format (version 4.0) as raw calls for all samples and sites flagged using the variant filtration module of GATK. Variant filtration was performed following best practice documentation of GATK version 4. The snpEFF software [28] together with the UMD3.1/bosTau Ensembl annotation was used to predict the functional effects of detected variants. The Delly package was used to detect larger deletions in cleaned BAM files [29]. Delly uses variation in pair-end reads distance and orientation to find deletions. Structural variation software that are based on coverage and orientation are unable to detect variations larger than the insert size as read mapping software usually requires the library insert size as an argument for aligning within range. Hence, in order to avoid missing large inserts, deletions and false positives all detected variants in the candidate region were also manually inspected by visual control of the BAM file using IGV browser [30].

Sanger sequencing

The *LAMC2* deletion was verified in the case and the available parents by re-sequencing of targeted PCR products using Sanger sequencing technology. PCR primers were designed using PRIMER3 [31]. PCR products were run on 0.8% agarose gel, 0.5 µg/ml ethidium bromide. PCR products were amplified using flanking primers for the *LAMC2* exon 1 deletion (F) GGCCTATAGAGAGT GGCATGA, (R) CAAATGAAGCCCTTTGAGGA and a second Reverse primer exclusive for the region deleted in the mutants TTCCTTCCCTCACCATCATC with Ampli-TaqGold360Mastermix (Life Technologies) and the products directly sequenced using the PCR primers on an ABI 3730 capillary sequencer (Life Technologies) after treatment with exonuclease I (N.E.B.) and rAPid alkaline phosphatase (Roche). Sequence data were analyzed using Sequencher 5.1 (GeneCodes).

Results and discussion

Phenotypes

Lesions in the skin were in principal similar in the two necropsied calves, but more widespread and severe in case 1 than in case 3 – probably reflecting the age difference (4 *vs.* 0 days of age). In case no. 3, skin lesions were restricted to bilateral absence of horn on the front limb dew claws and an area without horn affecting most of the hind limbs' lateral main digit (Figure 1a). The exposed dermis was hyperaemic but without exudation. The border was sharply demarcated and the adjacent epidermis seemed normal. The few days old case (no. 1) had skin lesions in the distal parts of all limbs. The horn wall was absent on all dew claws exposing a hyperaemic corium covered by crusts (Figure 1b) and the horn on all main digits was defective. The horn wall was totally absent in one hind limb digit and partly absent in the others and the exposed corium showed intense hyperaemia (Figure 1c).

The horn wall was loosened in both front limbs and separated from the corium in the coronet band with suppuration. Fistulas opened either in the coronet band or penetrated the sole. Skin ulcerations covered by crusts stretched proximally from the coronet band to the fetlock region in both hind limbs and were also found above the coronet band in the right front limb, in the left lateral metatarsal area and locally in the ventral part of the trunk.

Mucosal lesions were present in both necropsied cases. Case 3 had a large ulceration of the nasal plate with loosening of epidermis and stretching into the nostrils. In the oral cavity, both calves had extensive ulcerative lesions including a circular ulceration in the tongue around the anterior part of the torus (Figure 1d), and ulcerations in the palate, dental pad and adjacent area of the upper lip, gingiva, and cheeks.

Histopathological changes

Histopathological examination of the skin from the distal limbs of case 3, which died immediately after parturition, revealed an abrupt ulceration that was bordered by a hyperplastic epidermis. The skin proximal to the zone of epidermal hyperplasia was normal and without signs of dermoepidermal separation. The ulcerated area adjacent to the zone of epidermal hyperplasia showed acute mild suppurative inflammation, while more distant areas were dominated by an inflamed granulation tissue. Ulcerated areas where mostly without skin adnexa, i.e. glands and hair, although isolated hairs were rarely seen. Skin lesions of case 1 were dominated by ulcerations with superficial dermal necrosis, debris, and profound

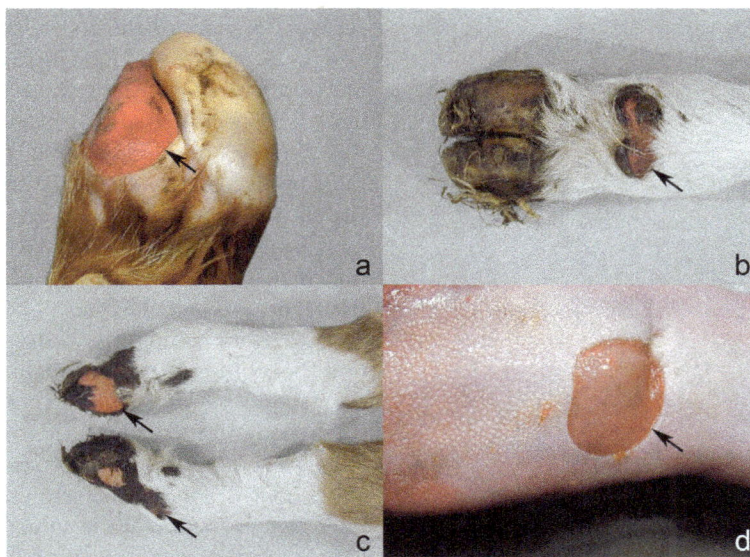

Figure 1 Gross lesions in Hereford calves with epidermolysis bullosa. a) Congenital absence of most of the hoof of a main digit (case 3); **b)** Loss of the horn of the dew claws with inflamed corium (case 1); **c)** Absence of part of the lateral aspect of the horn of the hind limb main digits exposing a hyperemic corium (case 1); **d)** Local absence of the lingual epithelium (case 1). The border of lesions is indicated by arrows.

suppurative inflammation. The epidermis adjacent to the ulcerative area was necrotic and separated from the dermis and the dermis had diffuse suppurative inflammation. This zone continued into areas with subepidermal blisters with a purulent content (Figure 2a) and in more distant areas by subepidermal blisters with just a few neutrophils and decreasing degrees of dermal inflammation (Figure 2b). Remnants of skin adnexa were present in the ulcerated areas.

Lesions of the dental pad and upper lip of case 3 were characterised by an abrupt transition from normal epithelium to an ulcer with peripheral acute inflammation and distant granulation tissue formation with sparse inflammation. Beneath ulcerated lesions, profoundly located merocrine sweat glands were present. In case 1, dental pad and nasal plate lesions were characterised by severe fibrinonecrotising and suppurative inflammation of the denuded

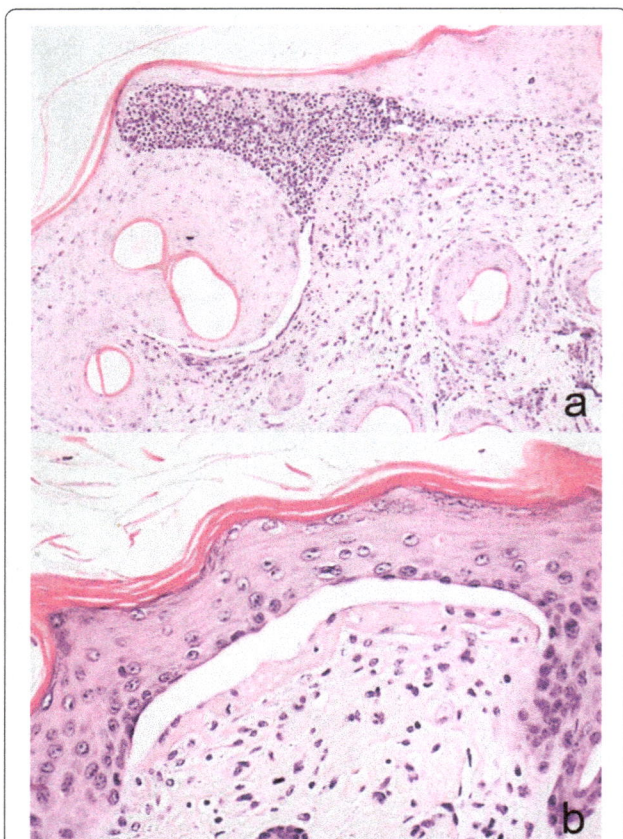

Figure 2 Microscopic lesions in Hereford calves with epidermolysis bullosa. a) Subepidermal blister with a purulent content and inflammation of the superficial dermis (case 1, hematoxylin and eosin, obj × 20); **b)** Subepidermal blister with just a few neutrophils, slight suppurative inflammation in the superficial dermis that is also covered by an eosinophilic material. The clear space may be artificial due to autolysis and tissue shrinkage during processing (case 1, hematoxylin and eosin, obj × 40).

dermis and bordered by areas with subepidermal blisters. In the tongue, lesions corresponded to those observed in the dental pad of cases 1 and 3, respectively. PAS staining revealed a basement membrane apparently located at the bottom of some blisters, while a distinct basement membrane was not present in others. An EB type/subtype was not established as appropriate materials were not available. Tissues were autolysed due to prolonged time between the death of the calves and necropsy and cryopreserved specimens for immunofluorescence antigen mapping were not sampled. Typing of EB is severely compromised if optimal specimens for immunofluorescence antigen mapping are not sampled and diagnostic based on formalin fixed tissues and suboptimal TEM examinations may be misleading [1,32] in microscopic typing of EB.

The calves had a severe congenital blistering disorder affecting the skin and mucous membranes, and the claws and dewclaws had either total or partial loss of horn. Histologically, blisters were present in the areas of the skin affected in EB although the precise localization of the spitting plane could not be determined. In combination, these findings are consistent with EB and the cases share many features with established or suspected cases of EB in cattle [6,16-20].

Pedigree analysis and mapping

The close familiar relationship between cases strongly indicated a genetic aetiology; we therefore decided to analyse the pedigree data to infer an inheritance mechanism. Pedigree data were not complete, but the available information regarding ancestors allowed us to draw a genealogical diagram (Figure 3). Analysis of the diagram indicated that inbreeding and the transmission of a recessive mutant allele from a common ancestor; either cow IV/A or Sire IV/B (Figure 3) could be the founder or the distributor of the responsible mutation. These animals had been mated and produced a son (III/A), who was bred to his own mother (IV/A). This inbreeding loop produced case 1; III/A was also bred to his sister (III/B) and produced case 2 and got a son (II/C) with a cow of unknown descent (III/C). The son II/C was mated to his mother (III/B), who gave birth to case 3. III/C and IV/A could share a common ancestor - presence of other common ancestors could not be excluded due to incomplete pedigree data. These data suggested a monogenic recessive inheritance mechanism; therefore, we hypothesized a simple Mendelian recessive inheritance was the most likely explanation for the condition. We initiated a positional cloning study to unravel the underlying genetics. We assumed that the affected calves were expected to be identical by descent (IBD) for the causative mutation and flanking chromosomal segments. We initially genotyped 777,961 evenly spaced SNPs one family trio (case 1 plus its parents). We searched for

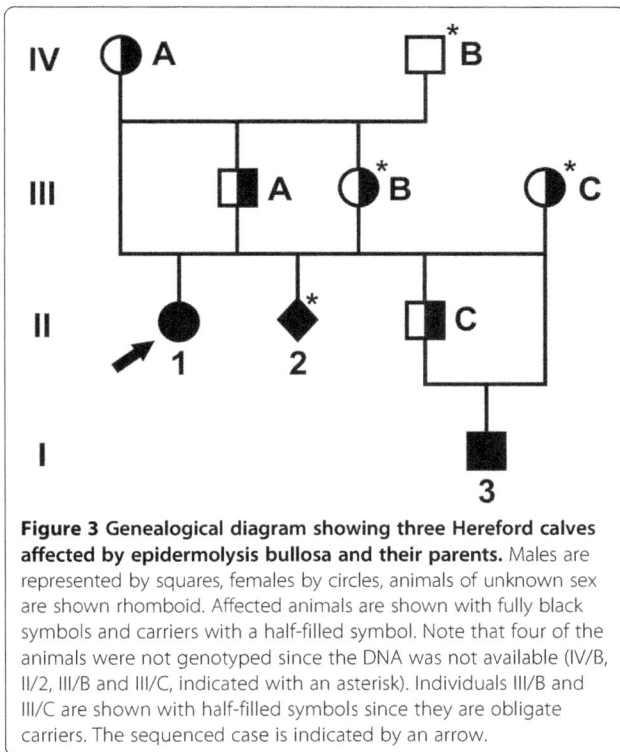

Figure 3 Genealogical diagram showing three Hereford calves affected by epidermolysis bullosa and their parents. Males are represented by squares, females by circles, animals of unknown sex are shown rhomboid. Affected animals are shown with fully black symbols and carriers with a half-filled symbol. Note that four of the animals were not genotyped since the DNA was not available (IV/B, II/2, III/B and III/C, indicated with an asterisk). Individuals III/B and III/C are shown with half-filled symbols since they are obligate carriers. The sequenced case is indicated by an arrow.

extended regions of homozygosity and compared the homozygous region between the case and the parents. Interestingly, in the genotyped affected animal about 37% of the genome is homozygous as expected in a consanguineous son-mother mating (Figure 3). We excluded any homozygous regions already present in the parents. Thereby, we found 40 genome regions greater than 1 Mb that fulfilled these criteria (Additional file 1).

In the light of the few reports of EB causing mutations in livestock we hypothesized that a causative variant might affect one of the known EB candidate genes. Eight out of 18 EB candidates mapped in the identified homozygous regions (Figure 4). We sequenced the whole genome of case 1 at 17.5× coverage of the genome and proceeded to screen the candidate genes present in the mapped homozygous intervals for possible variants. This allowed us to identify 118,014 single nucleotides and short insertion/deletion variants within the whole exome. From this point, we decided to use a candidate gene based approach. We carefully checked for all the variants present in the coding sequence of the 8 remaining EB candidate genes, which were located in the previously identified homozygous candidate regions (Figure 4). We found no homozygous private variant in all EB genes in the sequenced affected animal after comparison with available data of 40 sequenced control cattle genomes (Additional file 2), which were sequenced in the course of other

ongoing projects in our group (variants exclusive of the sequenced animal after this filtering step are reported in Additional file 3).

Using these controls genomes we went on searching for larger deletions and found a total of 349 private deletions occurring only in the genome of the affected calf (Additional file 4). Interestingly, among these deletions the only variant detected overlapping with an annotated coding region found was a 2,433 bp deletion on chromosome 16 (g.65,704,617_65,707,049del) affecting an EB candidate gene. This homozygous deletion encompasses the region more than 900 bp upstream and 1.1 kb downstream of the first exon of the annotated transcript *ENSBTAT00000061289*. This annotated bovine transcript corresponds to the human *LAMC2* gene encoding the laminin gamma 2 protein. The variant causes the complete deletion of the entire *LAMC2* exon 1 containing the start codon and the first 79 coding bases of the transcript (Figure 5). We genotyped the available family members (dam of case 1, IV/A; sire of case 1, III/A; sire of case 3, II/C) and found the mutation present in heterozygosity in these animals (Figure 5). This confirms the assumed recessive inheritance of the EB mutation within this cattle family. The mutant allele was absent in normal controls. A homozygous mutation completely removing the start codon of the evolutionary conserved *LAMC2* wildtype transcript is highly likely disruptive and almost certainly negates completely the presence of a functional LAMC2 protein. Alternatively, the possible usage of a second start codon located approximately 900 nucleotides further downstream is predicted to lead to a truncated protein lacking about 25% of the wildtype *LAMC2* including three conserved domains. Therefore we speculate that this mutant protein will, if really expressed, probably not compensate the physiological function of the wild type protein. The *LAMC2* loss of function mutation affects a well-known candidate gene associated with junctional EB in humans [33-40] and domestic animals like sheep and horse [8,9]. For this reason, we concluded that the observed EB type in this cattle family was caused by the detected *LAMC2* deletion.

Clinical and molecular characterization of EB

Diagnostic of EB in animals, including classification in major types, has been done in several studies based on histology and TEM. However, routine histological processing of skin is not recommended by human pathologists for EB diagnostic due to the difficulties in distinguishing at the light microscopy level between several types of EB [4]. Furthermore, correct sampling and processing of specimens is crucial to avoid artifactual blistering. Also fresh blisters should be induced by gently rubbing the skin rather that sampling older blisters as this may lead to a wrong diagnosis [41]. TEM examination has been used in

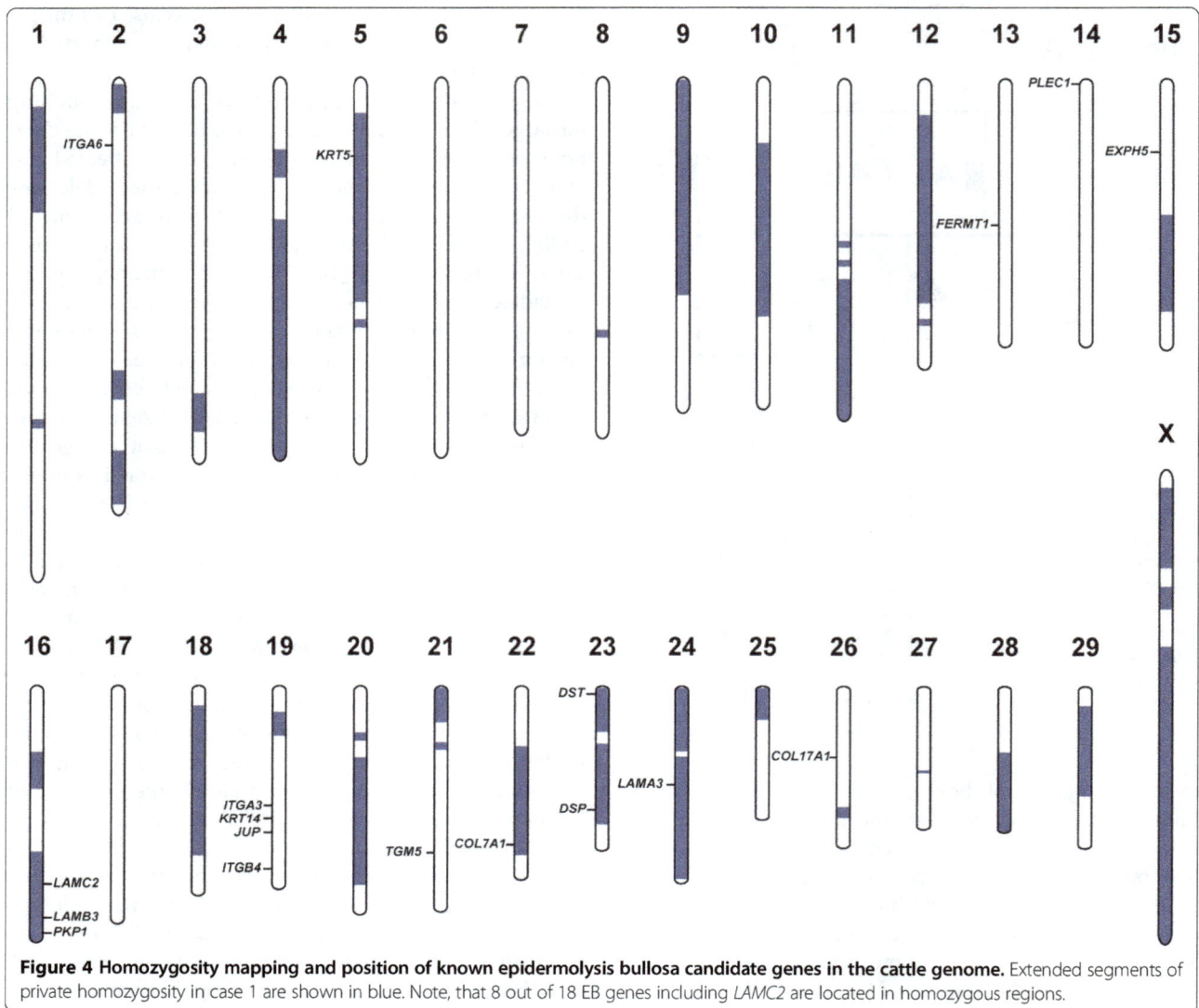

Figure 4 Homozygosity mapping and position of known epidermolysis bullosa candidate genes in the cattle genome. Extended segments of private homozygosity in case 1 are shown in blue. Note, that 8 out of 18 EB genes including *LAMC2* are located in homozygous regions.

several studies on EB in animals but require samples without autolysis. This may be difficult to achieve as animals often die or are euthanized on the farm by humane grounds before appropriate sampling is possible as for the cases reported here. Furthermore, processing of skin biopsy specimens for TEM and interpretation of EB ultrastructural changes require extensive experience and expertise that is available only in a very few recommended reference laboratories worldwide. Otherwise findings may be quite misleading and should be interpreted with caution [4]. Immunofluorescence mapping for antigens associated with EB in cryopreserved skin specimens taken from fresh spontaneous or traction-force induced blisters is the recommended diagnostic method, especially if samples are shipped to a reference laboratory [4]. The recommendations by experts in EB in

man [4] shows that there are many pitfalls in non-molecular diagnostic of EB that are obstacles in veterinary diagnostic, especially due to suboptimal materials and lack of experience with the highly specialised EB diagnostic.

Congenital localised absence of skin (CLAS) and mucosal epithelium was apparent in the calf that died immediately after parturition (case 3). CLAS has been reported as a manifestation of EB in man, e.g. Bart's Syndrome [42-44] and although CLAS and mucosal epithelium defects may be due inadequate development, CLAS in association with EB merely reflects intrauterine loss of tissue due to foetal development of EB [43].

Congenital blistering disorders in the mucous membranes, muzzle and skin, especially the distal part of the limbs, have been reported in cattle through decades and

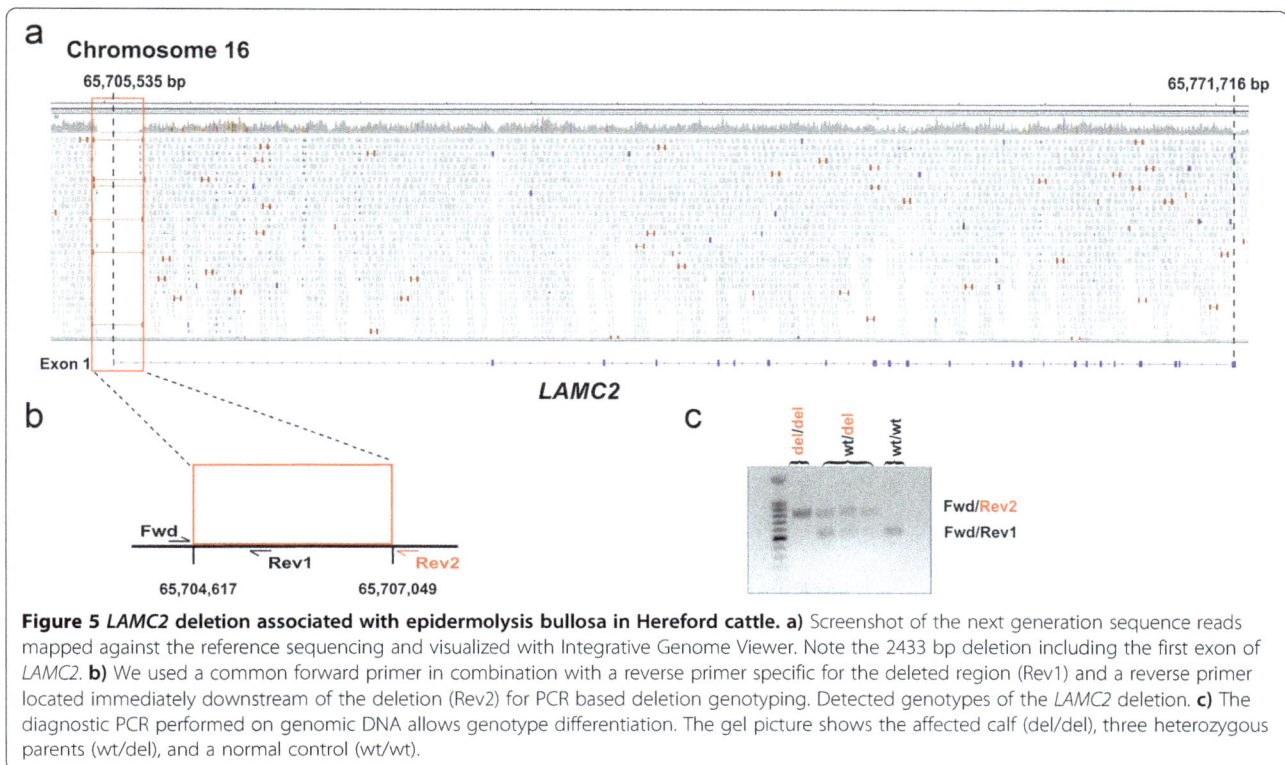

Figure 5 *LAMC2* **deletion associated with epidermolysis bullosa in Hereford cattle. a)** Screenshot of the next generation sequence reads mapped against the reference sequencing and visualized with Integrative Genome Viewer. Note the 2433 bp deletion including the first exon of *LAMC2*. **b)** We used a common forward primer in combination with a reverse primer specific for the deleted region (Rev1) and a reverse primer located immediately downstream of the deletion (Rev2) for PCR based deletion genotyping. Detected genotypes of the *LAMC2* deletion. **c)** The diagnostic PCR performed on genomic DNA allows genotype differentiation. The gel picture shows the affected calf (del/del), three heterozygous parents (wt/del), and a normal control (wt/wt).

usually referred to as "epitheliogenesis imperfecta" (EI) as proposed by Hadley [45]. Many of these cases have occurred in familial patterns associated with inbreeding and likely transmission of an autosomal recessive mutant allele from a founder animal [44-46] and many cattle breeds have been affected [15,45-51]. However, EI probably comprises of two distinct entities, namely congenital cutaneous aplasia (CCA) and EB and taking the current knowledge on the genetic background and variation even within subtypes of EB in man into consideration, the reported cases are likely to have different etiopathogeneses. Investigation of CCA has demonstrated that this is not a blistering disease and it is striking that cases resembling EI (except CCA cases) have turned out to be EB if investigated to the molecular level [5,6,9,10,52]. Furthermore, it is worth remembering that EI was introduced to veterinary medicine based on gross lesions only [44]. It is therefore proposed that EI is no longer used as a disease entity but replaced by either CCA or EB as also suggested by others [6,53].

EB is a rare disease known in man and many animal species. However, in livestock subtypes with recessive inheritance have the potential to become of significance if the defective allele is present in important sires used for artificial breeding through several years as seem for other genetic diseases in cattle [54-56]. It is therefore

important that cases are diagnosed to subtype level when the first cases are recognised to enable rapid development of genetic test that allows screening of the sire population. However, subtyping of EB is a task for clinicians and pathologists, but it starts with clinical examination and sampling and processing of adequate materials for microscopic and genomic analysis [41]. The quick identification of an highly disruptive mutation in a known candidate gene allowed us to unambiguously identify and classify the EB cases in Hereford and thus (I) allow for possible screening of the mutation in the Danish Hereford population as preventive measure (II) giving a new animal model for EB caused by a mutation in laminin gamma genes.

Conclusions

The study reports for the first time the occurrence of EB in Hereford cattle. Our investigation confirms the role of a recessively inherited *LAMC2* loss of function mutation in EB aetiology. Next-generation sequencing offers a powerful tool for understanding the genetic background of rare diseases in domestic animals with an available reference genome sequence. Verifying the causative mutation allowed us to confirm to the diagnosis of EB and allows breeders to eliminate this genetic defect from the population.

Additional files

Additional file 1: Private regions of homozygosity detected in epidermolysis bullosa case 1. Only homozygous regions exclusive for the case are shown.

Additional file 2: List of all the control cattle genomes and their breed.

Additional file 3: List of all the private homozygous variants of the sequenced epidermolysis bullosa case 1.

Additional file 4: Private larger deletions detected in epidermolysis bullosa case 1. Deletion in encompassing LAMC2 exon 1 is highlighted.

Abbreviations

Bp: Base pairs; CCA: Congenital cutaneous aplasia; CLAS: Congenital localised absence of skin; EB: Epidermolysis bullosa; EI: Epitheliogenesis imperfect; kb: Kilo bytes; PAS: Periodic acid-Schiff; PCR: Polymerase chain reaction; SNP: Single nucleotide polymorphism; TEM: Transmission electron microscopy.

Competing interests

The authors declare that they have no competing interests.

Authors' contributions

JSA necropsied case 1, evaluated pedigree information, did the histopathological analyses and drafted the manuscript. LKI necropsied case 3. LM and NW performed the genetic investigations and drafted the manuscript. VJ analysed the whole genome sequencing data. CD supervised the genetic project and edited the manuscript. All authors participated in discussion of results and critically revised the manuscript. All authors approved the final version of the manuscript.

Acknowledgements

The authors acknowledge Mr Ole R Kjærulf, Roskilde, Denmark for submission of the cases. The study was funded by the Danish Surveillance Programme for Genetic Diseases in Cattle. The authors wish to thank Michèle Ackermann and Muriel Fragnière for their precious technical assistance. We would like to express our appreciation to the University of Bern for the use of the Next Generation Sequencing Platform in performing the whole genome re-sequencing experiment and the Vital-IT high-performance computing center of the Swiss Institute of Bioinformatics for performing computationally intensive tasks (http://www.vital-it.ch/).

Author details

[1]Institute of Genetics, Vetsuisse Faculty, University of Bern, Bremgartenstrasse 109a, CH-3001 Bern, Switzerland. [2]Department of Veterinary Disease Biology, Section for Veterinary Pathology, Faculty of Health and Medical Sciences, University of Copenhagen, Ridebanevej 3, DK-1870 Frederiksberg C, Denmark. [3]Department of Large Animal Sciences, Section for Veterinary Reproduction and Obstetrics, Faculty of Health and Medical Sciences, University of Copenhagen, Dyrlaegevej 68, DK-1870 Frederiksberg C, Denmark.

References

1. Fine JD. Inherited epidermolysis bullosa: recent basic and clinical advances. Curr Opin Pediatr. 2010;22:453–8.
2. Ginn PE, Mansell JEKL, Rakich PM. Skin and appendages. In: Maxie MG, editor. Jubb, Kennedy and Palmer's pathology of domestic animals, vol. 1. 5th ed. Edinburgh: Saunders-Elsevier; 2007.
3. Fine JD, Bruckner-Tuderman L, Eady RA, Bauer EA, Bauer JW, Has C, et al. Inherited epidermolysis bullosa: updated recommendations on diagnosis and classification. J Am Acad Dermatol. 2014;70:1103–26.
4. Has C, Bruckner-Tuderman L. The genetics of skin fragility. Annu Rev Genomics Hum Genet. 2014;15:245–68.
5. Ford CA, Stanfield AM, Spelman RJ, Smits B, Ankersmidt-Udy AE, Cottier K, et al. A mutation in bovine keratin 5 causing epidermolysis bullosa simplex, transmitted by a mosaic sire. J Invest Dermatol. 2005;124:1170–6.
6. Menoud A, Welle M, Tetens J, Lichtner P, Drögemüller C. A COL7A1 mutation causes dystrophic epidermolysis bullosa in Rotes Höhenvieh cattle. PLoS One. 2012;7:e38823.
7. Baldeschi C, Gache Y, Rattenholl A, Bouillé P, Danos O, Ortonne JP, et al. Genetic correction of canine dystrophic epidermolysis bullosa mediated by retroviral vectors. Hum Mol Genet. 2003;12:1897–905.
8. Mömke S, Kerkmann A, Wöhlke A, Ostmeier M, Hewicker-Trautwein M, Ganter M, et al. A frameshift mutation within LAMC2 is responsible for Herlitz type junctional epidermolysis bullosa (HJEB) in black headed mutton sheep. PLoS One. 2011;6:e18943.
9. Milenkovic D, Chaffaux S, Taourit S, Guérin G. A mutation in the LAMC2 gene causes the Herlitz junctional epidermolysis bullosa (H-JEB) in two French draft horse breeds. Genet Sel Evol. 2003;35:249–56.
10. Graves KT, Henney PJ, Ennis RB. Partial deletion of the LAMA3 gene is responsible for hereditary junctional epidermolysis bullosa in the American Saddlebred Horse. Anim Genet. 2009;40:35–41.
11. Spirito F, Charlesworth A, Linder K, Ortonne JP, Baird J, Meneguzzi G. Animal models for skin blistering conditions: absence of laminin 5 causes hereditary junctional mechanobullous disease in the Belgian horse. J Invest Dermatol. 2002;119:684–91.
12. Capt A, Spirito F, Guaguere E, Spadafora A, Ortonne JP, Meneguzzi G. Inherited junctional epidermolysis bullosa in the German Pointer: establishment of a large animal model. J Invest Dermatol. 2005;124:530–5.
13. Bruckner-Tuderman L, McGrath JA, Robinson EC, Uitto J. Animal models of epidermolysis bullosa: update 2010. J Invest Dermatol. 2010;130:1485–8.
14. Deprez P, Maenhout T, De Cock H, Wullepit J, Charlier G, Muylle E, et al. Epidermolysis bullosa in a calf: a case report [in Dutch]. Vlaams Diergeneeskd Tijdschr. 1993;62:155–9.
15. Agerholm JS. Congenital generalized epidermolysis bullosa in a calf. Zentralbl Veterinarmed A. 1994;41:139–42.
16. Stocker H, Lott G, Straumann U, Rüsch P. Epidermolysis bullosa in a calf [in German]. Tierarztl Prax. 1995;23:123–6.
17. Medeiros GX, Franklin Riet-Correa F, Armién AG, Dantas AFM, de Galiza GJN, Simões SVD. Junctional epidermolysis bullosa in a calf. J Vet Diagn Invest. 2012;24:231–4.
18. Thompson KG, Crandell RA, Rugeley WW, Sutherland RJ. A mechanobullous disease with sub-basilar separation in Brangus calves. Vet Pathol. 1985;22:283–5.
19. Bassett H. A congenital bovine epidermolysis resembling epidermolysis bullosa simplex of man. Vet Rec. 1987;121:8–11.
20. Foster AP, Skuse AM, Higgins RJ, Barrett DC, Philbey AW, Thomson JR, et al. Epidermolysis bullosa in calves in the United Kingdom. J Comp Pathol. 2010;142:336–40.
21. Purcell S1, Neale B, Todd-Brown K, Thomas L, Ferreira MA, Bender D, et al. PLINK: a toolset for whole-genome association and population-based linkage analysis. Am J Hum Genet. 2007;81:559–75.
22. Murgiano L, Jagannathan V, Benazzi C, Bolcato M, Brunetti B, Muscatello LV, et al. Deletion in the EVC2 gene causes chondrodysplastic dwarfism in Tyrolean Grey Cattle. PLoS One. 2014;9:e94861.
23. Li H, Durbin R. Fast and accurate short read alignment with Burrows-Wheeler transform. Bioinformatics. 2009;25:1754–60.
24. Homepage Samtools. [http://samtools.sourceforge.net]
25. Picard. [http://sourceforge.net/projects/picard/]
26. McKenna A, Hanna M, Banks E, Sivachenko A, Cibulskis K, Kernytsky A, et al. The genome analysis toolkit: a MapReduce framework for analyzing next-generation DNA sequencing data. Genome Res. 2010;20:1297–303.
27. Homepage European Nucleotide Archive. [http://www.ebi.ac.uk/ena/data/view/PRJEB7527. Accessed 14 Juli 2014].
28. Cingolani P, Platts A, Wangle L, Coon M, Nguyen T, Wang L, et al. A program for annotating and predicting the effects of single nucleotide polymorphisms, SnpEff: SNPs in the genome of Drosophila melanogaster strain w1118; iso-2; iso-3. Fly. 2012;6:80–92.
29. Rausch T, Zichner T, Schlattl A, Stütz AM, Benes V, Korbel JO. DELLY: structural variant discovery by integrated paired-end and split-read analysis. Bioinformatics. 2012;28:i333–9.
30. Thorvaldsdóttir H, Robinson JT, Mesirov JP. Integrative Genomics Viewer (IGV): high-performance genomics data visualization and exploration. Brief Bioinform. 2013;14:178–92.
31. Untergrasser A, Cutcutache I, Koressaar T, Ye J, Faircloth BC, Remm M, et al. Primer3 - new capabilities and interfaces. Nucleic Acids Res. 2012;40:e115.

32. Ostmeier M, Kerkmann A, Frase R, Ganter M, Distl O, Hewicker-Trautwein M. Inherited junctional epidermolysis bullosa (Herlitz type) in German black-headed mutton sheep. J Comp Pathol. 2012;146:338–47.

33. Aumailley M, Bruckner-Tuderman L, Carter WG, Deutzmann R, Edgar D, Ekblom P, et al. A simplified laminin nomenclature. Matrix Biol. 2005;24:326–32.

34. Castiglia D, Posteraro P, Spirito F, Pinola M, Angelo C, Puddu P, et al. Novel mutations in the LAMC2 gene in non-Herlitz junctional epidermolysis bullosa: effects on laminin-5 assembly, secretion, and deposition. J Invest Dermatol. 2001;117:731–9.

35. Hartwig B, Borm B, Schneider H, Arin MJ, Kirfel G, Herzog V. Laminin-5-deficient human keratinocytes: defective adhesion results in a saltatory and inefficient mode of migration. Exp Cell Res. 2007;313:1575–87.

36. Mühle C, Jiang QJ, Charlesworth A, Bruckner-Tuderman L, Meneguzzi G, Schneider H. Novel and recurrent mutations in the laminin-5 genes causing lethal junctional epidermolysis bullosa: molecular basis and clinical course of Herlitz disease. Hum Genet. 2005;116:33–42.

37. Nakano A, Chao SC, Pulkkinen L, Murrell D, Bruckner-Tuderman L, Pfendner E, et al. Laminin 5 mutations in junctional epidermolysis bullosa: molecular basis of Herlitz vs. non-Herlitz phenotypes. Hum Genet. 2002;110:41–51.

38. Pulkkinen L, Uitto J. Mutation analysis and molecular genetics of epidermolysis bullosa. Matrix Biol. 1999;18:29–42.

39. Schneider H, Mühle C, Pacho F. Biological function of laminin-5 and pathogenic impact of its deficiency. Eur J Cell Biol. 2007;86:701–17.

40. Varki R, Sadowski S, Pfendner E, Uitto J. Epidermolysis bullosa. I. Molecular genetics of the junctional and hemidesmosomal variants. J Med Genet. 2006;43:641–52.

41. Intong LR, Murrell DF. How to take skin biopsies for epidermolysis bullosa. Dermatol Clin. 2010;28:197–200. vii.

42. Butler DF, Berger TG, James WD, Smith TL, Stanely JR, Rodman OG. Bart's syndrome: microscopic, ultrastructural, and immunofluorescent mapping features. Pediatr Dermatol. 1986;3:113–8.

43. Kanzler MH, Smoller B, Woodley DT. Congenital localized absence of the skin as a manifestation of epidermolysis bullosa. Arch Dermatol. 1992;128:1087–90.

44. Bart BJ, Lussky RC. Bart syndrome with associated anomalies. Am J Perinatol. 2005;22:365–9.

45. Hadley FB. Congenital epithelial defects of calves. J Hered. 1927;18:487–95.

46. Leipold HW, Mills JH, Huston K. Epitheliogenesis imperfecta in Holstein-Friesian calves. Can Vet J. 1973;14:114–8.

47. Dyrendahl S. Epitheliogenesis imperfecta in the Swedish Red and White breed [in Swedish]. Nord Vet Med. 1956;8:953–8.

48. Straub OC. Epitheliogenesis imperfecta in a calf [in German]. Vet Med Nachricht. 1969;3:189–93.

49. Yeruhama I, Goshen T, Lahav D, Perl S. Simultaneous occurrence of epitheliogenesis imperfecta with syndactyly in a calf and a lamb. Aust Vet J. 2005;83:149–50.

50. Jayasekara MU, Leipold HW. Epitheliogenesis imperfecta imperfecta in Shorthorn and Angus cattle. Zentralbl Veterinarmed A. 1979;26:497–501.

51. Hutt FB, Frost JN. Hereditary epithelial defects in Ayrshire cattle. J Hered. 1948;39:131–7.

52. Lieto LD, Swerczek TW, Cothran EG. Equine epitheliogenesis imperfecta in two american saddlebred foals is a lamina lucida defect. Vet Pathol. 2002;39:576–80.

53. Benoit-Biancamano MO, Drolet R, D'Allaire S. Aplasia cutis congenita (epitheliogenesis imperfecta) in swine: observations from a large breeding herd. J Vet Diagn Invest. 2006;18:573–9.

54. Agerholm JS. Inherited disorders in Danish cattle. APMIS. 2007;115 Suppl 122:1–76.

55. Murgiano L, Testoni S, Drögemüller C, Bolcato M, Gentile A. Frequency of bovine congenital pseudomyotonia carriers in selected Italian Chianina sires. Vet J. 2013;195:238–40.

56. Murgiano L, Drögemüller C, Sbarra F, Bolcato M, Gentile A. Prevalence of paunch calf syndrome carriers in Italian Romagnola cattle. Vet J. 2014;200:459–61.

3

Assessing the seasonal prevalence and risk factors for nuchal crest adiposity in domestic horses and ponies using the Cresty Neck Score

Sarah L Giles[1*], Christine J Nicol[1], Sean A Rands[2] and Patricia A Harris[3]

Abstract

Background: Nuchal crest adiposity in horses and ponies has been associated with an enhanced risk of metabolic health problems. However, there is no current information on the prevalence of, and risk factors specific to, nuchal crest adiposity in horses and ponies. In addition, the cresty neck score has not previously been utilised across different seasons within a UK leisure population, it is not know whether nuchal crest adiposity shows the same seasonal trends as general obesity.

Results: A Cresty Neck Score (CNS, 0–5) was given to 96 horses with access to pasture (>6 h per day) at the end of winter and at the end of summer in order to obtain two prevalence estimates. Risk factors were assessed using the single outcome cresty neck/no cresty neck in either season (binary), from owner questionnaires and analysed using a mixed effects logistic regression model (outcome variable CNS <3 or CNS ≥3/5). Agreement between winter and summer scores was assessed using weighted Kappa methods.
Winter CNS values were significantly higher than summer CNS values (p = 0.002) indicating a systematic bias. The prevalence of a CNS ≥ 3/5 was 45.83% at the end of winter, falling to 33.33% at the end of summer and was higher in ponies (<14.2 hh) than horses (≥14.2 hh) in both seasons. This may reflect a real winter increase in regional fat deposition, or an increased difficulty in obtaining an accurate estimate of regional adiposity in winter months. Breed was the strongest risk factor for CNS ≥3/5 in both seasons, with native UK breeds appearing to be most at risk (p < 0.001). In a separate, small validation study, the CNS showed good inter-observer reliability.

Conclusions: The prevalence of a CNS ≥3/5 was higher at the end of winter than at the end of summer, which was the opposite pattern seasonal variation to that observed for general obesity. Further studies are required to investigate the potential influence of time of year upon CNS interpretation and studies utilising the CNS should consider potential seasonal variability in nuchal crest adiposity.

Keywords: Horse, Pony, Equine, Cresty neck, Cresty neck score, Obesity, Season, Body condition, Prevalence, Risk factors

Background

It has become recognised in the human obesity literature that some patterns of regional fat accumulation have particularly damaging health consequences. Abdominal fat in humans has been linked to changes in circulating blood glucose levels, and fat accumulation in this area is a risk factor for insulin resistance, diabetes and other metabolic complications [1-4].

Increased fat deposits along the crest of the neck in horses and ponies (nuchal crest adiposity) has similarly been associated with an altered metabolic state [5,6] and an increased risk of certain metabolic disorders such insulin resistance [7-9]. A scoring system which targets this region specific adiposity has been developed by Carter and colleagues [5], named the 'Cresty Neck Score' (CNS), and in several studies a CNS score of ≥ 3/5 has been associated with an increased risk of laminitis [7,10,11]. It is not currently known whether this association with laminitis is due to the presence of additional fat in this nuchal crest region (potentially resulting in a

* Correspondence: sarah.giles@bristol.ac.uk
[1]School of Veterinary Science, University of Bristol, Langford, Bristol BS40 5DU, UK
Full list of author information is available at the end of the article

more inflammatory profile [12,13]) or whether nuchal crest adiposity is a proxy for e.g. increased abdominal fat (potentially leading to abnormal insulin dynamics [12]) which is not detected via external Body Condition Scoring (BCS) systems. It has been suggested that certain breeds may more at risk of nuchal crest adiposity and associated metabolic disorders [6,14], particularly pony breeds [15], but evidence is currently limited.

The Cresty Neck Score [5] has become the most commonly used method of distinguishing nuchal crest adiposity [16-19]. Whilst this method has not been formally validated using post-mortem methods, there is a lack of gold standard measure for this type of specific, regional adiposity. Previously authors have utilised a neck circumference [8,12,20], but due to a lack of reference as to what a cresty neck or non-cresty neck circumference should be for any particular breed or size of horse or pony, this measure is only really useful as a ratio to neck length, or basis for assessing change, and thus has obvious limitations.

Previous studies have explored the prevalence of and risk factors for obesity in horses and ponies [21-26]. The prevalence of general obesity has been shown to vary between winter and summer in UK horses and ponies, with lower values at the end of winter [25]. It is not known whether the prevalence of CNS ≥3/5 differs from general obesity, or whether there is similar seasonal variation. Our hypothesis is that there would thus be similar seasonal changes in neck crest adiposity, with higher values during summer months. Neck crest adiposity may be a site of long-term fat storage, with previous studies reporting that fat reserves in this region (along with the rump) appear not to vary greatly with short term changes in energy intake at different times of the year [26]. It is therefore possible that the pattern of seasonal change observed in neck crest adiposity may be different from that seen with more general measures of obesity.

The overall aims of this study were: 1) To assess the prevalence of CNS ≥3/5, both at the end of winter and at the end of summer in a domestic population with daily access to pasture; 2) To examine the risk factors associated with CNS ≥3/5; and 3) To use seasonal CNS measurements from the same individual horses and ponies, and the same human observer, to assess the between-season agreement of the CNS.

Methods
Animal and materials
The study population was outdoor, herd-living leisure horses in North Somerset, UK. Making the assumption that seasonal body condition trends are clearest in outdoor living animals, inclusion criteria specified that horses and ponies had to live outdoors on green pasture

for at least six hours per day. The target population was leisure horses and ponies in the UK, with daily access to pasture, the study population was thus likely to be fairly representative of this. The sampling frame consisted of horses and ponies whose owners attended a riding club membership renewals evening in January 2011. A cluster sampling strategy was used, where herds were randomly selected from the sampling frame using random number tables and all individuals were measured in that herd. 127 individual animals were initially recruited and measured between 5th February – 24th March 2011. Of these, 96 individuals remained with the same owners and were therefore were available for follow up. Second measurements were taken between 20th July – 1st September 2011 in these 96 individuals, which made up our study population.

Data on risk factors was obtained via two owner questionnaires which were completed at the same time as measurements were taken (for questionnaires see Additional file 1 in [25]). Owners completed risk factors questionnaires alone and in their own time to minimise observer bias. Questionnaires covered individual animal information such as breed and age, as well as management risk factors such as grazing and turnout routine, rug wearing, dental history, as well as a detailed breakdown of supplementary feed and exercise. Grass quality could not be measured due to horses moving pasture several times throughout the duration of the study and management routines such as strip grazing meant the quality of the grass forage varied daily. Height was measured at the withers using a measuring stick with spirit level. Horses and ponies were defined according to their height, where horses were >148 cm (equivalent to 14.2 hh) and ponies were ≤148 cm. Baseline descriptive statistics and study population demographics are presented in our related paper [25].

Nuchal adiposity was measured using the CNS [5] and scored by a single trained observer for both winter and summer measurements. This involved a visual assessment of the neck as well as a tactile assessment of the nuchal crest area. The Cresty Neck Score is shown in Figure 1. Animals were considered to be cases if they had a CNS of three or above in either season (a binary outcome variable), this is the cut-off value recommended by Carter et al. [5]. This binary variable was the outcome variable used for the risk factor analysis.

Statistical analysis
For the risk factor analysis, data were initially checked and missing values dealt with using complete case analysis, where incomplete units were removed. Response rate to the questionnaires was 100%. Age was considered as both a continuous variable and as a binary variable

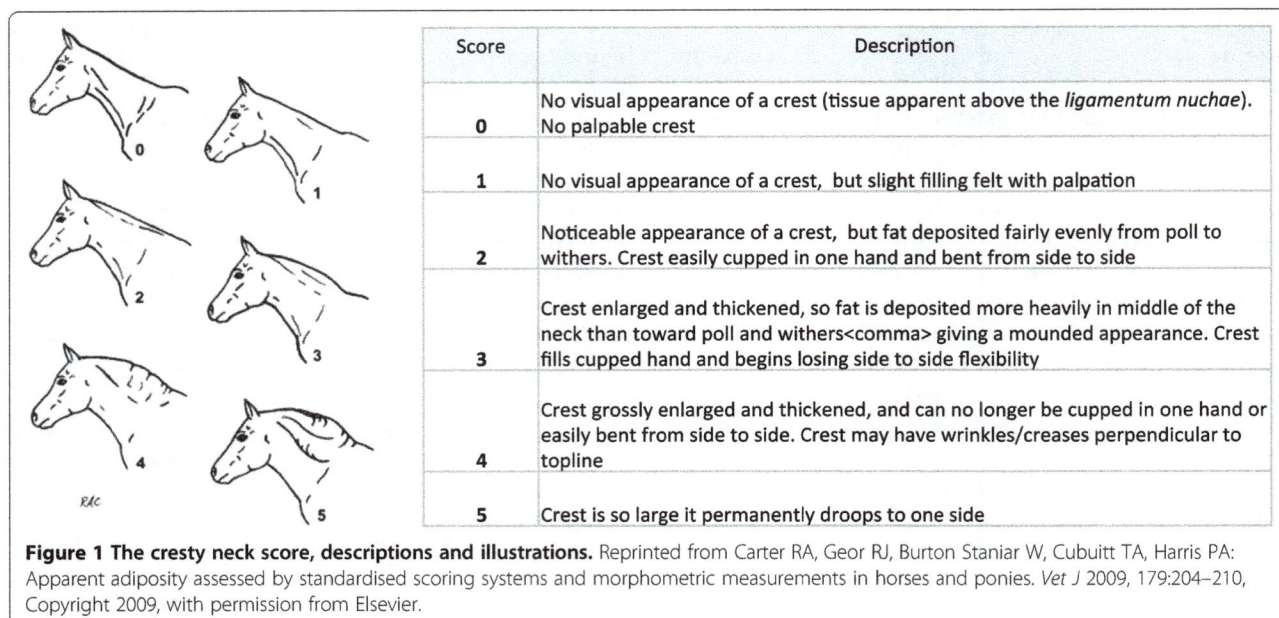

Score	Description
0	No visual appearance of a crest (tissue apparent above the *ligamentum nuchae*). No palpable crest
1	No visual appearance of a crest, but slight filling felt with palpation
2	Noticeable appearance of a crest, but fat deposited fairly evenly from poll to withers. Crest easily cupped in one hand and bent from side to side
3	Crest enlarged and thickened, so fat is deposited more heavily in middle of the neck than toward poll and withers<comma> giving a mounded appearance. Crest fills cupped hand and begins losing side to side flexibility
4	Crest grossly enlarged and thickened, and can no longer be cupped in one hand or easily bent from side to side. Crest may have wrinkles/creases perpendicular to topline
5	Crest is so large it permanently droops to one side

Figure 1 The cresty neck score, descriptions and illustrations. Reprinted from Carter RA, Geor RJ, Burton Staniar W, Cubuitt TA, Harris PA: Apparent adiposity assessed by standardised scoring systems and morphometric measurements in horses and ponies. *Vet J* 2009, 179:204–210, Copyright 2009, with permission from Elsevier.

('youngster'/'not youngster'), where not young was defined as an adult animal over four years of age). Height was also considered as both continuous and binary, so as to compare horses (≥148 cm) and ponies (<148 cm). Breed was initially coded into seven categories: native ponies (except Shetland), Shetlands and miniature breeds, lightweight breeds (Arabians and Thoroughbreds), heavyweight draught horses, cob types, sports horse breeds, and 'other'. Due to low sample size in both the heavyweight and miniature breed categories (just 4 individuals in each), Shetlands were added to the native ponies category and heavyweight breeds were added to 'other', giving five final breed categories.

Quantity of both supplementary feed and forage was coded into categories for analysis. The categories of supplementary feed represented: category 1, no supplementary feed at all; category 2, no energy-providing feed (concentrate) but vitamin and mineral supplements given; category 3, less than 1.5 kg day^{-1}) of 'concentrate' feed; and category 4, at least 1.5 kg day^{-1} of concentrate feed. These categories were analysed separately for horses and ponies, to account for the size of the animal. Hay was split into 3 categories, none, small amount (less than 5 kg day^{-1}), and large amount (at least 5 kg day^{-1}).

Risk factor variables were initially analysed univariably using χ^2 tests, analysis of variance (ANOVA) or linear regression (all two tailed). Variables with evidence of association with CNS ≥ 3/5 were taken forward into multivariable analysis (screening p value ≤ 0.07). A mixed effects logistic regression model was then forward-fitted using a positive stepwise approach, based on strength of univariable association. Explanatory variables were included as fixed effects and retained both on the basis of their p values and also on the strength of their contribution to the model fit, assessed

using the likelihood ratio test. Herd group was included as a random effect, to account for the clustered study design. Collinearity was assessed using pairwise correlations and the likelihood ratio test, and the possibility of non-linear or quadratic associations was also considered and assessed using the likelihood ratio test for all continuous explanatory variables.

Cresty neck score in summer and winter

The same animals were measured in both seasons ($n = 96$) by the same observer. The extent of agreement between these two sets of results was assessed, using a Bland-Altman plot on the paired winter and summer CNS scores. A Wilcoxon signed rank test was then used to assess whether or not the differences between winter and summer measurements were significant. A weighted Cohen's kappa statistic indicating level of agreement was also generated (using a squared weighting system equivalent to $1 - \{(i\text{-}j)/(k\text{-}1)\}^2$, where i and j refer to the row and column index, and k is the maximum number of possible ratings). All statistical analyses were performed in *Stata* 11.2 (Statacorp, College Station, Texas).

Inter-observer reliability of the cresty neck score

An additional 31 horses and ponies were recruited *post hoc* from the Royal Veterinary College, University of London, to obtain a measure of inter-observer reliability in summer CNS scores and to assess this as a potential source of error. Made up of 18 ponies, native types and 13 horses, mostly Thoroughbred types. Inter-observer agreement has not previously been reported for this score. These 31 horses were deliberately a mixture of ages, breeds and body condition scores. Three trained observers, including SLG (observer 2) assigned a CNS to the individual animals and all data collection was completed on the same day, 29/07/2014. One observer only assessed 29 animals. All observers were blinded to the results of the other observers. The agreement between the observers was then assessed using Cohen's kappa statistic using the weighting described above.

All experimental work was approved by the University of Bristol Ethical Review Group (university investigation number UB/10/049).

Results

Prevalence of CNS ≥ 3/5

The prevalence of CNS ≥3/5 within our study population ($n = 96$) varied between winter and summer measurements and there was strong evidence for a seasonal difference in nuchal crest adiposity ($\chi_1^2 = 16.45$, p < 0.001). The prevalence was 45.83% (95% CI 36.76% - 54.90%) at the end of winter, falling to 33.33% (95% CI 26.76% - 39.90%) at the end of summer. Of these 96 individuals, 20 (20.83%) had a CNS ≥3/5 in the winter and not in the summer, whereas only 8 (8.33%) had a CNS ≥3/5 in the summer and not in the winter.

The 20 individuals which had a CNS ≥3/5 in winter but not in summer were evenly spread across both height and breed categories.

Table 1 shows the observed differences between horses and ponies, ponies had a higher prevalence of CNS ≥3/5 during both seasons. At the end of the winter months ponies had twice (2.00) the odds of CNS ≥3/5 compared to horses, but this was not significant. There was however strong evidence of a difference in the number of cases between horses and ponies at the end of the summer months (OR 2.83 $p = 0.02$).

Risk factors for CNS ≥3/5

Risk factors which showed an initial univariable association with nuchal crest adiposity are summarised in Table 2. Height was associated with CNS ≥3/5, both as a categorical and binary (horses/ponies) variable ($p = 0.04$

and $p = 0.02$ respectively), where ponies, and more specifically ponies between 114–134 cm appear to be at greatest risk. Horses or ponies with a history of laminitis were more likely to have CNS ≥3/5 ($p = 0.04$). Breed showed strong evidence of association ($p < 0.001$), native UK breeds had the highest odds of CNS ≥3/5. Although feeding supplementary hay during the winter months was relatively rare in our study population (6.38%), this increased the odds of CNS ≥3/5 ($p = 0.06$). Those individuals with a complete change in feeding regimen between seasons showed the highest odds of CNS ≥3/5 ($p = 0.005$) however this is likely to be an issue of cause and effect, through owners attempting (and failing) to implement preventative strategies in at risk individuals. Herd size was also associated with cresty neck ($p = 0.01$), as herd size increased there were fewer cresty neck cases (CNS ≥3/5).

The final risk factor regression model for CNS ≥3/5 is presented in Table 3. The final model contained the variables, breed category and herd size. Native ponies had 19.72 times the odds of CNS ≥3/5 ($p = 0.006$), compared to lightweight breeds (as referent), and native cobs appear even more at risk with 31.48 times the odds ($p = 0.004$). As herd size increases, the odds of a CNS ≥3/5 are reduced by 18% per extra individual.

Cresty neck score in summer and winter

Figure 2 shows the Bland-Altman plot for the extent of agreement between winter and summer CNS measures. The mean winter CNS score was 2.5 and the mean summer score was 1.9. A mean difference above of 0.32 (95% CI 0.12 − 0.52) indicates a consistent tendency for winter CNS measurements higher than summer CNS measurements, indicating a systematic bias.

There was strong evidence of a difference between winter CNS and summer CNS measures using a Wilcoxon signed rank test ($T = 3.03$, $N = 96$, $p = 0.002$) confirming winter measurements were significantly higher. There was a moderate agreement between winter and summer CNS ($\kappa_w = 0.51$, $Z = 5.25$, $p < 0.001$).

Table 1 A comparison of CNS ≥3/5 prevalence between horses and ponies during winter and summer

Winter	Total number of subjects (%)	Number of cases (%)	Odds ratio (ponies/horses)	95% CI	χ^2	p
Horses	46 (47.92)	17 (38.64)	-	-		-
Ponies	50 (52.08)	27 (61.36)	2.00	0.87 – 4.61	2.77	0.09
Total	96 (100)	44 (45.83)				
Summer						
Horses	46 (47.92)	10 (31.25)	-	-		-
Ponies	50 (52.08)	22 (68.75)	2.83	112 – 7.14	5.29	0.02
Total	96 (100)	32 (33.33)				
Odds ratio (winter/summer)			0.71			

Table 2 Univariable risk factors associated with CNS ≥3/5

Exposure variables

		Total number of horses and ponies (%)	Number of CNS ≥3/5 cases (%)	Odds (CNS <3/5/ CNS ≥3/5)	95% CI	χ^2	p
Height (cm, categorical)	**≤113**	8 (8.33)	2 (6.25)	0.33	0.06 – 1.65		
	114 – 134	20 (20.83)	12 (37.5)	1.50	0.61 – 3.67		
	135 – 146	22 (22.92)	8 (25.0)	0.57	0.24 – 1.36		
	147– 159	22 (22.92)	5 (15.62)	0.29	0.11 – 0.80		
	≥160	24 (25.0)	5 (15.62)	0.26	0.09 – 0.70	9.91	0.04
Breed (categorical)	**Native ponies**	34 (35.42)	15 (46.88)	0.79	0.40 – 1.55		
	Lightweight	25 (26.04)	1 (3.12)	0.04	0.005 – 0.31		
	Native cobs	12 (12.50)	7 (21.88)	1.40	0.44 – 4.41		
	Sports horse	13 (13.54)	1 (3.12)	0.08	0.01 – 0.64		
	Other	12 (12.50)	8 (25.0)	2.0	0.60 – 6.64	–	<0.001*
Seasonal change in feeding regimen	**No change**	13 (13.98)	8 (25.0)	1.60	0.52 – 4.89		
	Reduction in quantity only	13 (13.98)	3 (9.38)	0.30	0.08 – 1.09		
	Change Parts	57 (61.29)	14 (43.75)	0.32	0.17 – 0.60		
	Complete Change	10 (10.75)	7 (21.88)	2.33	0.60 – 9.02	13.04	0.005
Laminitis	**No**	82 (89.13)	23 (79.31)	0.38	0.24 – 0.63		
	Yes	10 (10.87)	6 (20.69)	1.50	0.42 – 5.32	4.22	0.04
Fed hay or other supplementary forage during winter months	**No**	88 (93.62)	26 (86.67)	0.42	0.27 – 0.66		
	Yes	6 (6.38)	4 (13.33)	2.00	0.37 – 10.92	3.56	0.06
Height binary	**Pony (≤148 cm)**	50 (52.08)	22 (68.75)	0.78	0.44 – 1.37		
	Horse (>148 cm)	46 (47.92)	10 (31.25)	0.28	0.14 – 0.56	5.34	0.02
Herd size		96 (100)	-	-	-	-2.48	0.01**
Total		96 (100)	32 (100)				

*indicates probability estimated using Fisher's exact test. **continuous variable assessed for a univariable association using logistic regression.

Table 3 Final multivariable model for risk factors associated with CNS ≥3/5

Risk factor	Odds ratio	SE	95% CI	p
Breed				
Native ponies	19.72	26.42	2.31 – 168.73	0.006
Lightweight (baseline)	1	-	-	-
Native cobs	31.48	37.61	3.03 – 327.30	0.004
Sports horse	1.75	2.58	0.09 – 31.34	0.70
Other	40.03	48.21	3.78 – 424.31	0.002
*Herd size (number of individuals)**	0.87	0.05	0.77 – 0.98	0.02
Constant	0.10	0.12	0.01 – 0.92	0.04

*decrease CNS for every extra individual in the herd.

Inter-observer reliability of the cresty neck score

The inter-observer agreement of the three trained observers was good (Table 4), with moderate agreement between observers 1 and 2 and observers 1 and 3, and substantial agreement between observers 2 and 3. When the scores for horses and ponies were examined separately inter-observer reliability remained good, though agreement was lower for horses than ponies.

Discussion

The prevalence of CNS ≥3/5 was significantly higher at the end of the winter months, 45.83%, compared to 33.33% at the end of the summer. Nuchal neck adiposity therefore shows the opposite seasonal pattern to that previously demonstrated for general obesity in the same study population [25], where general obesity prevalence was found to be highest at the end of the summer

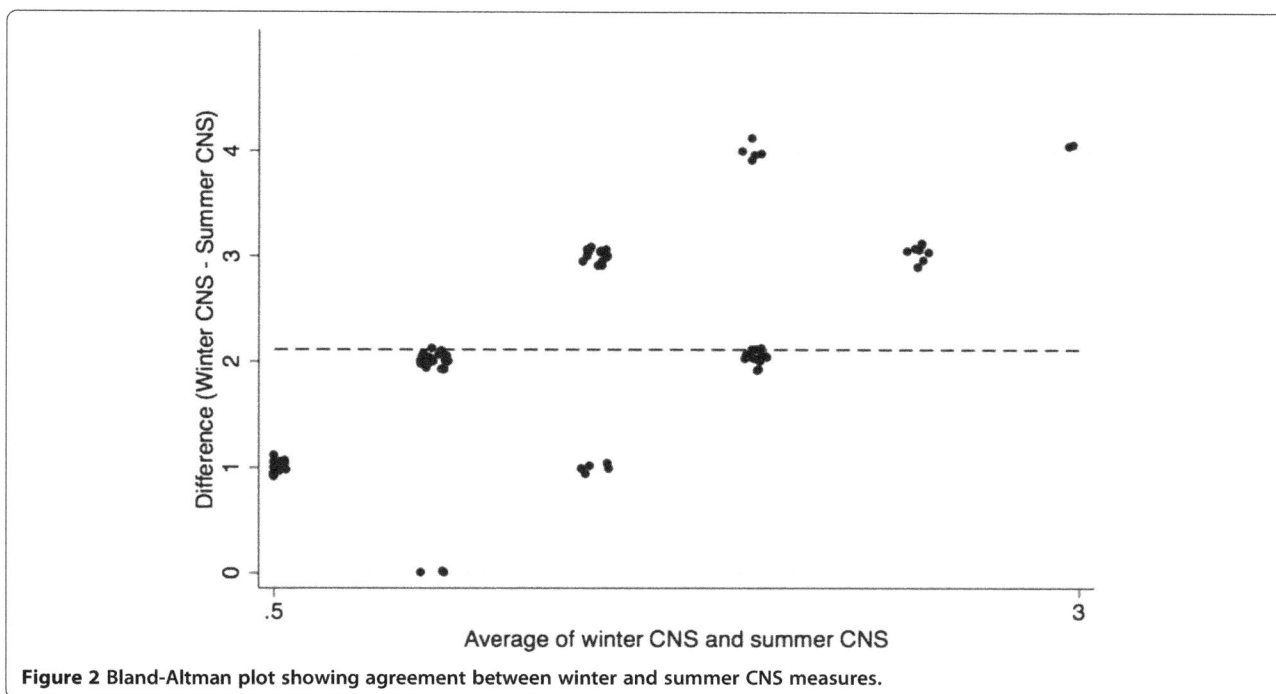

Figure 2 Bland-Altman plot showing agreement between winter and summer CNS measures.

months. This disproves our original hypothesis. There are two possible major reasons why neck crest adiposity differs to general adiposity in this way: this is either a real physiological effect, or a methodological anomaly with the Cresty Neck Score itself. First a potential methodological explanation will be considered, and then the biological results can be more clearly deliberated in light of this.

It is possible that the differences in the seasonal prevalences seen may be due to errors with our application of the CNS. There was a systematic variation between the winter and summer measures, where winter measures were significantly higher. Time of year appears to somehow affect the application and interpretation of this score. This was a non-blinded study, and so there is a potential that this could have biased the summer measurements, however even if observer bias did occur due to non-blinding, we would expect summer estimates to be an over rather than under-estimate, so this does not explain the results observed.

A lack of between-season agreement would not have been surprising in itself; it is the pattern of seasonal

variation observed here which was unexpected. We argue that observer error is ultimately unlikely to fully explain the extent of differences in the prevalence of cresty neck observed between seasons in this study population. However we do suggest that errors with the between-season repeatability of the score may partly contributed as a minor influence. It may be that the CNS is less effective at distinguishing neck adiposity during the winter months when horses and ponies have a fluffy winter coat (although measuring neck circumference using a tape measure would encounter similar issues). A large study conducted during the winter months, containing a number of different breeds with varying winter coat lengths and BCS systems, would be required to investigate this. This was beyond the scope of this particular study. As the CNS is a relatively new measure, and the seasonal variation in nuchal crest adiposity has not previously been investigated. These results may therefore have important implications for the future application of the CNS, particularly with regards to considering potential seasonal variability. Based on

Table 4 Weighted Cohen's kappa showing the inter-observer agreement results between the 3 trained observers assessing 31* horses and ponies

Observers compared	Observed agreement (%)	Expected agreement (%)	κ_w	SE	Z	p
Observer 1 and Observer 2	95.86	89.57	0.60	0.16	3.69	<0.001
Observer 2 and Observer 3	97.16	90.28	0.71	0.17	4.09	<0.001
Observer 1 and Observer 3	94.61	88.30	0.54	0.16	3.26	0.001

*note one observer only assessed 29 horses and ponies.

the between-season variability observed here , we would recommend that alongside an investigation of the influence of breed, the repeatability of the Cresty Neck Score be tested using test-retest methods at several key seasonal time points, to see if it is a suitable measure for such investigations. It may be that this measure is not appropriate to compare adiposity in outdoor living animals measured at different times of year.

As far as we are aware this is first study to have investigated the inter-observer reliability of the CNS score. Notably the agreement between observers, at a single moment in time, was greater than agreement between the results of the same observer at the two different seasonal time points. It was reassuring to discover that all observers had good agreement, indicating that the score has good inter-observer repeatability. However the systematic variation in scores observed may have other implications. Whilst discrepancies by just one scoring level would not contribute greatly to a perceived 'lack of agreement' using weighted kappa methods, they may have more serious clinical consequences. An observer that scores 2 instead of 3, or *vice versa*, could inadvertently alter the results of a clinical study dramatically if this is the cut-off criterion being used to distinguish a 'cresty neck' case from a non-'cresty neck' case. These two scores are the most commonly used by observers, occupying the middle of the scorable range. There is therefore still the possibility, regardless of the generally good agreement scores, that the final results were influenced by the cut-off used. Further investigations are certainly required to fully understand the possible implications of this.

Despite this systematic difference between winter and summer measures, our results suggest that the reliability of the CNS is generally good. It therefore is just as likely that there is a biological explanation for the pattern of seasonal variation observed in nuchal crest adiposity. It is possible that nuchal cresty adiposity could have a functional physiological role as an indicator of individuals coming out of winter in good breeding condition, but this is just speculation. Previous authors have suggested that tissue within the nuchal region in horses and ponies is akin to visceral abdominal fat in humans [10,27]. If nuchal fat is indeed similar to abdominal fat in humans, then the type of fat stored in the neck crest may be structurally different, and have different functional properties to that of fat stored elsewhere. In humans, visceral abdominal fat is more strongly associated with metabolic abnormalities such as type-2 diabetes mellitus, insulin resistance and hyperinsulinemia [1-4]. It has been suggested that adipose tissue in this region represents 'dysfunctional' adipose tissue in individuals unable to store excess energy effectively [28]. In humans this defect in energy partitioning leads to an altered metabolic profile and inflammatory state, and the same could be true in horses and ponies with excess nuchal crest adiposity.

Evidence regarding these physiological mechanisms in horses is still mixed. Burns and colleagues [12] found no evidence of a difference in gene expression for proinflammatory cytokines in the nuchal (neck crest) region between insulin resistant and insulin sensitive animals but did find higher levels of some interleukins (IL-1β and IL-6) in the nuchal crest region suggesting it was a more active proinflammatory cytokine depot. Bruynsteen and colleagues [13] found evidence of higher leptin mRNA expression in adipose tissue from the nuchal region compared to mesenteric adipose tissue, but in contrast to Burns et al. [12], the highest levels of IL-1β were found in abdominal adipose tissue, suggesting that this region, similarly to humans, may in fact be more important than the nuchal crest adipose tissue in determining circulating levels of cytokines. Potentially nuchal crest adiposity could simply be a proxy measure which is associated with increased internal abdominal adiposity not detectable by visual body condition scoring methods. Note that both of these studies rely on gene expression and thus results may be influenced by the reference genes chosen, studies relating directly to protein expression and circulating proinflammatory cytokines are clearly required to further investigate these mechanisms.

In horses and ponies, insulin resistance has been strongly associated with neck crest adiposity and generalised obesity [7,8,11]. Insulin sensitivity, like body condition, has also been suggested to vary seasonally [7,14,29,30] especially in hardy native pony breeds, in which the prevalence of nuchal crest adiposity was highest in the current study. Studies have shown a higher insulin sensitivity during the autumn and winter and a lower insulin sensitivity during the spring and summer [7,30]. Interestingly the results presented here show the same seasonal physiological pattern in nuchal crest adiposity. As we did not measure insulin sensitivity in these animals, any discussion of insulin responsiveness here is purely speculative.

The neck crest area of fat storage takes longer to develop and deplete than other fat storage sites in horses and ponies [6,26]. Changes in nuchal crest adiposity may therefore not fit within seasonal patterns of food availability and may instead reflect longer-term management trends. This could offer another explanation as to why the seasonal variation in nuchal crest adiposity is different to that of general obesity.

We examined whether the higher winter prevalence of CNS ≥3/5 could be explained by exercise. On average ponies carried out less exercise than horses and fewer ponies carried out any form of structured exercise (see [25]). It is possible this exacerbated the higher prevalence of CNS ≥3/5 in ponies over horses. On average, horses and ponies that were ridden received around 1.5 hours more exercise per week during the summer months than the winter months (see [25]). These seasonal changes in structured exercise may act to reduce nuchal crest adiposity during the summer months through a combination of higher amounts of exercise alongside increased metabolic rate and improved insulin sensitivity. Although exercise did not appear to explain variation within nuchal crest adiposity in our study population, but a high percentage (over 60%) did not carry out any regular structured exercise.

The prevalence of CNS ≥3/5 in ponies at the end of winter was 61%, representing a real potential welfare issue if a CNS ≥3/5 is shown to be truly associated with an increase risk of serious health consequences. Risk factor analysis revealed that native cobs as well as native ponies appear to have a strong breed predisposition to nuchal crest adiposity. This is similar to the breed association seen with general obesity [25]. This demonstrates that breed needs to be considered when CNS measurements are taken. Previous authors have also suggested a breed predisposition to an enlarged nuchal crest [6,15], and our results support this. Native UK breeds naturally live in nutritionally sparse winter environments, such as on mountains or moorland [31], and nuchal crest adiposity may therefore be an adaptive mechanism of fat storage for survival during periods of nutritional scarcity. These results support this, the described adaptive strategy may be less clear in domestically selected lines, with sports horse and lightweight breeds appearing to be at a lessened risk . It must be noted that lightweight breeds within this particular study population of UK leisure horses, refers mostly to Arabian and Thoroughbred types and there were few American stock horse or Spanish breeds, which previous authors have suggested may also be at higher risk of nuchal crest adiposity [6].

It must be considered however, that whilst the genetics of these native breeds may be similar to their wild or feral counterparts, and thus possess similar seasonal fluctuations in body condition, the management of domestic native breeds is often very different to their 'natural' environment, with food often plentiful year round. The seasonal pattern of nuchal crest variation observed here, could therefore just be a consequence of the unnaturally nutrient rich captive environment in which domestic native breeds are kept. It would certainly be of interest to investigate seasonal variation in nuchal crest adiposity in feral herds. The results of this study also focus purely on a study population with daily access to pasture, it is not know how applicable these results would be to horses and ponies kept in a predominantly stabled environment, which plausibly do not have the same seasonal variation in food supply and body condition.

The effect of herd size upon body condition in horses has not previously been reported. Our results suggest that as the number of horses in the herd increase, there is an apparent decrease in neck crest adiposity. With an increased group size there is likely to be greater competition between individuals for forage resources, individuals are likely to be interrupted from grazing more often due to socially mediated interference [32] and spontaneous activity levels may also be higher in larger groups. It was noted that generally large groups did have a larger pasture area, as would be expected, but this was not measured explicitly. An alternate management related explanation could be that laminitis prone horses and ponies, which are also likely to be those with the largest neck circumference, may be removed from the main herd or managed separately in smaller groups on smaller pasture areas.

Conclusions

Our study demonstrates that winter and summer cresty neck scores vary within the same population of animals. Several possible explanations for this have been outlined. These differences could represent a physiological phenomena, where neck crest fat is larger at the end of winter and depletes during the summer possibly due to a higher metabolic rate, higher activity and possibly a change in insulin sensitivity. Alternatively these results could represent an anomaly with the CNS itself. Further studies are required to validate the score for clinical research use, especially in outdoor living horses and ponies. Using the CNS system alongside the Henneke et al. [33] BCS system may enable potentially different types of obesity with different risks for health to be monitored more accurately.

Additional file

Additional file 1: Risk factor questionnaires.

Abbreviations
CNS: Cresty neck score; BCS: Body condition score.

Competing interests
Patricia A. Harris is an employee of WALTHAM Centre for Pet Nutrition. The authors have declared no competing interests.

Authors' contributions
SLG performed the studies, analysed the data, and wrote the paper. SAR prepared figures and tables. All authors conceived and designed the studies, and edited and commented on the manuscript. All authors read and approved the final manuscript.

Acknowledgements
Horseworld and the Blackdown Mendip Riding Club are thanked for their kind co-operation and use of horses and ponies. We also thank Dr Caroline McGregor-Argo for useful comments on the manuscript and Dr Nicola Menzies-Gow and Ms Liz Finding of the Royal Veterinary College for inter-observer reliability scoring. This study was funded by the Biotechnology and Biological Sciences Research Council [grant number BB/H01568X/1] and WALTHAM Centre for Pet Nutrition, and forms part of an Industrial CASE

studentship. The funders (other than Pat Harris as contributing author) had no role in study design, data collection and analysis, decision to publish, or preparation of the manuscript.

Author details
[1]School of Veterinary Science, University of Bristol, Langford, Bristol BS40 5DU, UK. [2]School of Biological Sciences, University of Bristol, Bristol Life Science Building, 24 Tyndall Avenue, Bristol BS8 1TQ, UK. [3]WALTHAM Centre for Pet Nutrition, Equine Studies Group, Freeby Lane, Waltham-on-the-Wolds, Leicestershire LE14 4RT, Melton Mowbray, UK.

References

1. Carey DG, Jenkins AB, Campbell LV, Freund J, Chisholm DJ. Abdominal fat and insulin resistance in normal and overweight women: direct measurements reveal a strong relationship in subjects at both low and high risk of NIDDM. Diabetes. 1996;45:633–8.
2. Cnop M, Landchild MJ, Vidal J, Havel PJ, Knowles NG, Carr DR, et al. The concurrent accumulation of intra-abdominal and subcutaneous fat explains the association between insulin resistance and plasma leptin concentrations: distinct metabolic effects of two fat compartments. Diabetes. 2002;51:1005–15.
3. Katsuki A, Sumida Y, Urakawa H, Gabazza EC, Murashima S, Maruyama N, et al. Increased visceral fat and serum levels of triglyceride are associated with insulin resistance in Japanese metabolically obese, normal weight subjects with normal glucose tolerance. Diabetes Care. 2003;26:2341–4.
4. Wagenknecht LE, Langefeld CD, Scherzinger AL, Norris JM, Haffner SM, Saad MF, et al. Insulin sensitivity, insulin secretion, and abdominal fat: the insulin resistance atherosclerosis study (IRAS) family study. Diabetes. 2003;52:2490–6.
5. Carter RA, Geor RJ, Burton Staniar W, Cubuitt TA, Harris PA. Apparent adiposity assessed by standardised scoring systems and morphometric measurements in horses and ponies. Vet J. 2009;179:204–10.
6. Johnson PJ, Wiedmeyer CE, LaCarrubba A, Ganjam VK, Messer NT. Laminitis and the equine metabolic syndrome. Vet Clin N Am-Equine. 2010;26:239–55.
7. Bailey SR, Habershon-Butcher JL, Ransom KJ, Elliott J, Menzies-Gow NJ. Hypertension and insulin resistance in a mixed-breed population of ponies predisposed to laminitis. Am J Vet Res. 2008;69:122–9.
8. Frank N, Elliott SB, Brandt LE, Keisler DH. Physical characteristics, blood hormone concentrations, and plasma lipid concentrations in obese horses with insulin resitance. J Am Vet Med Assoc. 2006;228:1383–90.
9. Johnson PJ. The equine metabolic syndrome: Peripheral Cushing's syndrome. Vet Clin N Am-Equine. 2002;18:271–93.
10. Carter RA, Treiber KH, Geor RJ, Douglass L, Harris PA. Prediction of incipient pasture-associated laminitis from hyperinsulinaemia, hyperleptinaemia and generalised and localised obesity in a cohort of ponies. Equine Vet J. 2009;41:171–8.
11. Geor RJ. Metabolic predispositions to laminitis in horses and ponies: obesity, insulin resistance and metabolic syndromes. J Equine Vet Sci. 2008;28:753–9.
12. Burns TA, Geor RJ, Mudge MC, McCutcheon LJ, Hinchcliff KW, Belknap JK. Proinflammatory cytokine and chemokine gene expression profiles in subcutaneous and visceral adipose tissue depots of insulin-resistant and insulin-sensitive light breed horses. J Vet Intern Med. 2010;24:932–9.
13. Bruynsteen L, Erkens T, Peelman LJ, Ducatelle R, Janssens GP, Harris PA, et al. Expression of inflammation-related genes is associated with adipose tissue location in horses. BMC Vet Res. 2013;9:240.
14. Frank N, Geor RJ, Bailey SR, Durham AE, Johnson PJ. Equine metabolic syndrome. J Vet Internal Med. 2010;24:467–75.
15. Alford P, Geller S, Richardson B, Slater M, Honnas C, Foreman J, et al. A multicenter, matched case–control study of risk factors for equine laminitis. Prev Vet Med. 2001;49:209–22.
16. Bamford N, Potter S, Harris P, Bailey S. Breed differences in insulin sensitivity and insulinemic responses to oral glucose in horses and ponies of moderate body condition score. Domest Anim Endocrin. 2014;47:101–7.
17. Morgan R, McGowan T, McGowan C. Prevalence and risk factors for hyperinsulinaemia in ponies in Queensland, Australia. Austral Vet J. 2014;92:101–6.
18. Laat MA, Patterson-Kane JC, Pollitt CC, Sillence MN, McGowan CM. Histological and morphometric lesions in the pre-clinical, developmental phase of insulin-induced laminitis in Standardbred horses. Vet J. 2013;195:305–12.
19. Brinkmann L, Gerken M, Riek A. Effect of long-term feed restriction on the health status and welfare of a robust horse breed, the Shetland pony (Equus ferus caballus). Res Vet Sci. 2013;94:826–31.
20. Pleasant R, Suagee J, Thatcher C, Elvinger F, Geor R. Adiposity, plasma insulin, leptin, lipids, and oxidative stress in mature light breed horses. J Vet Intern Med. 2013;27:576–82.
21. Stephenson HM, Green MJ, Freeman SL. Prevalence of obesity in a population of horses in the UK. Vet Rec. 2011;168:131.
22. Thatcher CD, Pleasant RS, Geor RJ, Elvinger F. Prevalence of overconditioning in mature horses in Southwest Virginia during the summer. J Vet Intern Med. 2012;26:1413–8.
23. Thatcher CD, Pleasant RS, Geor RJ, Elvinger F, Negrin KA, Franklin J, et al. Prevalence of obesity in mature horses: an equine body condition study. J Anim Physiol Anim Nutr. 2008;92:222–2.
24. Wyse CA, McNie KA, Tannahil VJ, Love S, Murray JK. Prevalence of obesity in riding horses in Scotland. Vet Rec. 2008;162(18):590–1.
25. Giles SL, Rands SA, Nicol CJ, Harris PA. Obesity prevalence and associated risk factors in outdoor living domestic horses and ponies. Peer J. 2014;2:e299.
26. Dugdale AHA, Curtis GC, Cripps PJ, Harris PA, Argo CM. Effects of season and body condition on appetite, body mass and body composition in ad libitum fed pony mares. Vet J. 2011;190:329–37.
27. Johnson PJ, Wiedmeyer CE, Messer NT, Ganjam VK. Medical implications of obesity in horses—lessons for human obesity. J Diabetes Sci Technol. 2009;3:163–74.
28. Després J-P, Lemieux I. Abdominal obesity and metabolic syndrome. Nature. 2006;444:881–7.
29. Beech J, Boston RC, McFarlane D, Lindborg S. Evaluation of plasma ACTH, α-melanocyte–stimulating hormone, and insulin concentrations during various photoperiods in clinically normal horses and ponies and those with pituitary pars intermedia dysfunction. J Am Vet Med Assoc. 2009;235:715–22.
30. Borer KE, Bailey SR, Menzies-Gow NJ, Harris PA, Elliott J. Effect of feeding glucose, fructose, and inulin on blood glucose and insulin concentrations in normal ponies and those predisposed to laminitis. J Anim Sci. 2012;90:3003–11.
31. Speed JG, Etherington MG. The Exmoor pony and a survey of the evolution of horses in Britain. Part 1. Brit Vet J. 1952;108:329–58.
32. Rands SA, Pettifor RA, Rowcliffe JMR, Cowlishaw G. Social foraging and dominance relationships: the effects of socially mediated interference. Behav Ecol Sociobiol. 2006;60:572–81.
33. Henneke DR, Potter GD, Kreider JL, Yeates BF. Relationship between condition score, physical measurements and body fat percentage in mares. Equine Vet J. 1983;15:371–2.

4

Changes in the equine fecal microbiota associated with the use of systemic antimicrobial drugs

Marcio C Costa[1*], Henry R Stämpfli[2], Luis G Arroyo[2], Emma Allen-Vercoe[3], Roberta G Gomes[4] and J Scott Weese[1]

Abstract

Background: The intestinal tract is a rich and complex environment and its microbiota has been shown to have an important role in health and disease in the host. Several factors can cause disruption of the normal intestinal microbiota, including antimicrobial therapy, which is an important cause of diarrhea in horses. This study aimed to characterize changes in the fecal bacterial populations of healthy horses associated with the administration of frequently used antimicrobial drugs.

Results: Twenty-four adult mares were assigned to receive procaine penicillin intramuscularly (IM), ceftiofur sodium IM, trimethoprim sulfadiazine (TMS) orally or to a control group. Treatment was given for 5 consecutive days and fecal samples were collected before drug administration (Day 1), at the end of treatment (Days 5), and on Days 14 and 30 of the trial. High throughput sequencing of the V4 region of the 16S rRNA gene was performed using an Illumina MiSeq sequencer. Significant changes of population structure and community membership were observed after the use of all drugs. TMS caused the most marked changes on fecal microbiota even at higher taxonomic levels including a significant decrease of richness and diversity. Those changes were mainly due to a drastic decrease of Verrucomicrobia, specifically the "5 genus *incertae sedis*". Changes in structure and membership caused by antimicrobial administration were specific for each drug and may be predictable. Twenty-five days after the end of treatment, bacterial profiles were more similar to pre-treatment patterns indicating a recovery from changes caused by antimicrobial administration, but differences were still evident, especially regarding community membership.

Conclusions: The use of systemic antimicrobials leads to changes in the intestinal microbiota, with different and specific responses to different antimicrobials. All antimicrobials tested here had some impact on the microbiota, but TMS significantly reduced bacterial species richness and diversity and had the greatest apparent impact on population structure, specifically targeting members of the Verrucomicrobia phylum.

Keywords: Horses, Antibiotics, Intestinal microbiota, Intestinal bacteria, Microbiome, Antimicrobial associated diarrhea

Background

The intestinal microbiota performs important roles in the maintenance of health and on the pathophysiology of several diseases [1]. In the horse, the intestinal bacterial microbiota is particularly important due to its role in cellulose fermentation and short chain fatty acid production, which comprise the main energy sources for this animal species [2]. Gastrointestinal disease is one of the leading causes of morbidity and mortality in the horse [3], yet, despite its importance, the equine intestinal microbiota has not been extensively investigated. However, new

molecular technologies, especially next-generation sequencing methods, have become more available of late, and recently a number of publications have brought new insights into this complex microbial community [4-9]. Yet, much about the equine intestinal microbiota remains to be discerned.

Several factors have been shown to induce profound changes on the gastro-intestinal microbiota of horses including diet [10,11], intestinal disease [5], fasting [12,13] and transportation [14]. Of special interest are the effects of antimicrobials, as this group of drugs can have major impact on the intestinal microbiota of horses [15], and colitis is an important (and potentially life-threatening) complication of antimicrobial exposure in this species [16-18].

* Correspondence: costamc@gmail.com
[1]Department of Pathobiology, Ontario Veterinary College, University of Guelph, Guelph, Canada
Full list of author information is available at the end of the article

Changes in the intestinal microbiota induced by the use of antibiotics can be present as soon as 24 hours after administration of the drug in humans, with profound changes around 4 days [19,20] and partial recovery of the intestinal microbiota occurring around 30 to 40 days after treatment [19,21,22]. However, structural changes in bacterial communities may take years to return to pre-treatment baseline following antibiotic induced disturbance [23].

To date, many investigations of the effects of antimicrobial usage in horses have been limited to culture-based studies [15,24,25], which have yielded conflicting results. Gustafsson et al. [25] found no effect on the fecal microbiota of horses treated with oral or intravenous trimethoprim-sulfadiazine (TMS). Conversely, Harlow et al. [15] showed dramatic disruption of the culturable microbiota concurrent with increased shedding of enteropathogens after administration of TMS or ceftiofur sodium in horses. Moreover, a study using DGGE failed to detect changes caused by the use of antibiotics [26]; however, it is unclear whether there was no true difference or whether results simply reflect the limited resolution of this technique. While culture-dependent methods are necessary to characterize new bacterial species and can give better resolution for the identification of microorganisms, sequencing methods have become the elective choice for a broader characterization of the intestinal microbiota.

The objective of this study was to evaluate changes in the intestinal microbiota of healthy horses in response to administration of commonly used antimicrobials using next generation sequencing.

Results

Metrics

A total of 4,275,413 reads from 96 samples (mean: 47,431; SD: 29,796) passed all quality filters and were assigned into operational taxonomic units (OTUs). A subsample of 10.482 reads per sample was taken in order to normalize the number of reads across all samples and six samples were excluded from analysis because of low read numbers. These belonged to the groups: penicillin (Day 30), TMS (Day 1: two samples and Day 14: two samples) and control (Day 5). The number of OTUs in the subsampled population varied between 1,333 and 3,628 per sample (mean: 2,671; SD: 488). The number of OTUs found in each sample is presented in Additional file 1.

The average of the number of reads found in each group after subsampling of 10,000 reads is represented by rarefaction curves in Figure 1. Results from the Good's coverage achieved after subsampling are presented in Additional file 1 (mean: 85%; SD: 4%) and are also supportive of good coverage.

Relative abundances

The relative abundances at the phylum, class and genus levels found in each group at the different sampling times are represented in Figure 2. Sequences were classified into 25 different phyla, of which, only eight accounted for more than 1% of sequences. The majority of bacteria found in all groups throughout the trial were assigned to the Firmicutes phylum. Verrucomicrobia represented the second main phylum, followed by bacteria that were unclassified at the phylum level. At the genus level, "5 genus incertae sedis", a genus from the Subdivision 5 class of the Verrucomicrobia phylum, predominated followed by bacteria unclassified at the phylum level. Figure 3 represents variation of the main genera overtime in each treatment group.

No statistical changes in relative abundances were observed at the phylum level in response to ceftiofur administration. A decrease of Spirochetes followed by a significant increase on Day 14 (P = 0.017) was observed after treatment with penicillin. Oral TMS significantly reduced the relative abundance of Verrucomicrobia (P = 0.012), unclassified bacteria (P = 0.025) and a trend to reduce Proteobacteria (P = 0.052) and increased the abundance of Firmicutes (P = 0.012) after 5 days of treatment.

Population analysis

Results of Simpson's index estimating samples' diversity, and of Catchall estimation of richness are presented in Additional file 1. Table 1 contains results from the comparison of those results at different sampling times within each group. There was a significant decrease in richness (P = 0.017) and diversity (P = 0.018) after the use of TMS (Day 1 × Day 5), but after 30 days, both estimates were similar to the beginning of the trial. No other differences in diversity or richness were identified.

Figures 4A and B represent the dendrograms obtained with the Yue and Clayton and the Classic Jaccard analyses that respectively represent population structure (taking into account the number of OTUs and their relative abundances) and community membership (taking into account the number of OTUs). Figure 4A indicates that samples collected before treatment had more similar microbial population structure to each other and to samples collected on Day 14 and 30. In general, samples collected after treatment (Day 5) are observed at the lower part of the tree and interestingly, samples tended to cluster by the drug administered, indicating a somewhat consistent effect of each antibiotic, with the exception of animals treated with penicillin. Conversely, penicillin and ceftiofur seemed to have a strong effect on community membership, as represented by Figure 4B, in which samples from animals receiving those drugs were more distinct from other samples, even at Day 14. The changes caused by TMS and ceftiofur administration on

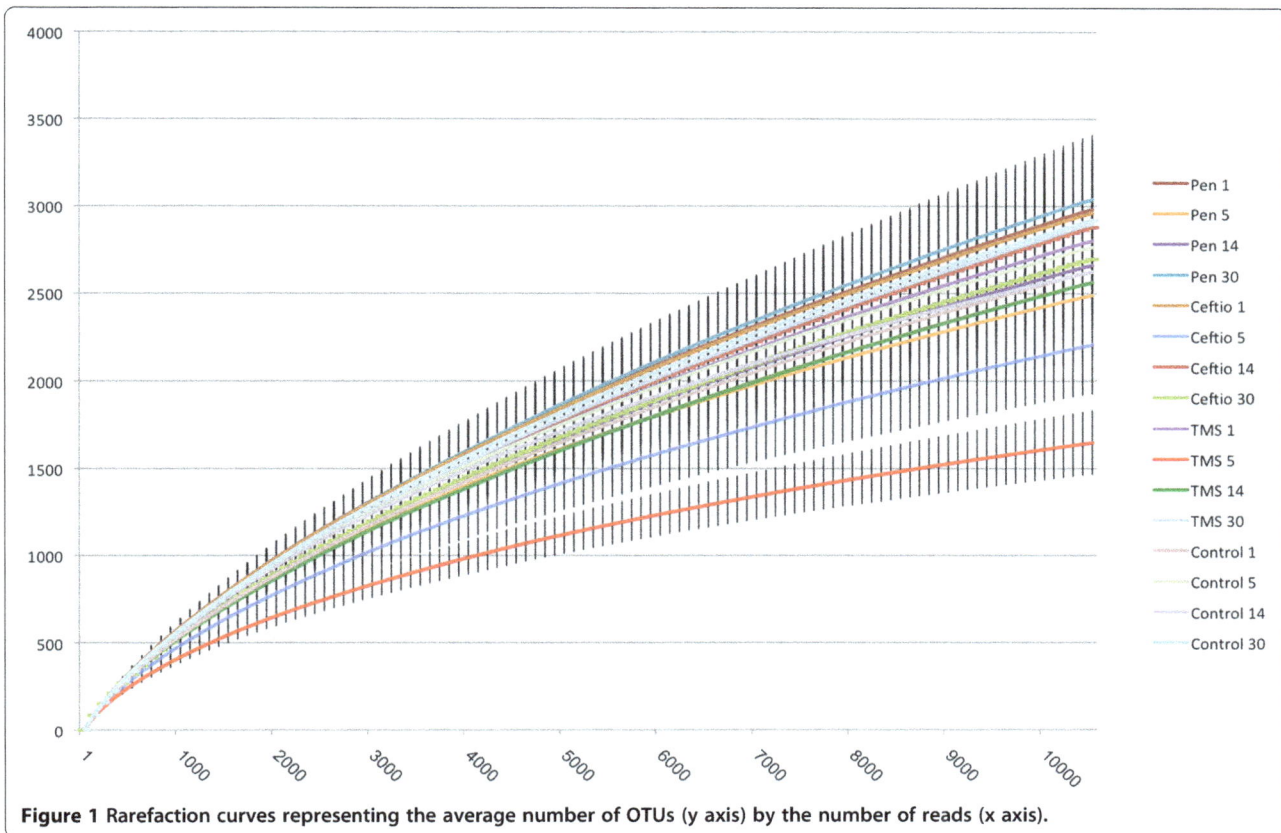

Figure 1 Rarefaction curves representing the average number of OTUs (y axis) by the number of reads (x axis).

community membership were also consistent, as samples after drug administration (Day 5) tended to cluster together.

Results from the Parsimony and AMOVA tests comparing each group at the different sampling times for either population structure and community membership are presented in Table 1. Overall, population structure and community membership were significantly different after the use of antimicrobials, regardless of the statistical test applied. The results also indicate that after 14 and 30 days population structures were still different from the beginning of the trial. Considering each group individually, penicillin had no impact on population structure and community membership evaluated by the Parsimony test, but a significant difference was identified using AMOVA. Ceftiofur and TMS induced significant changes 5 days after drug administration, but changes tended not to last for more than 14 days, indicating a recovery of population structure and community membership in the studied animals.

The graphical representation of the PCoA is shown in Figure 5A and B, for the Yue and Clayton and the Classic Jaccard respectively. Despite the two first axes of the PCoA explained only 28% and 3.7% of the dissimilarities between samples respectively for the Yue and Clayton and

the Classic Jaccard, clustering of samples by date of sampling and by drug administered is still evident, reinforcing the strong impact caused by antibiotics administration on the intestinal microbiota of those animals, which is further supported by the significant results from the AMOVA test (Table 1).

Potential confounding factors

A moderate lameness was noticed in one mare in the penicillin group on Day 4 of the trial due to a sole abscess on the right front limb. The mare was transported (approximately 10 km) to the Ontario Veterinary College Health Sciences Centre (OVCHSC) after collection of the Day 5 sample and the last antimicrobial treatment was given at the hospital. The diet of that horse was unchanged (with the exception of feeding from a different batch of hay). Treatment with 2 g of phenylbutazone was given and the mare returned to the research station on Day 9. Another dose of phenylbutazone was given on Day 15, as the mare became mildly lame again. On Day 22 of the trial, another mare from the ceftiofur group was found with a deep laceration on her chest and was therefore shipped to the OVCHSC for treatment. Cleaning with topical antiseptic solution was started with no systemic antimicrobials required. The mare recovered well

A

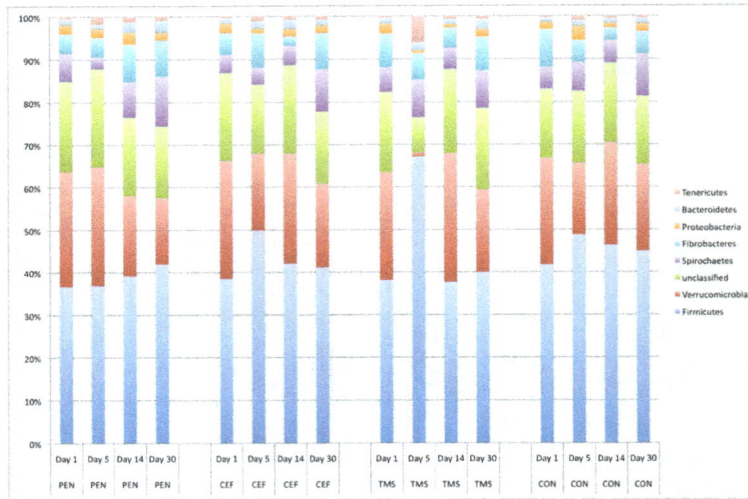

B

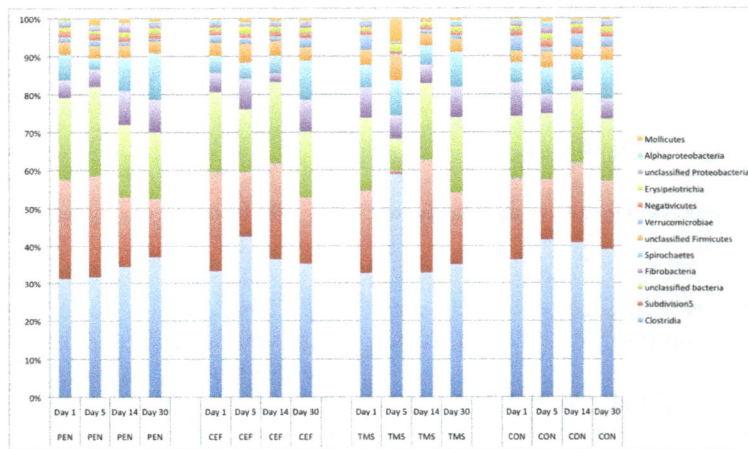

C

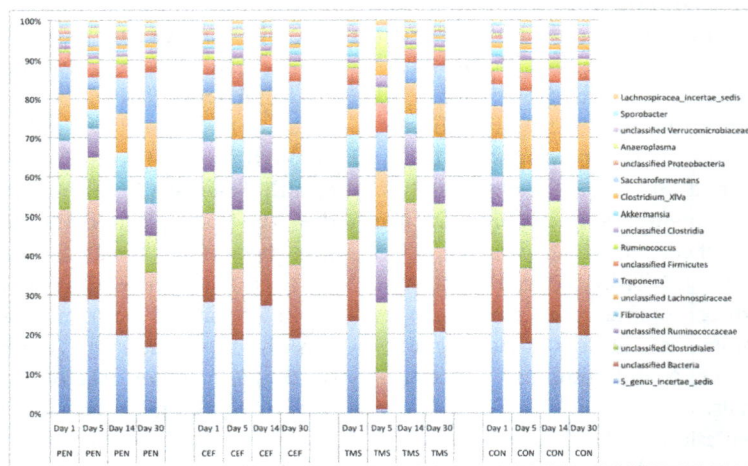

Figure 2 Relative abundance of predominant bacteria at the phylum (A), class (B) and genus (C) levels. Figure legend: penicillin (PEN), ceftiofur (CEF) and sulfa trimethoprin (TMS) and control group (CON). Day 0: before treatment; Day 5: last day of treatment.

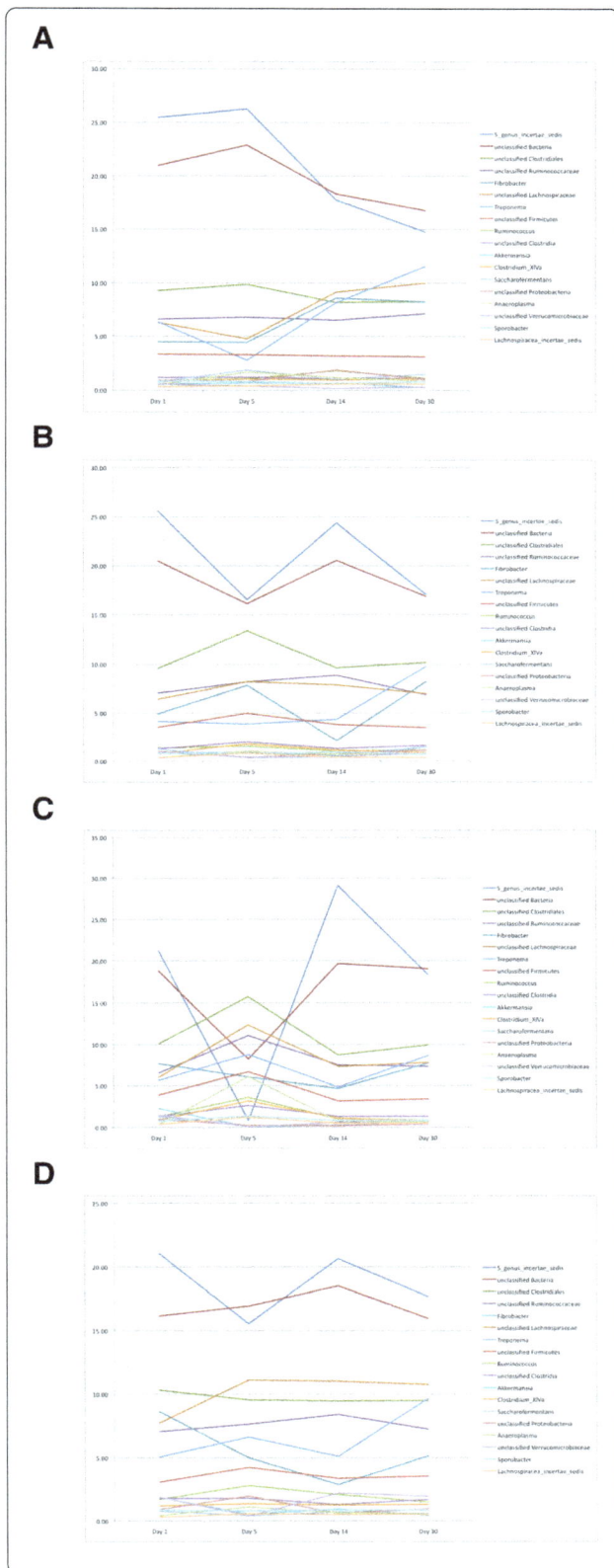

Figure 3 Variation in relative abundance of predominant bacteria in feces of healthy horses treated with antibiotics. Figure legend: **A**: penicillin; **B**: ceftiofur; **C**: sulfa trimethoprin; **D**: control group. Day 0: before treatment; Day 5: last day of treatment.

and was discharged from the hospital after the end of the trial.

Discussion

Antimicrobial administration produced variable but detectable changes in the fecal microbiota. Differences were noted in specific taxonomic comparisons as well as broader evaluation of community membership (organisms present) and population structure (that takes into account the organisms present and their relative abundances). The presence of an impact of antimicrobial administration of a bacterial population is not unexpected, but the types of changes, the differences between different antimicrobials and the duration of impact are noteworthy and provide important insight.

The composition of the microbiota before antibiotic administration was not surprising, as the predominance of Firmicutes is in agreement with other studies [5,6,8,9]. The "5 genus *incertae sedis*" was the most abundant genus. This unculturable organism has been recently classified and it has been found in high abundances in feces of healthy adult horses [8,9], but its role on the equine GI tract remains to be elucidated.

The most profound effects of antimicrobials on the intestinal microbiota were observed immediately after treatment (Day 5), which is in agreement with reports in humans [20,27] and horses [15]. It was not surprising to see the main effect during antimicrobial treatment. Cessation of antimicrobial administration did not result in an immediate return to the baseline microbiota, as significant changes were still present 9 days after the end of treatment (Day 14). A similar effect has been previously observed after the use of ampicillin in humans [22] and of TMS or ceftiofur in horses [15]. By day 30 the microbiota was more similar to baseline than it was in the day 5 or day 14 samples, yet a discernable difference was still present, also evidenced by the significantly different AMOVA comparison in the group treated with penicillin (P = 0.021) and a trend in the group treated with TMS (P = 0.066). Immediate restoration of the microbiota was not expected, based on human data [21,22,27]. There was also limited apparent clustering of the day 1 and day 30 samples in the treatment group based on the dendrograms, as opposed to the control group, but further statistical comparison were not possible due to the low number of animals in the control group.It is assumed that there is more inter- than intra-individual variation and serial samples from the same individual typically cluster together

Table 1 P values from the Parsimony, AMOVA and t tests comparing groups at different sampling times

Treatment	Day 1- 5	Day 5- 14	Day 14- 30	Day 1- 14	Day 1- 30
Yue and Clayton					
Overall					
Parsimony	<0.001	<0.001	0.137	0.005	0.053
AMOVA	<0.001	<0.001	<0.001	0.060	<0.001
Penicillin					
Parsimony	0.263	0.052	0.865	0.059	0.114
AMOVA	0.042	0.010	0.272	0.141	0.021
Ceftiofur					
Parsimony	0.004	0.065	0.704	0.305	0.298
AMOVA	0.786	0.038	0.024	0.786	0.141
TMS					
Parsimony	0.002	<0.001	0.214	0.858	0.674
AMOVA	<0.001	0.002	0.028	0.119	0.066
Control					
Parsimony	1	1	1	1	1
AMOVA	1	1	1	1	1
Jaccard					
Overall					
Parsimony	<0.001	0.003	0.753	0.068	0.054
AMOVA	<0.001	<0.001	0.007	<0.001	<0.001
Penicillin					
Parsimony	0.063	0.714	0.836	0.698	0.408
AMOVA	<0.001	0.012	0.669	0.172	0.260
Ceftiofur					
Parsimony	<0.001	<0.001	0.701	0.281	0.683
AMOVA	<0.001	0.006	0.140	0.037	0.074
TMS					
Parsimony	<0.001	<0.001	0.682	0.878	0.67
AMOVA	0.003	0.003	0.033	0.025	0.096
Control					
Parsimony	1	1	1	1	1
AMOVA	1	1	1	1	1
t test					
Penicillin					
Simpson's	0.181	0.898	0.607		
CatchAll	0.163	0.172	0.794		
Ceftiofur					
Simpson's	0.628	0.370	0.321		
CatchAll	0.385	0.068	0.206		
TMS					
Simpson's	0.018	0.008	0.876		
CatchAll	0.017	0.002	0.508		

Table 1 P values from the Parsimony, AMOVA and t tests comparing groups at different sampling times (Continued)

Control			
Simpson's	0.400	0.554	0.495
CatchAll	0.278	0.680	0.266

[13,28], and clustering of control horse samples was evident. Here, the lack of clustering of day 1 and 30 samples from the same horse provides further evidence of an ongoing impact of antimicrobials. This provides more evidence of an ongoing impact on the microbiota, as intra-individual similarity would be expected in serial samples if the microbiota had reverted to its baseline.

Among the antimicrobials chosen for this study, TMS induced the most marked changes in population structure. Possible reasons for this are the route of administration used for this drug (oral) and its broader spectrum of action, especially when compared to penicillin, which has a narrower spectrum and is mainly excreted by the urinary tract. Oral administration can result in delivery of a large amount of active drug to the intestinal tract; however, the degree of absorption and local inactivation would have a major impact on exposure to the microbiota of the distal hindgut. Conversely, parenterally administered drugs can potentially achieve high intestinal concentrations, particularly those that undergo extensive hepatic excretion. Indeed, several classes of antimicrobials have been shown to induce changes on the luminal bacteria after intramuscular administration [29,30] and some of the horses receiving penicillin and ceftiofur in this study had marked changes observed on community membership (Figure 4B). It is worth mentioning that the dose of ceftiofur sodium used in this study is an extra-label dose, but it was used as it reflects common dosing in the field. Further studies comparing oral versus parenteral administration of TMS would help answer the question of whether changes observed here were induced by route of administration or by the spectrum of action of this drug.

Factors such as the antimicrobial spectrum, drug levels in the gut and inactivation of the antimicrobial in the gut could all influence the impact of individual antimicrobials. TMS is one of the few drugs that horses tolerate after oral administration, and it is also available as a parenteral formulation, so comparison of the parenteral and oral routes would be useful in a future study to determine the impact of route of administration of this drug.

While TMS produced the most identifiable impacts, some degree of change was noted with all of the tested antimicrobials. A lack of understanding of the pathophysiology of antimicrobial-associated colitis and the clinical relevance of the gut microbiota hamper direct clinical assessment of the relevance of these changes. It is reasonable to postulate that more profound microbiota changes

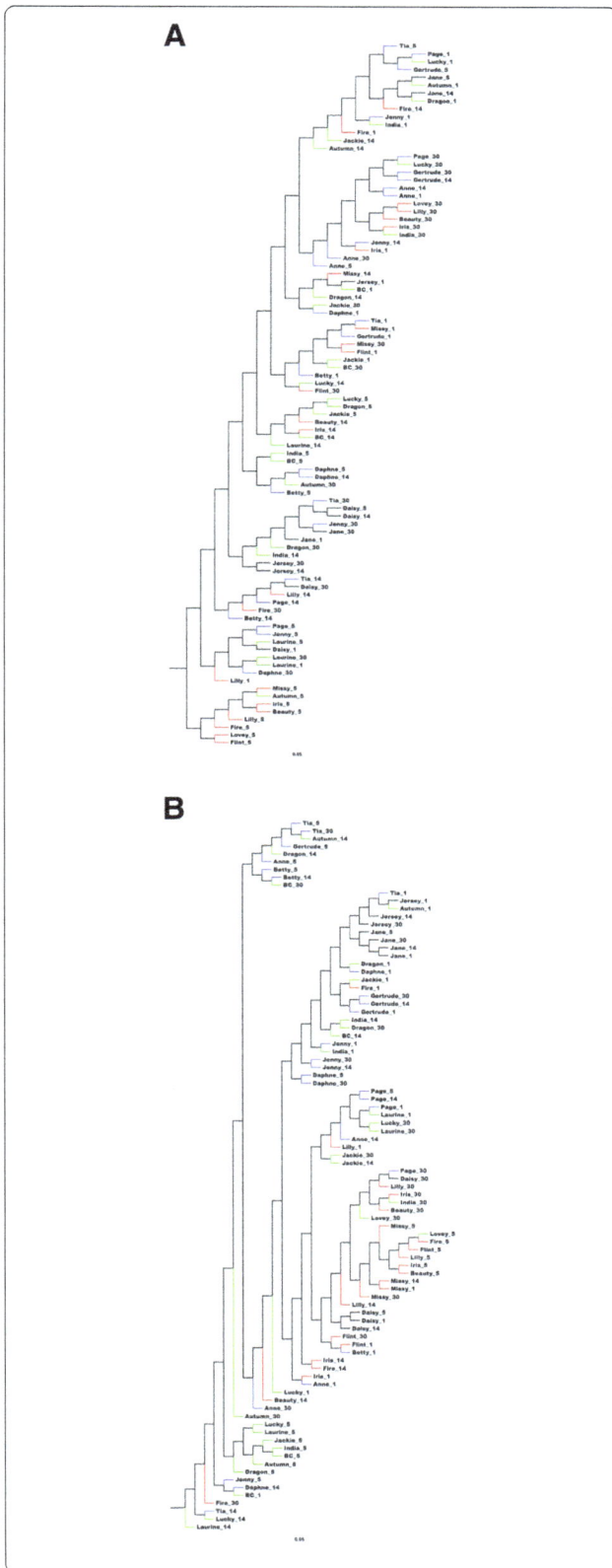

Figure 4 Dendrograms representing the similarities between population structure addressed by the Yue and Clayton analysis (A) and community membership addressed by the Classic Jaccard (B). Figure legend: Dendrograms were generated based on phylip-formatted distance matrixes using the UPGMA algorithm. The number after the name of the horse represents the day of sampling and the color of the tree brunch represents the drug used: Penicillin = blue, Ceftiofur = green, TMS = red and Control = black.

result in a greater risk of disease, yet 'change' and 'clinically relevant change' are not necessarily the same thing, and it is certainly possible that some less evident changes could be more relevant clinically. This highlights the need for more study of the intestinal microbiota in health and disease, to identify specific populations or population changes that have a greater influence.

The methods used in the present study allowed for differentiation between population structure addressed by the Yue and Clayton measure of dissimilarity that takes into account relative abundance in each sample and community membership addressed by the classic Jaccard index that takes into account the number of species. Interestingly, as it can be observed on the dendrograms, there was greater alteration of population structure compared to community membership. Thus, changes that were encountered were less likely to be addition or loss of specific community members, but rather changes in the relative abundance of existing members. This is consistent with the concept of 'overgrowth' of certain members in response to antimicrobial exposure.

Significant changes in the relative abundances at the phylum level observed in horses treated with penicillin and especially TMS, emphasize the potential those drugs have in causing disruption of the normal resident intestinal microbiota. Interestingly, the dramatic decrease (from 21.2% to 0.8%) of organisms classified as "5 genus *incertae sedis*" and unclassified Verrucomicrobia after the used of TMS is suggestive that this drug has a strong action against Verrucomicrobia, which allowed several genera belonging to Firmicutes to increase in abundance and it may be related to the resilience of the intestinal microbiota during recovery from severe disturbances [31]. The degree of change noted here is in contrast with earlier culture-dependent or DGGE studies, something that is not surprising because of the much greater depth that high throughput sequencing technologies allow. For instance, Gustafsson et al. [25] reported minimal effect of TMS on streptococci, Bacteroides and Veillonella counts in feces of horses, with a concurrent decrease in total coliforms. White and Prior [24] found no impact of this drug in coliforms, but a large increase of coliforms, Bacteroides, *Clostridium perfringens*, and streptococci after treatment with oxytetracycline. Moreover, Grønvold et al.

A

B

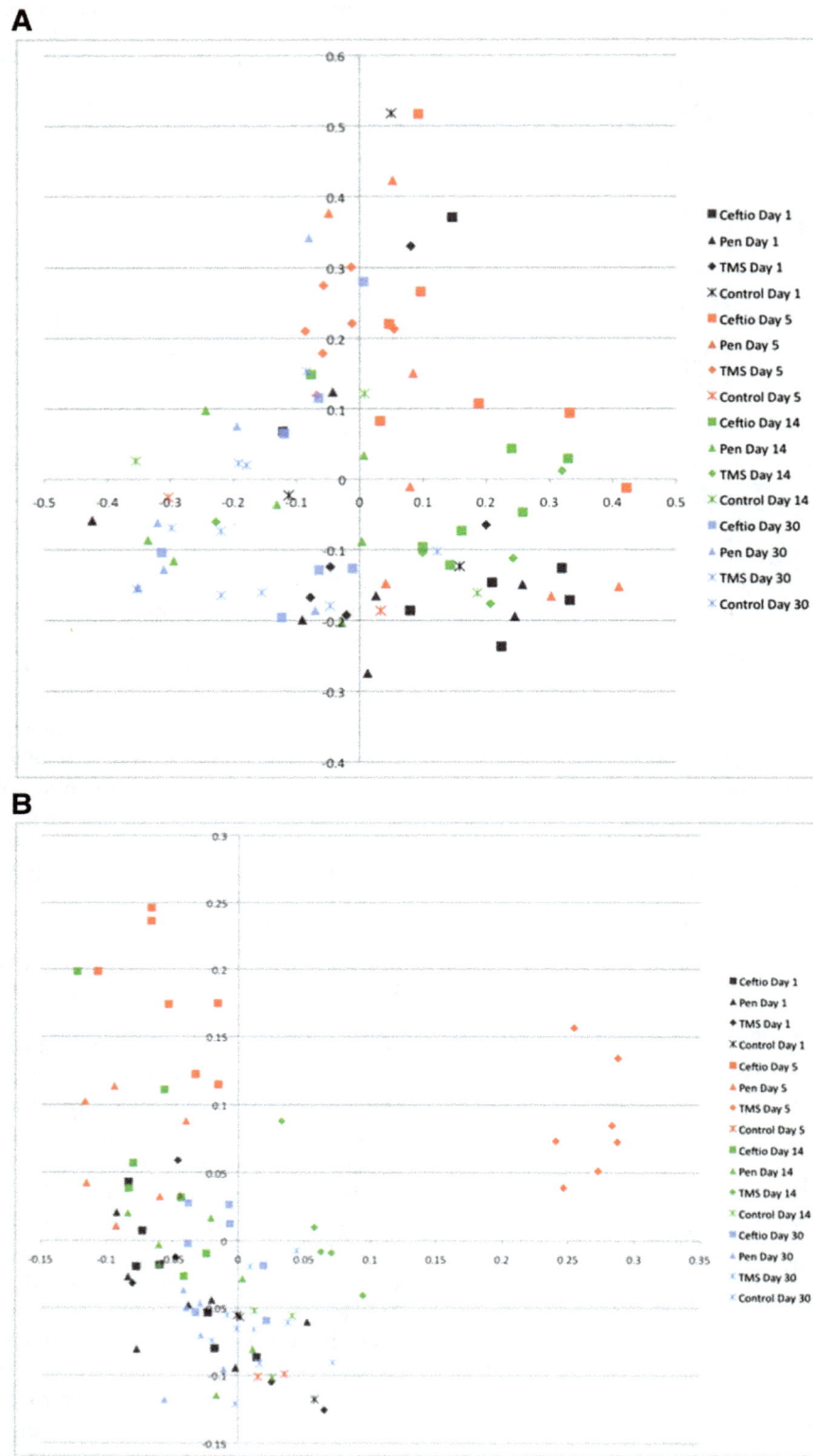

Figure 5 (See legend on next page.)

(See figure on previous page.)
Figure 5 Principal coordinate analysis (PCoA) of bacterial communities present in feces of horses treated with antibiotics. Figure legend: Bidimentional representation of the principal coordinate analysis of bacterial communities structure addressed by the Yue and Clayton analysis **(A)** and bacterial membership addressed by the Classic Jaccard analysis **(B)** found in feces of healthy horses before (Day 1), after (Day 5) treatment with antibiotics and at Days 14 and 30.

[26] found no significant differences in the DGGE profile of horses after treatment with penicillin, but differences in specific bacterial groups were present in the same study when investigated by qPCR. Therefore, the conflicting results found in the literature may reflect differences based on drugs used, horse characteristics or geography, but are more likely a result of variable fidelity of the chosen methods.

Conflicting results can be found in the literature regarding the predictability of changes induced by specific antimicrobial drugs. Vancomycin has been reported to induce consistent changes on intestinal microbial structures of humans treated with that drug [32], but another study reported unpredictable changes caused by the same drug [33]. Another report [27] found different individual responses to antimicrobial therapy despite identical dosing. This disagreement might be related to the presence of other factors impacting the intestinal microbiota in those subjects. Further, since there tends to be some variability in the microbiota between individuals, it is possible that some individual microbiotas are more or less susceptible to alteration by individual antimicrobials. This study used horses that were co-housed, fed an identical diet and with other management similarities (e.g. exercise, environmental exposures), something that might minimize the inter-individual variability.

A few limitations must be considered. While consistent with many other microbiota studies, the sample size was low, which may have affected the ability to identify certain differences through limitations in statistical power. However, numerous changes were still identified. Also, we used a carefully controlled population in order to minimize other effects on the gut microbiota of these horses; therefore, caution is required for the extrapolation of our results to horses managed differently or living in different regions. In addition, it would have been interesting to continue to sample the horses in our cohort for a longer period to see when, or if, the microbiota would return to 'normal' for the individual animals. Finally, despite the fact that fecal microbiota have been suggested to represent the microbiota present in the large colon of horses [6], use of fecal samples may limit the study of changes occurring in more proximal compartments of the GI tract.

Conclusions

The use of systemic antimicrobials leads to changes in the intestinal microbiota, with different and specific responses to different antimicrobials. All antimicrobials tested here had some impact on the microbiota, but TMS significantly reduced bacterial richness and diversity and had the greatest apparent impact on bacterial structures, specifically targeting members of the Verrucomicrobia phylum.

Methods
Animal selection

Twenty-one healthy adult horses and three ponies with no history of gastrointestinal diseases or antimicrobial administration during the previous six months were enrolled. The animals were kept on pasture and fed grass hay twice a day. All horses received hay from the same batch throughout the trial and were moved into a pen 5 days before the beginning of the trial for acclimatization. Seven horses were randomly assigned to each of three treatment groups that received procaine penicillin (20.000 UI/kg intramuscularly (IM), q12h (Pen Aqueous®, Wyeth, ON, Canada)), ceftiofur sodium (2.2 mg/kg IM, q12h (Excenel® Pfizer Animal Health, QC, Canada)) or trimethoprim sulfadiazine (TMS) (30 mg/kg orally, q12h (Uniprim Powder®, Macleod Pharmaceuticals Inc., CO, USA)) for 5 days. The sites of intra muscular injections were alternated with a maximum volume of 20 mL per site. Trimethoprim sulfadiazine was mixed with approximately 20 mL of warm corn syrup in order facilitate administration. Three individuals (one pony, one Belgian and one Thoroughbred) were assigned to the control group, which received no antimicrobials. The date of sampling, breed, age and treatment given for each horse used for the trial are presented in Table 2.

Fecal samples were collected by rectal palpation using one rectal sleeve per animal. Samples were stored in plastic sterile containers and frozen at −80°C within 2 hours after collection until DNA extraction. Samples were collected before drug administration (Day 1), on the third and fifth day of treatment and again on Days 7, 14, 23 and 30 after the onset of treatment.

Table 2 lists the breed, group of treatment and dates when the trial was performed in each group. The study was approved by the University of Guelph Animal Care Committee.

DNA extraction, 16S rRNA gene PCR and sequencing

DNA extraction was performed using a commercial kit (E.Z.N.A. Stool DNA Kit, Omega Bio-Tek Inc., USA) following the manufacturer's "stool DNA protocol for pathogen detection".

Table 2 Breed, age, treatment group, and date of sampling of each studied horse

	Breed	Year of birth	Treatment	Date
Anne	Standardbred	2006	Pen	Nov 12 – Dec 12
Betty	Standardbred	2003	Pen	Oct 9 –Nov 8
Daphne	Standardbred	2000	Pen	Sep 4 – Oct 4
Gertrude	Standardbred	2006	Pen	Sep 4 – Oct 4
Jenny	Standardbred	2000	Pen	Sep 4 – Oct 4
Paige	Standardbred	2003	Pen	Nov 12 – Dec 12
Tia	Pony	2006	Pen	Sep 4 – Oct 4
Autumn	Pony	2006	Ceftio	Sep 4 – Oct 4
Butter Cup	Standardbred	2003	Ceftio	Sep 4 – Oct 4
Dragon	Standardbred	2003	Ceftio	Sep 4 – Oct 4
India	Thoroughbred	1996	Ceftio	Sep 4 – Oct 4
Jackie	Standardbred	2007	Ceftio	Oct 9 –Nov 8
Lauryn	Standardbred	2004	Ceftio	Nov 12 – Dec 12
Lucky	Standardbred	2001	Ceftio	Nov 12 – Dec 12
Beauty	Standardbred	2004	TMS	Nov 12 – Dec 12
Fire	Standardbred	unknown	TMS	Oct 9 –Nov 8
Finch	Standardbred	1999	TMS	Oct 9 –Nov 8
Iris	Standardbred	2004	TMS	Nov 12 – Dec 12
Lilly	Belgian/Paint	2005	TMS	Nov 12 – Dec 12
Lovie	Standardbred	1997	TMS	Oct 9 –Nov 8
Missy	Standardbred	unknown	TMS	Oct 9 –Nov 8
Daisy	Belgian/Paint	2005	Control	Nov 12 – Dec 12
Jane	Standardbred	2002	Control	Sep 4 – Oct 4
Jersey	Pony	2005	Control	Sep 4 – Oct 4

PCR amplification of the V4 region of the 16S rRNA gene was designed based on Klindworth et al. [34] study using the primers forward S-D-Bact-0564-a-S-15 (5′-AY TGGGYDTAAAGNG-3′) and reverse S-D-Bact-0785-b-A-18 (5′-TACNVGGGTATCTAATCC-3′). The forward and reverse primers were designed containing an overlapping region of the forward and reverse Illumina sequencing primers (TCGTCGGCAGCGTCAGATGTGT ATAAGAGACAG and GTCTCGTGGGCTCGGAGAT GTGTATAAGAGACAG, respectively) in order to anneal them to primers containing the Illumina adaptors plus the 8 bp identifiers indices (AATGATACGGCGACCACCG AGATCTACAC-index-TCGTCGGCAGCGTC forward and CAAGCAGAAGACGGCATACGAGAT-index-GT CTCGTGGGCTCGG reverse). For a final volume of 50 μL, 2 μL of each DNA sample was added to a solution containing 18.7 μL of water, 25 μL of Fast HotStart ReadyMix 2X (KapaBiosystems, USA), 1.3 μL of BSA (Invitrogen, USA), and 0.5 μL of each 16S primer and 1 μL of each Illumina primers (100 pmol/μL). The mixture was subjected to the following PCR conditions: 5 min at 94°C for denaturing, and 25 cycles of 30 sec at

94°C for denaturing, 30 sec at 46°C for annealing and 30 sec at 72°C for elongation followed by a final period of 7 min at 72°C and kept at 4°C until purification.

PCR products were evaluated by electrophoresis in 2% agarose gel and purified with the Agencourt AMPure XP (Beckman Coulter Inc, Mississauga, ON) by mixing 22 μL of amplicon with 72 μL of AMPure on a 96 well plate. After 5 min at room temperature, beads were separated and washed twice with 80% ethanol and eluted in 30 μL of water. After purification samples were quantified by spectrophotometry using the NanoDrop® (Roche, USA) and normalized to a final concentration of 2 nM. The library pool was sequenced with an Illumina MiSeq for 250 cycles from each end at the University of Guelph Genomics Facility.

Data was made publicly available at the NCBI Sequence Read Archive under the accession number PRJNA264726.

Sequence analysis and statistical analysis

Bioinformatic analysis was performed using the Mothur (version 1.31.2) package of algorithms [35] following the MiSeq SOP accessed in January 2014 [36]. Briefly, original fastq files were assembled into contigs and sequences that were longer than 275 bp in length, contained any ambiguous base pairs or had runs of homopolymers greater than 8 bp were removed. Sequences were aligned using the SILVA 16S rRNA reference database [37]. Chimeras were identified and removed using uchime [38]. Sequences were then assigned into operational taxonomic units (OTUs) using a cutoff of 0.03 for the distance matrix and into phylotypes by clustering all sequences belonging to the same genus. Taxonomic classification was obtained from the Ribosomal Database Project (RDP – March 2012) [39].

A subsample from the main dataset was used for richness and diversity calculation in an attempt to decrease bias caused by non-uniform sequence depth and some low sequence number samples. The minimum number of reads that would not compromise coverage and would eliminate the fewest samples as possible from the analysis was used (10.482 reads per sample). Good's coverage after sub-sampling was calculated in order to ensure representative sub-samples. Diversity was estimated by the inverse Simpson diversity index and richness by using CatchAll [40]. Comparison among groups was performed using a t-test. Sampling effort was evaluated by calculation of Good's coverage and visual assessment by rarefaction curves.

The dissimilarity between groups was measured by a phylip-formated distance matrix using the Yue & Clayton measure of dissimilarity (taking into account the relative abundance of OTUs present in each group: population structure) and the classical Jaccard index (taking into account the number of shared OTUs between the groups: community membership). Dendrograms comparing the similarity of the bacterial profiles among all samples were generated using the Jaccard index and Yue & Clayton measures and figures were generated using FigTree (version 1.4.0). Population membership and structure present in the dendrograms were compared by the parsimony test.

Clustering of samples was evaluated by plotting the resultant vector of the Principal Coordinate Analysis (PCoA) with 2 dimensions. Analysis of molecular variance (AMOVA) was used to determine significance of clustering between the groups.

Bar charts representing the relative abundance at the phylum, class and genus levels of each group at the different sampling times were generated for visualization of population structure and relative abundances were compared at the different sampling times by the Steel-Dwass test controlling for multiple comparison error.

Additional file

Additional file 1: Table S1. Good's coverage, and alpha diversity indices after subsampling of 10.482 reads per sample.

Competing interests
The authors declare that they have no competing interests.

Authors' contributions
Study design: MCC, HRS, EAV, JSW. Antimicrobial administration and sampling: MCC, HRS, LGA, RGG. Sample processing: MCC. Data analysis: MCC, JSW. Writing of manuscript: MCC. Critical review of manuscript: HRS, LGA, EAV, RGG, JSW. All authors read and approved the final manuscript.

Acknowledgements
Source funding: Equine Guelph.

Author details
[1]Department of Pathobiology, Ontario Veterinary College, University of Guelph, Guelph, Canada. [2]Department of Clinical Studies, Ontario Veterinary College, University of Guelph, Guelph, Canada. [3]Department of Molecular and Cellular Biology, College of Biological Sciences, University of Guelph, Guelph, Canada. [4]Department of Clinical Studies, "Universidade Estadual de Londrina", Londrina, Brazil.

References
1. Blaser MJ, Falkow S. What are the consequences of the disappearing human microbiota? Nat Publishing Group. 2009;7:887–94.
2. Glinsky MJ, Smith RM, Spires HR, Davis CL. Measurement of volatile fatty acid production rates in the cecum of the pony. J Anim Sci. 1976;42:1465–70.
3. Jassim Al RAM, Andrews FM. The bacterial community of the horse gastrointestinal tract and its relation to fermentative acidosis, laminitis, colic, and stomach ulcers. Vet Clin North Am Equine Pract. 2009;25:199–215.
4. Bordin AI, Suchodolski JS, Markel ME, Weaver KB, Steiner JM, Dowd SE, et al. Effects of administration of live or inactivated virulent *Rhodococccus equi* and Age on the fecal microbiome of neonatal foals. PLoS One. 2013;8:e66640.
5. Costa MC, Arroyo LG, Allen-Vercoe E, Stampfli HR, Kim PT, Sturgeon A, et al. Comparison of the fecal microbiota of healthy horses and horses with colitis by high throughput sequencing of the V3-V5 region of the 16S rRNA gene. PLoS One. 2012;7:e41484.
6. Dougal K, la Fuente de G, Harris PA, Girdwood SE, Pinloche E, Newbold CJ. Identification of a core bacterial community within the large intestine of the horse. PLoS ONE. 2013; 8:e77660.
7. O' Donnell MM, Harris HMB, Jeffery IB, Claesson MJ, Younge B, O' Toole PW, Ross RP. The core faecal bacterial microbiome of Irish Thoroughbred racehorses. Lett Appl Microbiol. 2013; 57:492–501.
8. Shepherd ML, Swecker WSJ, Jensen RV, Ponder MA. Characterization of the fecal bacteria communities of forage-fed horses by pyrosequencing of 16S rRNA V4 gene amplicons. FEMS Microbiol Lett. 2012;326:62–8.
9. Steelman SM, Chowdhary BP, Dowd S, Suchodolski J, Janecka JE. Pyrosequencing of 16S rRNA genes in fecal samples reveals high diversity of hindgut microflora in horses and potential links to chronic laminitis. BMC Vet Res. 2012;8:1–1.
10. Willing BP, Voros A, Roos S, Jones C, Jansson A, Lindberg JE. Changes in faecal bacteria associated with concentrate and forage-only diets fed to horses in training. Equine Vet J. 2009;41:908–14.
11. Daly K, Proudman CJ, Duncan SH, Flint HJ, Dyer J, Shirazi-Beechey SP. Alterations in microbiota and fermentation products in equine large intestine in response to dietary variation and intestinal disease. Br J Nutr. 2012;107:989–95.
12. Kuhn M, Guschlbauer M, Feige K, Schluesener M, Bester K, Beyerbach M, et al. Feed restriction enhances the depressive effects of erythromycin on equine hindgut microbial metabolism in vitro. Berl Munch Tierarztl Wochenschr. 2012;125:351–8.
13. Perkins GA, den Bakker HC, Burton AJ, Erb HN, McDonough SP, McDonough PL, et al. Equine stomachs harbor an abundant and diverse mucosal microbiota. Appl Environ Microbiol. 2012;78:2522–32.
14. Faubladier C, Chaucheyras-Durand F, da Veiga L, Julliand V. Effect of transportation on fecal bacterial communities and fermentative activities in horses: Impact of *Saccharomyces cerevisiae* CNCM I-1077 supplementation. J Anim Sci. 2013;91:1736–44.

15. Harlow BE, Lawrence LM, Flythe MD. Diarrhea-associated pathogens, lactobacilli and cellulolytic bacteria in equine feces: Responses to antibiotic challenge. Vet Microbiol. 2013;166:225–32.

16. Chapman AM. Acute diarrhea in hospitalized horses. Vet Clin North Am Equine Pract. 2009;25:363–80.

17. Barr BS, Waldridge BM, Morresey PR, Reed SM, Clark C, Belgrave R, et al. Antimicrobial-associated diarrhoea in three equine referral practices. Equine Vet J. 2013;45:154–8.

18. Cohen ND, Woods AM. Characteristics and risk factors for failure of horses with acute diarrhea to survive: 122 cases (1990–1996). J Am Vet Med Assoc. 1999;214:382–90.

19. Cochetière MF, Durand T, Lalande V, Petit JC, Potel G, Beaugerie L. Effect of antibiotic therapy on human fecal microbiota and the relation to the development of Clostridium difficile. Microb Ecol. 2008;56:395–402.

20. Dethlefsen L, Relman DA. Incomplete recovery and individualized responses of the human distal gut microbiota to repeated antibiotic perturbation. Proc Natl Acad Sci U S A. 2011;108 Suppl 1:4554–61.

21. Janczyk P, Pieper R, Souffrant WB, Bimczok D, Rothkötter H-J, Smidt H. Parenteral long-acting amoxicillin reduces intestinal bacterial community diversity in piglets even 5 weeks after the administration. ISME J. 2007;1:180–3.

22. Perez-Cobas AE, Gosalbes MJ, Friedrichs A, Knecht H, Artacho A, Eismann K, et al. Gut microbiota disturbance during antibiotic therapy: a multi-omic approach. Gut. 2013;62:1591–601.

23. Jakobsson HE, Jernberg C, Andersson AF, Sjölund-Karlsson M, Jansson JK, Engstrand L. Short-term antibiotic treatment has differing long-term impacts on the human throat and Gut microbiome. PLoS One. 2010;5:e9836.

24. White G, Prior SD. Comparative effects of oral administration of trimethoprim/sulphadiazine or oxytetracycline on the faecal flora of horses. Vet Rec. 1982;111:316–8.

25. Gustafsson A, Baverud V, Franklin A, Gunnarsson A, Ogren G, Ingvast-Larsson C. Repeated administration of trimethoprim/sulfadiazine in the horse–pharmacokinetics, plasma protein binding and influence on the intestinal microflora. J Vet Pharmacol Ther. 1999;22:20–6.

26. GrÃ nvold A-MR, L'AbÃ e-Lund TM, SÃ rum H, Skancke E, Yannarell AC, Mackie RI. Changes in fecal microbiota of healthy dogs administered amoxicillin. FEMS Microbiol Ecol. 2010; 71:313–326.

27. La Cochetiere De MF, Durand T, Lepage P, Bourreille A, Galmiche JP, Doré J. Resilience of the dominant human fecal microbiota upon short-course antibiotic challenge. J Clin Microbiol. 2005;43:5588–92.

28. Blackmore TM, Dugdale A, Argo CM, Curtis G, Pinloche E, Harris PA, et al. Strong stability and host specific bacterial community in faeces of ponies. PLoS One. 2013;8:e75079.

29. Ferran AA, Bibbal D, Pellet T, Laurentie M, Gicquel-Bruneau M, Sanders P, et al. Pharmacokinetic/pharmacodynamic assessment of the effects of parenteral administration of a fluoroquinolone on the intestinal microbiota: comparison of bactericidal activity at the gut versus the systemic level in a pig model. Int J Antimicrob Agents. 2013;42:429–35.

30. Tanayama S, Yoshida K, Adachi K, Kondo T. Metabolic fate of SCE-1365, a new broad-spectrum cephalosporin, after parenteral administration to rats and dogs. Antimicrob Agents Chemother. 1980;18:511–8.

31. Peris-Bondia F, Latorre A, Artacho A, Moya A, D'Auria G. The active human Gut microbiota differs from the total microbiota. PLoS One. 2011;6:e22448.

32. Robinson CJ, Young VB. Antibiotic administration alters the community structure of the gastrointestinal micobiota. Gut Microbes. 2010;1:279–84.

33. Morotomi N, Fukuda K, Nakano M, Ichihara S, Oono T, Yamazaki T, et al. Evaluation of intestinal microbiotas of healthy Japanese adults and effect of antibiotics using the 16S ribosomal RNA gene based clone library method. Biol Pharm Bull. 2011;34:1011–20.

34. Klindworth A, Pruesse E, Schweer T, Peplies J, Quast C, Horn M, et al. Evaluation of general 16S ribosomal RNA gene PCR primers for classical and next-generation sequencing-based diversity studies. Nucleic Acids Res. 2013;41:e1.

35. Schloss PD, Westcott SL, Ryabin T, Hall JR, Hartmann M, Hollister EB, et al. Introducing mothur: open-source, platform-independent, community-supported software for describing and comparing microbial communities. Appl Environ Microbiol. 2009;75:7537–41.

36. Kozich JJ, Westcott SL, Baxter NT, Highlander SK, Schloss PD. Development of a dual-index sequencing strategy and curation pipeline for analyzing amplicon sequence data on the MiSeq illumina sequencing platform. Appl Environ Microbiol. 2013;79:5112–20.

37. Quast C, Pruesse E, Yilmaz P, Gerken J, Schweer T, Yarza P, et al. The SILVA ribosomal RNA gene database project: improved data processing and web-based tools. Nucleic Acids Res. 2013;41:D590–6.

38. Edgar RC, Haas BJ, Clemente JC, Quince C, Knight R. UCHIME improves sensitivity and speed of chimera detection. Bioinformatics. 2011;27:2194–200.

39. Cole JR, Wang Q, Fish JA, Chai B, McGarrell DM, Sun Y, et al. Ribosomal database Project: data and tools for high throughput rRNA analysis. Nucleic Acids Res. 2014;42:D633–42.

40. Bunge J: Estimating the number of species with CatchAll. Pac Symp Biocomput 2011;121–130.

5

Natural *Besnoitia besnoiti* infections in cattle: hematological alterations and changes in serum chemistry and enzyme activities

Martin C Langenmayer[1]*, Julia C Scharr[2], Carola Sauter-Louis[3], Gereon Schares[4] and Nicole S Gollnick[3]

Abstract

Background: The emerging disease bovine besnoitiosis is caused by the apicomplexan parasite *Besnoitia besnoiti*. Clinical signs of acute besnoitiosis are pyrexia, anorexia and subcutaneous edema. In subacute and chronic besnoitiosis parasitic cysts arise in a variety of tissues and affected cattle display skin lesions and weight loss. In all stages of bovine besnoitiosis, lesions can be found in many organ systems and therefore presumably alter a variety of laboratory parameters. In this study, the impact of naturally acquired acute, subacute and chronic bovine besnoitiosis on hematologic parameters, serum chemistry, and enzyme activities was investigated. Laboratory parameters of two Simmental heifers and two Limousin cows were monitored during acute, subacute and chronic besnoitiosis and in another Simmental heifer during subclinical besnoitiosis. To determine aberrations of laboratory parameters, values were compared with reference ranges obtained from *B. besnoiti* negative Simmentals (224 samples of nine animals) and Limousins (41 animals). Further, laboratory parameters of *B. besnoiti* seropositive Limousin cows (54 animals; 32 of these showing clinical signs) and healthy *B. besnoiti* seronegative Limousin cows (41 animals) were compared.

Results: During acute and subacute besnoitiosis, a reduction of leukocyte and erythrocyte concentrations, hematocrit, serum albumin, urea, magnesium, and calcium concentrations were observed. Serum total protein, globulin, total bilirubin and creatinine concentrations were increased and aspartate transaminase (AST) and creatine kinase (CK) activities were elevated. In chronic besnoitiosis, erythrocyte parameters were statistically significantly lower, and total protein and globulin concentrations were significantly higher in *B. besnoiti* seropositive compared with *B. besnoiti* seronegative Limousin cows.

Conclusions: In this study, altered laboratory parameters during the course of naturally acquired acute, subacute and chronic bovine besnoitiosis are described for the first time. Only a few animals were examined in acute and subacute besnoitiosis, however the alterations of laboratory parameters during these stages reflected i) the acute inflammatory state (*e.g.* high levels of serum globulin fractions), ii) clinical findings such as disturbed condition (*e.g.* bilirubin concentrations), and iii) lesions such as muscle necroses described in the literature (*e.g.* AST or CK activities). Chronic besnoitiosis led to typical alterations of chronic inflammatory diseases like hyper-(gamma)-globulinemia or reduced erythrocyte concentrations.

Keywords: Bovine besnoitiosis, Besnoitia besnoiti, Hematological and biochemical parameters, Cattle

* Correspondence: langenmayer@patho.vetmed.uni-muenchen.de
[1]Institute of Veterinary Pathology at the Centre for Clinical Veterinary Medicine, Ludwig-Maximilians-Universitaet Muenchen, Munich, Germany
Full list of author information is available at the end of the article

Background

Besnoitia besnoiti, a cyst-forming apicomplexan protozoon, is the causative agent of bovine besnoitiosis. Bovine besnoitiosis has spread within Europe in the past few years, with latest outbreaks in Hungary [1], Switzerland [2], Italy [3], and Germany [4]. In 2010, the disease has been classified as "emerging disease" by the European Food Safety Authority [5]. Clinical signs of infected cattle in the early stage of the disease include fever, edema, enlarged lymph nodes, anorexia, weight loss and, in bulls, swollen and painful testes [6-8]. In the chronic stage, parasitic cysts arise in various organs, including skin, vascular walls, scleral *conjunctivae*, and other non-intestinal mucous membranes [9-11].

Clinical signs, morphological changes, pathological lesions, parasitological examinations and diagnosis of bovine besnoitiosis have been in the focus of researchers [6,9,12-16]. However, the effects of the parasitic infection on laboratory parameters during acute and chronic stages of the disease were not investigated.

B. caprae, a parasite very closely related to *B. besnoiti* [17,18], causes similar clinical signs in goats [19,20] and data on altered laboratory parameters in caprine besnoitiosis are already available. In naturally acquired caprine besnoitiosis in Iran, alterations of various hematological and biochemical parameters as well as enzyme activities have been observed [20,21]. However, similar examinations regarding bovine besnoitiosis are missing, and metabolic disturbances caused by tachyzoites and bradyzoites are unknown.

We hypothesized that pathological alterations during the acute stage like hemorrhages, necroses or degenerative lesions in different organs, for example muscle and liver cells, and activation of lymphatic tissues [15] lead to alterations of laboratory parameters connected to those lesions. Hemorrhages may affect erythrocyte parameters, muscle and liver necroses may lead to an increase in organ specific enzyme activities, and alterations of lymphatic tissues or multifocal inflammation may affect leukocyte parameters.

In the chronic stage, we hypothesized that emaciation and the huge number of tissue cysts partially surrounded by chronic granulomatous inflammation in different organs [4,9,22] may negatively affect serum albumin concentrations (emaciation) or elevate serum globulin concentrations (chronic inflammation).

The objective of the present study was to monitor laboratory parameters during acute, subacute and chronic naturally acquired bovine besnoitiosis and to connect those findings to already obtained clinical and serological findings in the same animals [13,23,24]. In addition, we aimed to compare these findings with laboratory parameters of *B. besnoiti* seronegative cattle and altered parameters of a larger group of chronically infected seropositive Limousin cattle from a German cow-calf-operation (Herd-BbGER1) [13,23].

Methods

Animals

Chronology of acute, subacute, and chronic bovine besnoitiosis monitoring infected Simmental and Limousin cattle

Animals were part of a longitudinal study focusing on the different stages and disease progression of naturally acquired bovine besnoitiosis [13,23]. Permission for this study was granted by the responsible authorities (Animal ethics committee, regional government of Upper Bavaria, TV Az. 55.2-54-2531-83-09). The study consisted of a 12-week cohabitation period (August 18, 2009, until November 9, 2009). Five healthy German Simmental heifers (Study Animal [SA] 3, SA 4, SA 6, SA 8, and SA 9) and one healthy German Simmental bull (SA 1) were kept on a pasture with three chronically infected and *B. besnoiti* seropositive Limousin cows. Six healthy Simmental heifers (SA 2, SA 5, SA 7, SA 10, SA 11, and SA 12) between 11 and 20 months of age were kept on a paddock 20 m away as a control group [23]. Prior to the trial, the Simmentals tested negative for *B. besnoiti* and *Neospora caninum* antibodies in immunoblots and IFAT [24].

On trial day (td) 3 and td 51, two Limousin cows (SA 20 and SA 22) of Herd-BbGER1 suspected to be in the acute stage of bovine besnoitiosis, were added to the pasture. Infection of SA 4, SA 6, SA 20, and SA 22 was confirmed clinically, histologically, and serologically. In the case of SA 8, infection was confirmed serologically (Table 1) [23]. Although SA 22 had already seroconverted on the day of admission, this day was regarded as day of seroconversion to make inter-animal comparison possible for data analyses.

The acute stage was classified according to clinical criteria. Animals had to show fever (body temperature > 39.0°C) or at least two of the following clinical signs/

Table 1 Overview of *B. besnoiti* affected Simmental (SA 4, SA 6, and SA 8) and Limousin (SA 20 and SA 22) cattle

Animal ID	SA 4	SA 6	SA 8	SA 20	SA 22
Breed	S	S	S	L	L
Age (months)	20	19	13	53	49
Pregnancy status	np	np	np	p	p
Study entry (td)	1	1	1	3	51
Acute stage: start (td)	36	29	-	unknown	unknown
Acute stage: end (td)	47	41	-	7	51
Seroconversion (td)	45	35	73	4	-
Chronic stage: start (td)	64	67	-	27	63
Course of disease	mild	mild	subclinical	severe	severe

SA = Study animal, S = Simmental, L = Limousin, np = non pregnant, p = pregnant, td = trial day.

diagnoses of acute besnoitiosis: depression, conjunctivitis, subcutaneous edema, lymphadenitis, lameness. As soon as cysts were clinically observed in the scleral *conjunctivae*, the term 'chronic stage' was used (Table 1). The subacute stage was defined as stage between the end of the acute and the beginning of the chronic stage.

Blood samples were collected twice a week during the whole trial period and daily for 21 days after animals showed signs of acute besnoitiosis. On day 225, SA 4, SA 6, SA 8, SA 20, and SA 22 were bled during a routine herd health status examination.

In total, 224 samples collected from the control heifers and SA 1, SA 3, and SA 9 were used to determine reference ranges for Simmental hematology, serum chemistry and enzymes activities. Values outside of three times interquartile range from the 25th and 75th percentile were defined as outliers and eliminated. Thereafter, the reference ranges were determined non-parametrically as interval between the 2.5th and 97.5th percentile.

Hematological and biochemical parameters of SA 4, SA 6, and SA 8 were compared with these reference ranges. Values of SA 20 and SA 22 were compared with those of *B. besnoiti* seronegative Limousin cattle (see below).

Herd-BbGER1: monitoring of B. besnoiti seropositive Limousin cattle

In total, 75 samples were collected from 54 female Limousin cattle (one to eleven years old) during routine herd health status examinations in the years 2008, 2011, and 2012. The sampling of these animals was conducted according to international guidelines and national law concerning animal welfare. Limousin cattle were free of BHV-1 and BVD infection and did not show clinical signs of gastrointestinal helminthoses or lung worm disease. All animals were seropositive for *B. besnoiti* antibodies in immunoblots and IFAT [24] and 32 animals displayed cysts in the scleral *conjunctivae* and/or vaginal *vestibula*. Only single animals showed large numbers of parasitic cysts in the vaginal *vestibula* and the scleral *conjunctivae* as well as visible and palpable lesions in the skin of the trunk, limbs and udder.

Values outside of three times interquartile range from the 25th and 75th percentile were defined as outliers and eliminated. After that, the 2.5th and 97.5th percentiles were determined non-parametrically.

Herd-BbGER1: monitoring of B. besnoiti negative Limousin cattle

Samples were collected from two groups of female adult cattle of Herd-BbGER1. Fifteen samples from 14 healthy female Limousin cattle (one to eight years old) were collected during routine herd health status examinations in 2008, 2011 and 2012. The sampling of these animals was conducted according to international guidelines and national law concerning animal welfare.

Twenty-seven Limousin cows (two to 14 years old) without a history of bovine besnoitiosis were introduced into Herd-BbGER1 in spring 2013. Samples from these animals were collected as part of the quarantine health check. Limousin cattle from both groups were free of BHV-1 and BVD infection and did not show clinical signs of gastrointestinal helminthoses or lung worm disease and sera were negative for *B. besnoiti* antibodies in immunoblots and IFAT as previously described [24].

To determine Limousin reference ranges, values outside of three times interquartile range from the 25th and 75th percentile were defined as outliers and eliminated. After that, reference ranges were determined non-parametrically as interval between the 2.5th and 97.5th percentiles.

Blood sample collection and processing

Blood samples were collected from the tail or jugular veins. Immediately after sampling, a blood smear was performed on a glass slide for differentiation count of cells. All blood samples were stored at approximately 8°C for up to 6 hours until transferred to the laboratory. Sera for antibody detection and serum protein electrophoresis were frozen at −80°C until transferred to the Friedrich-Loeffler-Institut (Wusterhausen, Germany) and Vet Med Labor GmbH (Division of IDEXX Laboratories, Ludwigsburg, Germany) for further examination. Samples for serum chemistry, hematology and enzyme activities were kept overnight at 8°C and were processed the next day.

Biochemical analysis and hematological examination

Urea, creatinine, total protein (TP), albumin, total bilirubin, conjugated bilirubin, calcium, magnesium, phosphor, sodium, chloride and potassium concentrations, aspartate transaminase (AST), glutamate dehydrogenase (GLDH), gamma-glutamyl transpeptidase (GGT), creatine kinase (CK) activities were analyzed in sera with a Hitachi 912 Chemistry Analyzer (Boehringer Mannheim, Mannheim, Germany) in the laboratory of the Clinic for Ruminants. Globulin, albumin/globulin (A/G) ratio and unconjugated bilirubin were determined arithmetically.

A complete blood cell count was performed using EDTA-anticoagulated blood, analyzed with a hematological analyzer (pocH-100iV DIFF, Sysmex, Norderstedt, Germany). Air-dried slides for differential blood count were stained using a Pappenheim stain (Haema Schnellfaerbung, LT-SYS® Labor + Technik Eberhard Lehmann GmbH, Berlin, Germany). Mean corpuscular hemoglobin concentration (MCHC), mean corpuscular volume (MCV) and mean corpuscular hemoglobin (MCH) were determined arithmetically.

Serum protein gel electrophoresis

Sera from SA 4, SA 6, and SA 20 were examined on the day of seroconversion, 2 days post seroconversion (*dps*), 5 *dps* and on day 225. Sera from SA 8 and SA 22 were examined likewise with the exception of serum from 2 *dps*. In addition, three sera from SA 4 and two sera from SA 6 were analyzed during the febrile phase before seroconversion. Serum protein gel electrophoresis was performed at Vet Med Labor GmbH (Division of IDEXX Laboratories, Ludwigsburg, Germany) with a semiautomated agarose gel electrophoresis system (HYDRA-SIS®2, Sebia, Norcross, USA).

Reference ranges were calculated from the 24 samples of SA 1 to SA 12 from the beginning and the mid of the trial as described above. In order to exclude possible effects of parasite circulation on the determined parameters in SA 4, SA 6, and SA 8, only samples taken before the calculated incubation period of 13 days [6] were used.

Serological examinations

To detect *B. besnoiti* antibodies in serum, three tests were performed as previously described: one IFAT and two immunoblots either based on *B. besnoiti* tachyzoite or bradyzoite antigen. A reciprocal positive cut-off titer of 200 was used in IFAT and recognition of at least four of ten bands in both immunoblots was regarded specific [24]. Animals were regarded as positive if two of the three serological tests yielded a positive result.

Statistical analysis

Hematological results, serum chemistry and enzyme activities of *B. besnoiti* seronegative and *B. besnoiti* seropositive Limousin cattle were compared statistically. Additionally, the same parameters of *B. besnoiti* seropositive subclinically affected and *B. besnoiti* seropositive clinically affected animals were compared statistically. To assess normality, D'Agostino and Pearson omnibus normality test was applied. To compare the two groups, the non-parametric Mann–Whitney-Test was performed. *P* values below 0.01 where considered significant. Data were analyzed using the software Graphpad Prism 5.04 for Windows.

Results

Chronology of hematologic alterations during acute, subacute, and chronic bovine besnoitiosis

Shortly before seroconversion, infected animals SA 4, SA 6, and SA 8 showed a period of decline in white blood cell (WBC) concentration followed by an increase. SA 20 and SA 22 showed only a consistent increase in WBC concentrations after seroconversion. In SA 4 and SA 6, the decline was below the Simmental reference range (Table 2) for four days shortly after entering the acute

Table 2 Mean, SD and percentiles for laboratory parameters of *B. besnoiti* negative Simmental cattle (9 animals, 224 samples)

Hematology	Mean ± SD	Percentiles	
		2.5th	97.5th
RBCs (T/l)	7.45 ± 0.8	6.28	9.29
Hemoglobin (mmol/l)	6.5 ± 0.5	5.6	7.6
HCT (%)	32.6 ± 2.8	27.9	38.3
MCV (fl)	43.8 ± 3.1	36.1	48.9
MCH (fmol)	0.9 ± 0.1	0.7	1.0
MCHC (mmol/l)	20.0 ± 0.7	18.6	21.6
WBCs (G/l)	7.90 ± 1.7	3.80	10.70
Serum chemistry			
Total protein (g/l)	75.2 ± 4.7	66.3	83.0
Albumin (g/l)	34.8 ± 2.5	30.5	39.2
Globulin (g/l)	40.4 ± 5.2	29.2	49.3
A/G ratio	0.86 ± 0.16	0.64	1.24
Urea (mmol/l)	5.2 ± 0.9	3.5	6.8
Creatinine (µmol/l)	97.5 ± 16.5	70.4	128.2
Total bilirubin (µmol/l)	1.4 ± 0.7	0.1	2.8
Sodium (mmol/l)	142.3 ± 2.6	137.0	147.0
Potassium (mmol/l)	4.2 ± 0.4	3.4	5.0
Calcium (mmol/l)	2.4 ± 0.1	2.3	2.7
Phosphorus (mmol/l)	2.4 ± 0.3	1.8	3.1
Magnesium (mmol/l)	0.9 ± 0.1	0.8	1.1
Chloride (mmol/l)	100.8 ± 2.6	96.0	106.0
Enzymes			
AST (IU/l)	70.4 ± 9.7	50.6	89.4
GGT (IU/l)	18.9 ± 4.8	11.0	27.8
GLDH (IU/l)	12.5 ± 7.4	4.2	31.5
CK (IU/l)	217.0 ± 65.0	133.2	377.0

SD = standard deviation.

stage (Figure 1A). Reduced WBC concentrations consisted of an equal reduction in the concentrations of neutrophils and lymphocytes.

A decline in red blood cell (RBC) concentration was observed in SA 4 lasting for 20 days (Figure 1B). RBC concentrations of SA 20 fluctuated below the lower limit of the Limousin reference range (Table 3) for the whole trial period.

SA 4 and SA 6 showed a decline in hemoglobin concentration and HCT shortly before seroconversion. SA 20 showed strong fluctuation below or around the lower limit of the reference range for the whole trial period (Figure 1C and D).

Mean corpuscular hemoglobin concentration (MCHC) showed strong fluctuations above the lower limit of reference range in all infected animals (data not shown). Mean corpuscular volume (MCV) and mean corpuscular

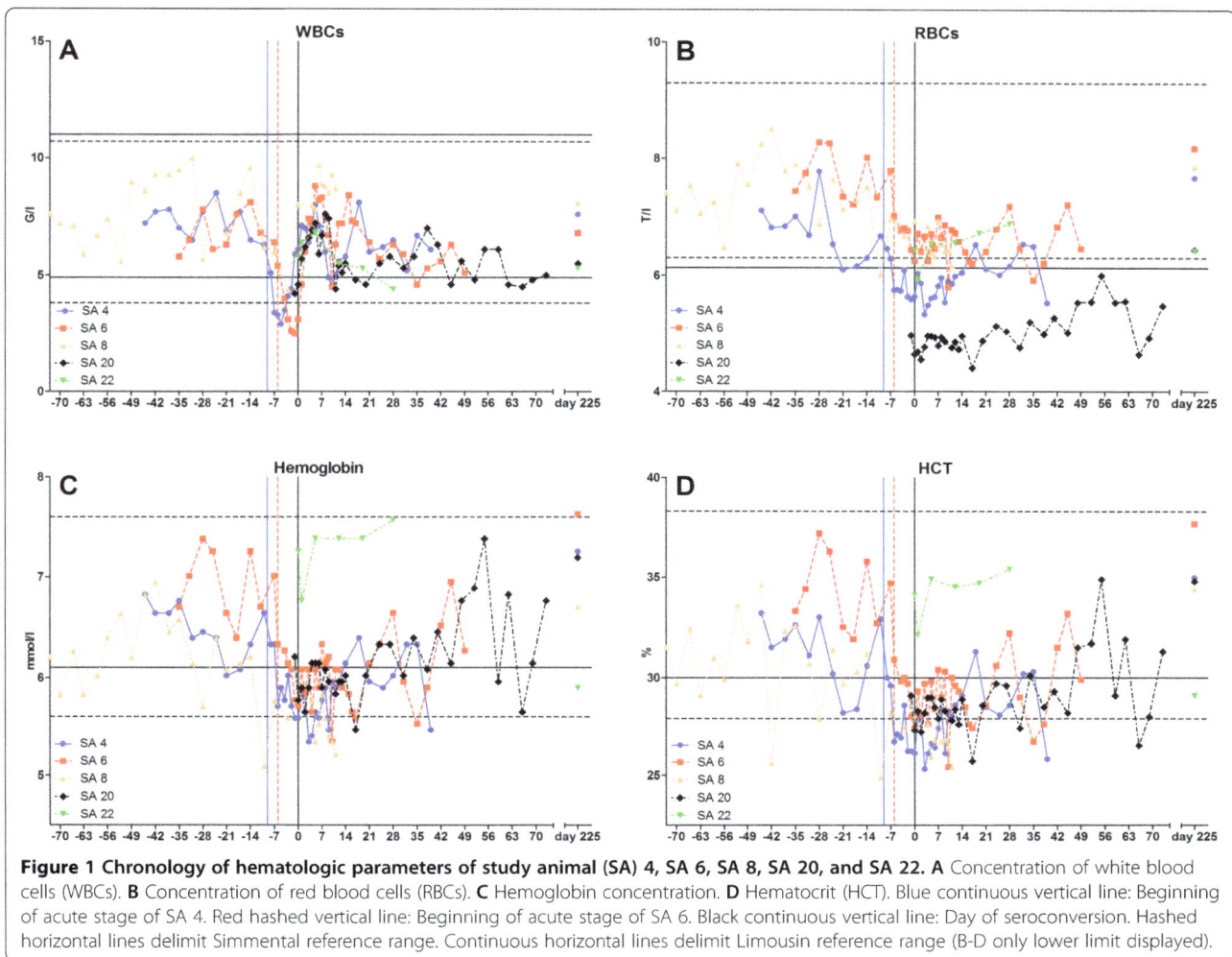

Figure 1 Chronology of hematologic parameters of study animal (SA) 4, SA 6, SA 8, SA 20, and SA 22. A Concentration of white blood cells (WBCs). **B** Concentration of red blood cells (RBCs). **C** Hemoglobin concentration. **D** Hematocrit (HCT). Blue continuous vertical line: Beginning of acute stage of SA 4. Red hashed vertical line: Beginning of acute stage of SA 6. Black continuous vertical line: Day of seroconversion. Hashed horizontal lines delimit Simmental reference range. Continuous horizontal lines delimit Limousin reference range (B-D only lower limit displayed).

hemoglobin (MCH) concentrations were within the reference range in all infected animals with few borderline values (data not shown).

Chronology of changes in serum chemistry during acute, subacute, and chronic bovine besnoitiosis

Elevations of TP and globulin concentrations plus decline in A/G ratio were detectable shortly after seroconversion in SA 4, SA 6, SA 20, and SA 22 (Figure 2A and B).

Albumin concentration declined within reference range shortly after the beginning of the acute stage in SA 4. SA 20 displayed fluctuating albumin concentrations around the lower limit of the reference range during the whole trial period. SA 20 and SA 22 showed increasing albumin concentrations for few days after seroconversion.

On day 225, albumin concentrations were within reference range in SA 20 and SA 22 and borderline in SA 4, SA 6, and SA 8.

Total bilirubin concentrations were above the reference range in SA 4, SA 20, and SA 22 (Figure 2C). In SA 20 and SA 22, this elevation was mainly caused by an elevated unconjugated bilirubin concentration (data not shown).

Urea concentrations were below the reference range for five days in SA 4 starting 4 days *ante* seroconversion (*das*) and for four days in SA 6 starting 4 *dps*. Lowest values were 2.8 mmol/l for SA 4 and 3.1 mmol/l for SA 6. SA 20 displayed an increased urea concentration on 1 *das* (7.9 mmol/l). SA 22 showed decreased urea concentration (2.4 mmol/l) for one day 5 *dps* (data not shown).

Creatinine concentrations were above the reference range in SA 4 for five days starting 8 *das* (147 µmol/l) and for three days starting 3 *das* in SA 6 (135 µmol/l). On day 225, total bilirubin, urea and creatinine concentrations were within the respective reference ranges in all animals except creatinine concentration in SA 22 (100.8 µmol/l) (data not shown).

Concentrations of magnesium (except SA 4, see below), phosphate, potassium, sodium and chloride displayed

Table 3 Mean, SD and percentiles of laboratory parameters of _B. besnoiti_ seronegative and _B. besnoiti_ seropositive Limousin cattle

	Seronegative			Seropositive		
	Mean ± SD	Percentiles		Mean ± SD	Percentiles	
Hematology		2.5th	97.5th		2.5th	97.5th
RBCs (T/l)	8.44 ± 1.9[a]	6.13	13.70	**7.08 ± 1.2[a,b]**	5.08	9.76
Hemoglobin (mmol/l)	7.5 ± 0.7	6.1	8.9	7.9 ± 1.3[a]	5.8	10.7
HCT (%)	35.5 ± 3.5	30.0	41.3	36.3 ± 5.6[a]	23.0	45.4
MCV (fl)	43.9 ± 9.4	25.9	58.1	**52.2 ± 3.9[b]**	43.9	58.8
MCH (fmol)	0.9 ± 0.2	0.5	1.3	**1.1 ± 0.1[b]**	0.9	1.3
MCHC (mmol/l)	21.2 ± 0.9	19.8	23.2	21.5 ± 1.4[a]	19.2	24.6
WBCs (G/l)	7.34 ± 1.6	4.90	11.00	7.31 ± 2.94[a]	2.83	14.44
Serum chemistry						
Total protein (g/l)	68.4 ± 5.9	60.1	81.7	**76.0 ± 6.9[b]**	63.1	89.1
Albumin (g/l)	32.9 ± 4.4	26.0	41.2	**36.4 ± 2.7[b]**	31.5	41.3
Globulin (g/l)	35.3 ± 4.3	28.7	43.8	**40.3 ± 7.0[a,b]**	28.5	55.5
A/G ratio	0.95 ± 0.18[a]	0.73	1.39	0.94 ± 0.19[a]	0.63	1.38
Urea (mmol/l)	3.9 ± 1.3[a]	2.6	7.0	**5.2 ± 1.9[a,b]**	2.2	9.6
Creatinine (µmol/l)	163.6 ± 21.2	124.7	207.7	164.4 ± 27.1[a]	125.4	214.6
Total bilirubin (µmol/l)	2.6 ± 0.9	1.0	4.4	2.9 ± 1.2[a]	0.9	5.5
Sodium (mmol/l)	145.8 ± 3.4	139.0	153.0	**141.1 ± 3.1[b]**	135.5	146.5
Potassium (mmol/l)	5.3 ± 0.9	3.6	6.7	**4.8 ± 0.7[b]**	3.4	6.0
Calcium (mmol/l)	2.3 ± 0.1	2.1	2.6	2.3 ± 0.2	1.9	2.6
Phosphorus (mmol/l)	1.6 ± 0.3	1.1	2.3	**1.9 ± 0.4[b]**	1.3	2.8
Magnesium (mmol/l)	0.6 ± 0.2	0.3	1.1	**0.9 ± 0.1[a,b]**	0.7	1.1
Chloride (mmol/l)	99.2 ± 2.3	95.6	103.2	**96.7 ± 2.6[b]**	91.6	101.5
Enzymes						
AST (IU/l)	155.1 ± 61.9[a]	68.9	323.4	**102.2 ± 31.6[a,b]**	58.2	166.0
GGT (IU/l)	16.6 ± 6.6	6.8	28.7	19.5 ± 9.1	1.7	35.4
GLDH (IU/l)	14.7 ± 7.1[a]	5.2	29.6	12.7 ± 8.1[a]	4.0	33.2
CK (IU/l)	702.8 ± 466.8[a]	78.0	2092.0	**331.9 ± 283.1[a,b]**	106.5	885.0

Samples from _B. besnoiti_ seronegative Limousins comprise 41 samples from 41 animals, samples from _B. besnoiti_ seropositive Limousins comprise 75 samples (hematology) respectively 65 samples (serum chemistry/enzymes) from 54 animals. SD = standard deviation, [a] = normality test not passed, [b] = significantly (P < 0.01) different versus seronegative Limousins (Mann–Whitney-Test) highlighted in bold.

strong fluctuations within the respective reference ranges in all infected animals, with single values lying outside the upper or lower limits (data not shown). SA 4 displayed a decline of magnesium concentrations starting 6 _das_ for four days below reference range. Calcium concentrations declined in all three Simmentals shortly before seroconversion and were below the reference range in SA 4 and SA 20 (Figure 2D).

Chronology of serum protein gel electrophoresis during acute, subacute, and chronic bovine besnoitiosis

During the acute stage, SA 4 displayed no alterations of serum protein fractions compared with the Simmental reference range (Table 4). SA 6 displayed a slightly elevated α_1-globulin-fraction (7.1 g/l) and a diminished α_2-globulin-fraction (2.4 g/l) 7 _das_. Alterations of serum protein fractions on the day of seroconversion and thereafter are depicted in Figure 3A-D.

Chronology of enzyme activities during acute, subacute, and chronic bovine besnoitiosis

AST activities are depicted in Figure 4.

CK activities were elevated for one day 3 _dps_ in SA 4 (1,115 U/l) and 1 _das_ in SA 20 (2,900 U/l). Serum activities of GGT and GLDH remained below the upper limit of the reference range in all infected animals.

On day 225, activities of GGT, GLDH, and CK remained below the upper limit of the reference range in all animals.

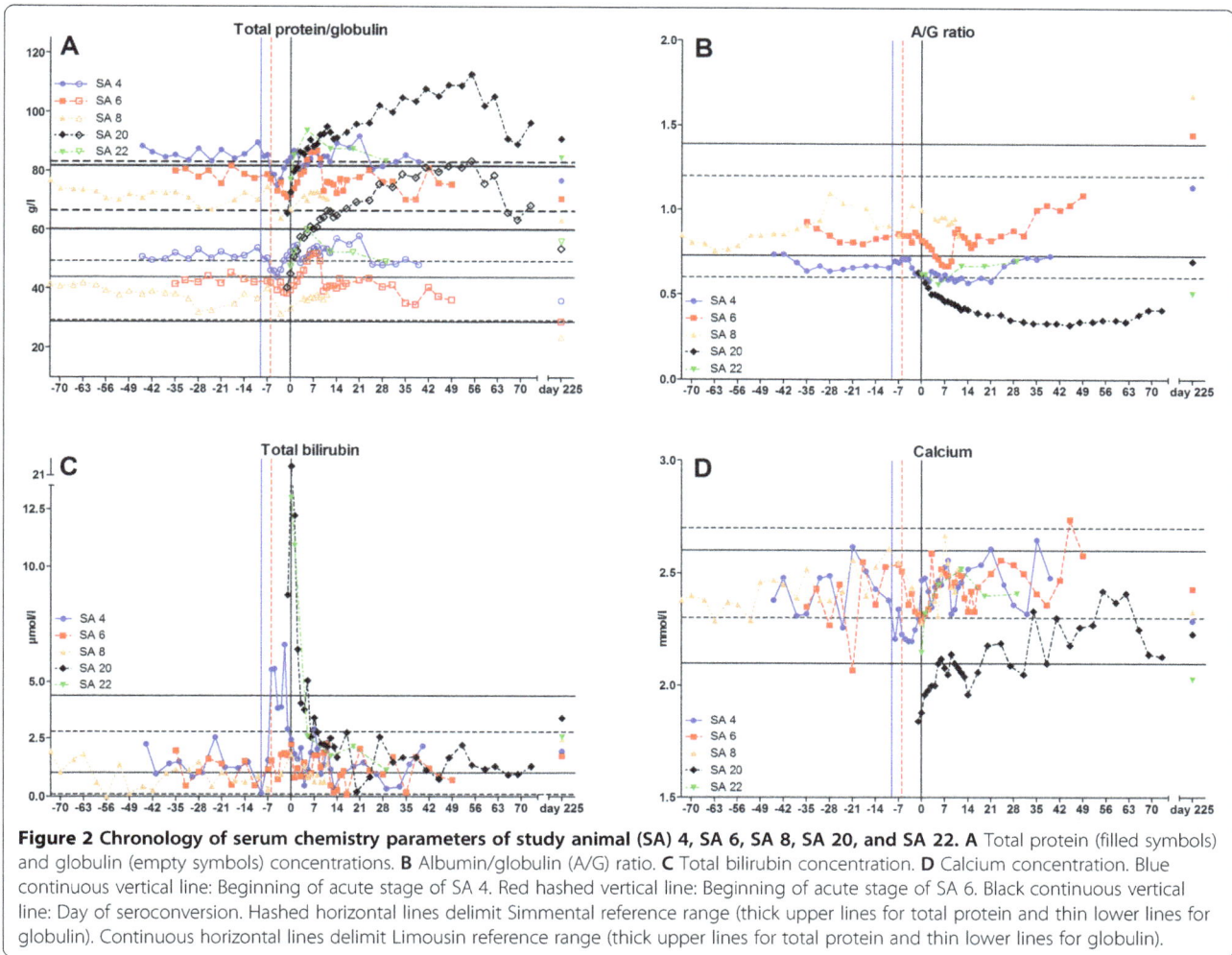

Figure 2 Chronology of serum chemistry parameters of study animal (SA) 4, SA 6, SA 8, SA 20, and SA 22. **A** Total protein (filled symbols) and globulin (empty symbols) concentrations. **B** Albumin/globulin (A/G) ratio. **C** Total bilirubin concentration. **D** Calcium concentration. Blue continuous vertical line: Beginning of acute stage of SA 4. Red hashed vertical line: Beginning of acute stage of SA 6. Black continuous vertical line: Day of seroconversion. Hashed horizontal lines delimit Simmental reference range (thick upper lines for total protein and thin lower lines for globulin). Continuous horizontal lines delimit Limousin reference range (thick upper lines for total protein and thin lower lines for globulin).

Herd-BbGER1 monitoring: significant differences in laboratory parameters between *B. besnoiti* seronegative and *B. besnoiti* seropositive Limousin cattle

Means, standard deviations and percentiles of hematology, serum chemistry and enzyme activities for *B. besnoiti* seronegative and *B. besnoiti* seropositive Limousin cattle are shown in Table 3.

The RBC concentration was significantly higher and MCV and MCH were significantly lower in *B. besnoiti* seronegative Limousins. TP, albumin and globulin concentrations were significantly higher in *B. besnoiti* seropositive Limousins.

AST and CK activities were significantly lower in *B. besnoiti* seronegative Limousins (Table 3).

There were no statistical significant differences between parameters of *B. besnoiti* seropositive subclinically affected and *B. besnoiti* seropositive clinically affected Limousin cattle.

During chronic besnoitiosis, laboratory parameters of SA 20 and SA 22 were within the percentiles of the *B.* *besnoiti* seropositive Limousin group, except RBC and albumin concentrations which were lower in SA 20 and globulin concentration which was higher in SA 20.

Discussion

The results of this study present the chronology of laboratory parameters during a longitudinal clinical trial monitoring five cattle with naturally acquired acute, subacute, and chronic bovine besnoitiosis. In addition, the laboratory parameters of *B. besnoiti* seronegative and *B. besnoiti* seropositive chronically infected Limousin cattle from a herd naturally affected by bovine besnoitiosis are compared.

Variations exist between reference ranges of different laboratories, cattle breeds, age groups, lactation and pregnancy status [26-31]. Thus, reference ranges for the evaluation of laboratory parameters of *B. besnoiti* infected Simmental cattle were calculated from values of healthy *B. besnoiti* negative Simmental study animals. Although larger animal cohorts are usually used for

Table 4 Mean, SD and percentiles of serum gel electrophoresis of B. besnoiti negative Simmental cattle (12 animals, 24 samples) and comparison with results from the *2-year-group (24 animals) of Alberghina et al. [25]

Serum Gel Electrophoresis	Data obtained in the present study			Literature data*
	Mean ± SD	Percentiles		Mean ± SD
		2.5th	97.5th	
Total protein (g/l)	64.92 ± 3.55	59.58	70.85	68.10 ± 10.13
Albumin (%)	49.4 ± 4.6	40.3	56.1	Not given
α1-globulins (%)	5.7 ± 0.8	4.5	7.3	Not given
α2-globulins (%)	9.4 ± 1.4	6.5	11.2	Not given
β-globulins (%)	13.2 ± 2.1	8.2	16.7	Not given
γ-globulins (%)	22.4 ± 6.0	14.3	36.1	Not given
Albumin (g/l)	32.04 ± 3.35	25.45	36.85	31.79 ± 5.12
α1-globulins (g/l)	3.67 ± 0.42	3.06	4.54	5.92 ± 2.54
α2-globulins (g/l)	5.96 ± 0.68	4.68	7.19	5.77 ± 1.73
β-globulins (g/l)	8.54 ± 1.47	5.58	11.43	7.50 ± 1.16
γ-globulins (g/l)	14.55 ± 4.22	9.45	23.85	16.81 ± 3.72

SD = standard deviation.

calculation, these reference ranges were regarded representative for this study, because housing, feeding and handling were similar and examination of cattle samples of the same breed were examined in the same laboratories. For the same reason, laboratory parameters of SA 20 and SA 22 were compared with reference ranges calculated from healthy *B. besnoiti* seronegative female Limousin cattle of Herd-BbGER1. Furthermore, we could not find appropriate up-to-date reference values for adult Limousin cows in the literature and application of older data could have caused misinterpretations because reference values may change due to genetic and environmental factors [32].

The effect of bovine besnoitiosis on hematological parameters

Several hematological parameters were altered during acute bovine besnoitiosis. In the acute stage, leukopenia was observed in SA 4, SA 6, and SA 20. Leukopenia is a common finding in cattle with viral, bacterial and protozoan infections [33,34] and is due to the low storage neutrophil pool of adult cattle as well as increased margination and tissue emigration during acute inflammation.

For the low RBC concentrations in SA 4 and SA 20 there are two possible explanations: First, multifocal hemorrhages, which have been described in acute besnoitiosis [15] and were also clinically observed in SA 4 [23] and in multiple consecutive histological skin sections taken during acute besnoitiosis in these animals [35]. However, total bilirubin concentrations - although

of limited value as a confirmation of hemorrhages in sick cattle (see below) - returned to the normal range after a few days, indicating that hemorrhages are not the only reason contributing to this finding. Second, anemia can also be a result of a chronic inflammatory disease [36,37]. The constantly low RBC concentrations of SA 20 and the lower RBC concentrations in the seropositive Limousin group are most likely caused by the chronic inflammatory state. Reticulocyte stains of blood smears to assess the origin of anemia were not performed and reticulocytes were not observed in conventionally stained smears. Similar significant differences in hematological parameters, namely increased MCV and MCH and decreased RBC concentrations were also observed in Iranian goats infected by *B. caprae* [21].

The effect of bovine besnoitiosis on serum chemistry values

The initial hypothesis of increased globulin concentrations during chronic bovine besnoitiosis proved true. However, the effect of besnoitiosis on albumin concentrations was different than expected.

A decrease in albumin synthesis, albumin loss or hemodilution can be the cause of SA 20´s hypoalbuminemia [38]. However, clinical examinations and the results of laboratory tests did not reveal evidence for albumin loss or hemodilution. Two effects probably caused the decreased albumin synthesis in SA 20: inflammation and a negative energy balance. Albumin is a negative acute phase protein and inflammatory hypoalbuminemia can develop after ongoing inflammatory states and is usually expected to be mild [38]. Moreover, it is tempting to speculate that the massive development of numerous *B. besnoiti* cysts in the tissues of SA 20 led to an increased demand in nutrients and subsequently to a negative energy balance. The hypocalcemia in this animal is very likely associated with hypoalbuminemia [39], as clinical signs of hypocalcemia were not observed.

The increased globulin concentrations are most likely due to increased antibodies against *B. besnoiti*, since reciprocal IFAT titers displayed a similar increase post seroconversion [23]. This hypothesis is supported by the electrophoresis findings displaying increased γ-globulin fractions 5 *dps* in SA 20 and on day 225 in SA 20 and SA 22.

The increase in the α_1-fraction (α_1-lipoprotein, α_1-antitrypsin, and α_1-antichymotrypsin) during the febrile phase of SA 6 and the increase in both α_1- and α_2-fractions (α_2-macroglobulin and haptoglobins) of SA 4, SA 6, SA 20, and SA 22 shortly after seroconversion are most likely a response to the acute inflammation. Interestingly, the α-fraction was only elevated during the febrile phase in SA 6 on one day. A reason for this may be the rather mild clinical course of the disease in SA 4 and

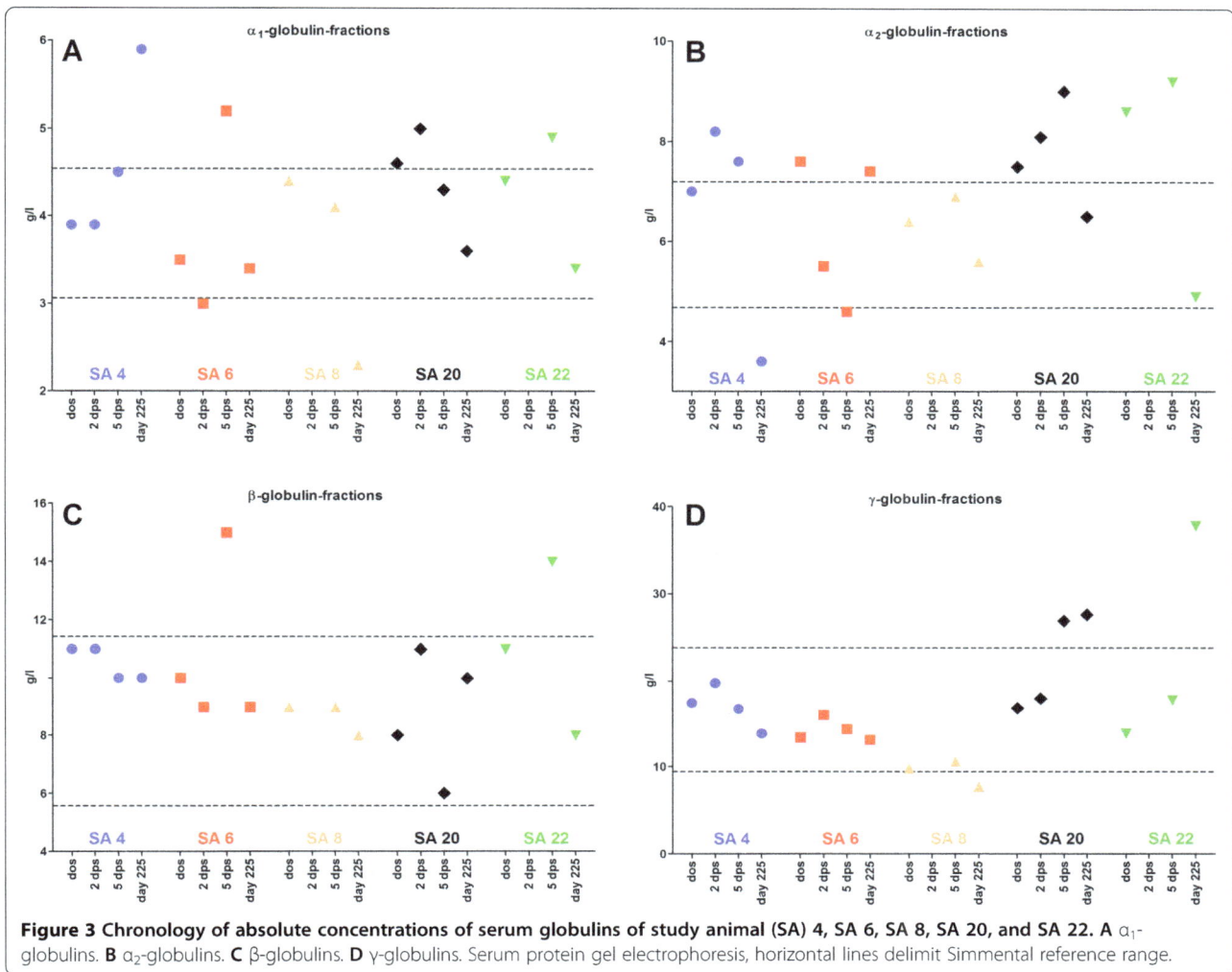

Figure 3 Chronology of absolute concentrations of serum globulins of study animal (SA) 4, SA 6, SA 8, SA 20, and SA 22. **A** α_1-globulins. **B** α_2-globulins. **C** β-globulins. **D** γ-globulins. Serum protein gel electrophoresis, horizontal lines delimit Simmental reference range.

SA 6. The increase in the β-fraction of SA 6 and SA 22 on 5 *dps* is most likely due to an increase in IgM-antibodies or complement proteins, because transferrin, a main part of the β-fraction is expected to be low during acute inflammation [40]. SA 20's elevated γ-globulin fraction (mainly IgG) displayed a two-peak pattern 5 *dps*, and elevated γ-globulin fractions of the other days displayed only one peak. This is indicative of a polyclonal hypergammaglobulinemia shortly after seroconversion changing into a monoclonal or oligoclonal gammoglobulinemia in the chronic stage.

The significant hyperproteinemia of *B. besnoiti* seropositive Limousin cows of Herd-BbGER1 compared with *B. besnoiti* seronegative Limousin cows is mainly caused by hyperglobulinemia. These findings correlate with the results obtained from the trial animals. Elevation of γ-globulin concentration is common during chronic inflammatory diseases [38], and similar results have also been reported in goats suffering from natural chronic caprine besnoitiosis [20]. Unexpectedly, albumin

concentrations were higher in *B. besnoiti* seropositive Limousins. Albumin tends to decrease during inflammatory states (see above), and decreased albumin concentrations have also been found in cases of caprine besnoitiosis [41]. Maybe the higher albumin concentrations are due to a slight dehydration of these animals, which is also indicated by slightly higher urea concentrations of *B. besnoiti* seropositive Limousins compared with *B. besnoiti* seronegative Limousins. Severely infected Limousins in this study had a tendency to have higher total protein and globulin concentrations as well as lower A/G ratios. The former two observations were also made in goats naturally infected with *B. caprae* in Iran [20].

The hyperbilirubinemia of SA 4, SA 20, and SA 22 most likely has two main causes: A prehepatic icterus following hemorrhages (see above), or anorexia and sickness, which are common reasons for hyperbilirubinemia in different species (including cattle) and can include elevated unconjugated bilirubin concentrations [42-45].

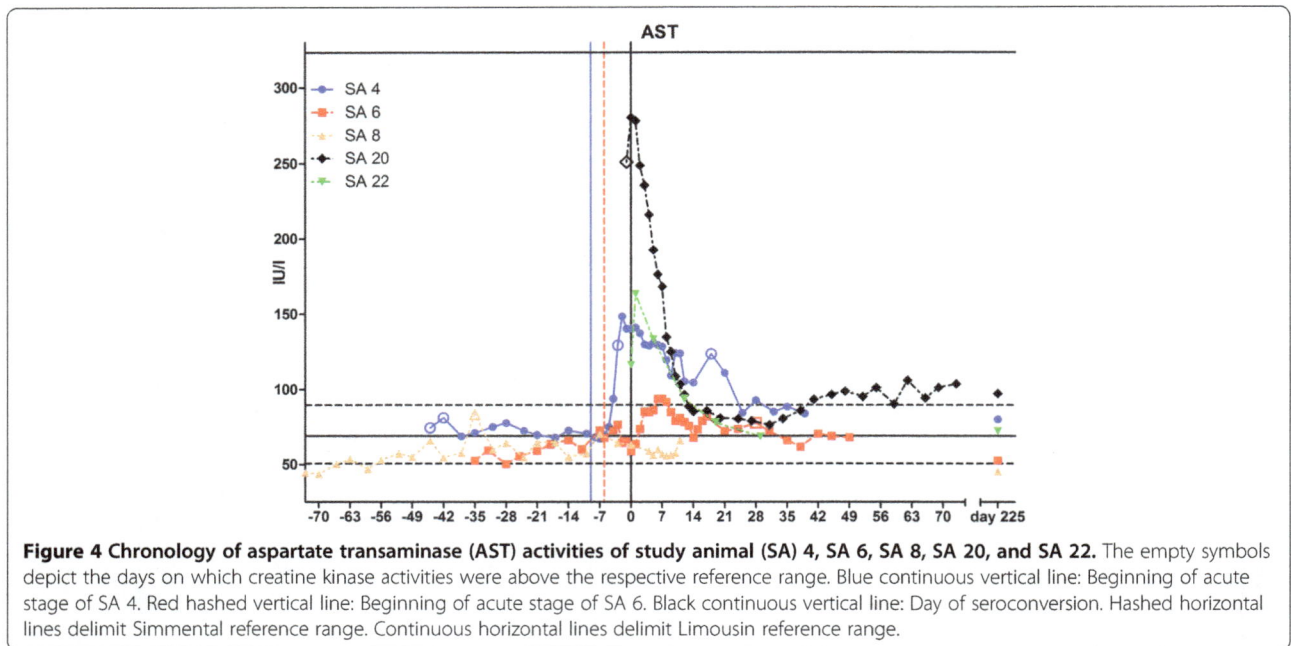

Figure 4 Chronology of aspartate transaminase (AST) activities of study animal (SA) 4, SA 6, SA 8, SA 20, and SA 22. The empty symbols depict the days on which creatine kinase activities were above the respective reference range. Blue continuous vertical line: Beginning of acute stage of SA 4. Red hashed vertical line: Beginning of acute stage of SA 6. Black continuous vertical line: Day of seroconversion. Hashed horizontal lines delimit Simmental reference range. Continuous horizontal lines delimit Limousin reference range.

The decrease in urea concentrations in SA 4 and SA 6, as well as low and borderline magnesium concentrations observed for 7 *das* in SA 4 can be associated with a period of anorexia in these animals, too. The elevation of creatinine concentrations in SA 4 and SA 6 are most likely due to dehydration [46]. SA 4 and SA 6 showed clinical dehydration on several days and the dehydration period coincides with the anorectic period [23]. Urea/ creatinine ratio to further assess azotemia was not helpful in these cases, because urea concentrations were reduced.

Electrolyte concentrations in blood are influenced by feed intake, hydration status or sweating and are subject to daily change, as it was observed in the trial animals. These factors are also a plausible explanation for the occasional changes observed in the two Limousin groups. Using our data to conclude that bovine besnoitiosis affects electrolyte concentrations seems inappropriate at this point and further studies should be conducted to assess the importance of these alterations.

The effect of bovine besnoitiosis on enzyme activities
The increased AST activities of SA 4 and SA 20 are most likely associated with a loss of muscle fiber integrity, because CK activities were elevated at the same time and GLDH and GGT displayed no elevated activities. The longer half-life of AST [47,48] explains the relatively rapid decline of CK activities and the slow removal of AST from serum. Muscle fiber damage may be caused by prolonged recumbence, because *B. besnoiti* affected cattle show apathy and are more likely to lie down and rest [49]. Or elevated AST activities could be a result of

mild muscular degeneration and necrosis, lesions which are described in cattle during acute besnoitiosis after experimental infection with high parasite doses [15].

Although lower AST and CK activities are of little clinical significance, it is surprising that AST and CK activities were lower in *B. besnoiti* seropositive Limousins compared with *B. besnoiti* seronegative Limousins. Tissue cysts surrounded by severe chronic inflammatory reaction can be found in the musculature of diseased cattle [9], and loss of muscle fiber integrity due to cysts or inflammation seems likely. Maybe the effect of tissue cysts on muscle fiber integrity is too low to get noticed or leads to mild, gradual release of muscle enzymes, which cannot be detected due to the short half-life of CK. In comparison with the results obtained from the trial animals, loss of muscle fiber integrity seems to play only a role during acute and subacute besnoitiosis.

Conclusions
This study provides detailed results of laboratory parameters obtained during the course of naturally acquired acute, subacute and chronic bovine besnoitiosis for the first time. Even though a low number of animals were examined in acute and subacute besnoitiosis, it could be shown that hematologic parameters were altered especially during acute and subacute besnoitiosis, leading to reduced red and white blood cell concentrations. Furthermore, during acute and subacute besnoitiosis, elevation of serum globulin fractions reflected the acute inflammatory state, clinical parameters like disturbed condition resulted in increased bilirubin concentrations and lesions like muscle necroses, which are described in

the literature led to increased aspartate transaminase and creatine kinase activities. Chronic besnoitiosis led to reduced concentrations of red blood cells and to hyper-(gamma)-globulinemia most likely due to the chronic inflammatory condition caused by the parasite.

Abbreviations
A/G ratio: Albumin/globulin ratio; AST: Aspartate transaminase; CK: Creatine kinase; das: Days ante seroconversion; dps: Days post seroconversion; GGT: Gamma-glutamyl transpeptidase; GLDH: Glutamate dehydrogenase; HCT: Hematocrit; Herd-BbGER1: First German cattle herd diagnosed with cases of bovine besnoitiosis; IFAT: Immunofluorescent antibody test; MCH: Mean corpuscular hemoglobin; MCHC: Mean corpuscular hemoglobin concentration; MCV: Mean corpuscular volume; RBCs: Red blood cells; SA: Study animal; td: Trial day; WBCs: White blood cells.

Competing interests
The authors declared no potential conflicts of interest with respect to the research, authorship, and/or publication of this article. Prionics AG, Schlieren, Switzerland funded parts of the study but had no influence on the design of the experiment, data collection and analysis and was not involved in writing the manuscript.

Authors' contributions
MCL collected the samples, performed the data management and analysis and wrote the manuscript. JCS collected the samples and performed data management. CS did the statistical workup and revised the manuscript. GS designed and coordinated the serological investigations and performed the respective data analysis. NSG was involved in sample collection, data analysis, study design and helped drafting the manuscript. All authors read and approved the final manuscript.

Acknowledgements
We acknowledge the excellent technical assistance of Ingrid Hartmann, Christina Beyer, and Monika Altmann. We also like to express our gratitude to the owner of the animals for his collaboration and support. Partial financial support for this study was provided by Prionics AG (Schlieren, Switzerland) and Vet Med Labor GmbH (Division of IDEXX Laboratories, Ludwigsburg, Germany).

Author details
[1]Institute of Veterinary Pathology at the Centre for Clinical Veterinary Medicine, Ludwig-Maximilians-Universitaet Muenchen, Munich, Germany. [2]Rammingen, Germany. [3]Clinic for Ruminants with Ambulatory and Herd Health Services at the Centre for Clinical Veterinary Medicine, Ludwig-Maximilians-Universitaet Muenchen, Oberschleissheim, Germany. [4]Friedrich-Loeffler-Institut, Federal Research Institute for Animal Health, Institute of Epidemiology, Greifswald-Isle of Riems, Germany.

References
1. Hornok S, Fedak A, Baska F, Hofmann-Lehmann R, Basso W. Bovine besnoitiosis emerging in Central-Eastern Europe, Hungary. Parasit Vectors. 2014;7(1):20.
2. Lesser M, Braun U, Deplazes P, Gottstein B, Hilbe M, Basso W. [First cases of besnoitiosis in cattle in Switzerland]. Schweiz Arch Tierheilkd. 2012;154(11):469–74.
3. Gentile A, Militerno G, Schares G, Nanni A, Testoni S, Bassi P, et al. Evidence for bovine besnoitiosis being endemic in Italy - first *in vitro* isolation of *Besnoitia besnoiti* from cattle born in Italy. Vet Parasitol. 2012;184(2–4):108–15.
4. Rostaher A, Mueller RS, Majzoub M, Schares G, Gollnick NS. Bovine besnoitiosis in Germany. Vet Dermatol. 2010;21(4):329–39.
5. EFSA. European food safety authority - Bovine Besnoitiosis: an emerging disease in Europe. EFSA J. 2010;8(2):1499.
6. Bigalke RD. New concepts on the epidemiological features of bovine besnoitiosis as determined by laboratory and field investigations. Onderstepoort J Vet Res. 1968;35(1):3–137.
7. Pols JW. Studies on bovine besnoitiosis with special reference to the aetiology. Onderstepoort J Vet Res. 1960;28:265–356.
8. Schulz KCA. A report on naturally acquired besnoitiosis with special reference to its pathology. J S Afr Vet Med Assoc. 1960;31:21–35.
9. McCully RM, Basson PA, Van Niekerk JW, Bigalke RD. Observations on *Besnoitia* cysts in the cardiovascular system of some wild antilopes and domestic cattle. Onderstepoort J Vet Res. 1966;33:245–76.
10. Majzoub M, Breuer W, Gollnick NS, Rostaher A, Schares G, Hermanns W. Ein Ausbruch von Besnoitiose bei Rindern in Deutschland: pathomorphologische, ultrastrukturelle und molekularbiologische Untersuchungen. Wien Tieraerztl Mschr. 2010;97:9–15.
11. Franko EE, Borges I. Sur la sarcosporidiose bovine. Arq Inst Bac Camera Pestana. 1915;269–289
12. Garcia-Lunar P, Ortega-Mora LM, Schares G, Gollnick NS, Jacquiet P, Grisez C, et al. An inter-laboratory comparative study of serological tools employed in the diagnosis of *Besnoitia besnoiti* infection in bovines. Transbound Emerg Dis. 2012.
13. Schares G, Langenmayer MC, Scharr JC, Minke L, Maksimov P, Maksimov A, et al. Novel tools for the diagnosis and differentiation of acute and chronic bovine besnoitiosis. Int J Parasitol. 2013;43(2):143–54.
14. Basso W, Schares G, Gollnick NS, Rutten M, Deplazes P. Exploring the life cycle of *Besnoitia besnoiti* - Experimental infection of putative definitive and intermediate host species. Vet Parasitol. 2011;178(3–4):223–34.
15. Basson PA, McCully RM, Bigalke RD. Observations on the pathogenesis of bovine and antelope strains of *Besnoitia besnoiti* (Marotel, 1912) infection in cattle and rabbits. Onderstepoort J Vet Res. 1970;37(2):105–26.
16. Dubey JP, Shkap V, Pipano E, Fish L, Fritz DL. Ultrastructure of *Besnoitia besnoiti* tissue cysts and bradyzoites. J Eukaryot Microbiol. 2003;50(4):240–4.
17. Ellis JT, Holmdahl OJ, Ryce C, Njenga JM, Harper PA, Morrison DA. Molecular phylogeny of *Besnoitia* and the genetic relationships among *Besnoitia* of cattle, wildebeest and goats. Protist. 2000;151(4):329–36.
18. Namazi F, Oryan A, Sharifiyazdi H. Genetic characterization of the causative agent of besnoitiosis in goats in Iran on the basis of internal transcribed spacer rDNA and its comparison with *Besnoitia* species of other hosts. Parasitol Res. 2011;108(3):633–8.
19. Njenga JM, Bwangamoi O, Mutiga ER, Kangethe EK, Mugera GM. Preliminary findings from an experimental study of caprine besnoitiosis in Kenya. Vet Res Commun. 1993;17(3):203–8.
20. Oryan A, Nazifi S, Mohebbi H. Pathology and serum biochemical changes in natural caprine besnoitiosis. Rev Med Vet. 2008;159(1):27–32.
21. Nazifi S, Oryan A, Mohebbi M. Evaluation of Hematological Parameters in Caprine Besnoitiosis. J Appl Anim Res. 2002;21:123–8.
22. Besnoit C, Robin V. Sarcosporidiose cutanée chez une vache. Rev Vét. 1912;37:649–63.
23. Gollnick NS, Scharr JC, Schares G, Langenmayer MC. Natural *Besnoitia besnoiti* infections in cattle: chronology of disease progression. BMC Vet Res. accepted 2015.
24. Schares G, Basso W, Majzoub M, Rostaher A, Scharr J-C, Langenmayer MC, et al. Comparative evaluation of immunofluorescent antibody and new immunoblot test for the specific detection of antibodies against *Besnoitia besnoiti* tachyzoites and bradyzoites in bovine sera. Vet Parasitol. 2010;171(1–2):32–40.
25. Alberghina D, Giannetto C, Vazzana I, Ferrantelli V, Piccione G. Reference intervals for total protein concentration, serum protein fractions, and albumin/globulin ratios in clinically healthy dairy cows. J Vet Diagn Invest. 2011;23(1):111–4.
26. Brun-Hansen HC, Kampen AH, Lund A. Hematologic values in calves during the first 6 months of life. Vet Clin Pathol. 2006;35(2):182–7.
27. Doornenbal H. Physiological and endrocine parameters in beef cattle: breed, sex and year differences. Can J Comp Med. 1977;41(1):13–8.
28. Doornenbal H, Tong AK, Murray NL. Reference values of blood parameters in beef cattle of different ages and stages of lactation. Can J Vet Res. 1988;52(1):99–105.
29. Monke DR, Kociba GJ, DeJarnette M, Anderson DE, Ayars Jr WH. Reference values for selected hematologic and biochemical variables in Holstein bulls of various ages. Am J Vet Res. 1998;59(11):1386–91.
30. Yokus B, Cakir UD. Seasonal and physiological variations in serum chemistry and mineral concentrations in cattle. Biol Trace Elem Res. 2006;109(3):255–66.
31. Knowles TG, Edwards JE, Bazeley KJ, Brown SN, Butterworth A, Warriss PD. Changes in the blood biochemical and haematological profile of neonatal calves with age. Vet Rec. 2000;147(21):593–8.
32. George JW, Snipes J, Lane VM. Comparison of bovine hematology reference intervals from 1957 to 2006. Vet Clin Pathol. 2010;39(2):138–48.
33. Andresen HA. Evaluation of leukopenia in cattle. J Am Vet Med Assoc. 1970;156(7):858–66.

34. Glass EJ, Preston PM, Springbett A, Craigmile S, Kirvar E, Wilkie G, et al. Bos taurus and Bos indicus (Sahiwal) calves respond differently to infection with Theileria annulata and produce markedly different levels of acute phase proteins. Int J Parasitol. 2005;35(3):337–47.

35. Langenmayer MC, Gollnick NS, Majzoub-Altweck M, Scharr JC, Schares G, Hermanns W. Naturally acquired bovine besnoitiosis: histological and immunohistochemical findings in acute, subacute and chronic disease. Vet Pathol. 2014; doi: 101177/0300985814541705.

36. Stockham SL, Scott MA. Erythrocytes. In: Fundamentals of Veterinary Clinical Pathology. 2nd ed. Ames: Blackwell Publishing; 2008. p. 107–222.

37. Thrall MA. Classification of and diagnostic approach to anemia. In: Troy DB, editors. Veterinary Hematology and Clinical Chemistry. Lippincott Williams & Wilkins; 2004. p. 83–8

38. Stockham SL, Scott MA. Proteins. In: Fundamentals of Veterinary Clinical Pathology. 2nd ed. Ames: Blackwell Publishing; 2008. p. 369–414.

39. Stockham SL, Scott MA. Calcium, phosphorus, magnesium, and their regulatory hormones. In: Fundamentals of Veterinary Clinical Pathology. 2nd ed. Ames: Blackwell Publishing; 2008. p. 593–638.

40. O'Connell TX, Horita TJ, Kasravi B. Understanding and interpreting serum protein electrophoresis. Am Fam Physician. 2005;71(1):105–12.

41. Nazifi S, Oryan A, Namazi F. Hematological and serum biochemical analyses in experimental caprine besnoitiosis. Korean J Parasitol. 2011;49(2):133–8.

42. Cakala S, Bieniek K. Bromosulphthalein clearance and total bilirubin level in cows deprived of food and water. Zentralbl Veterinaermed A. 1975;22(7):605–10.

43. Gronwall R, Engelking LR. Effect of glucose administration on equine fasting hyperbilirubinemia. Am J Vet Res. 1982;43(5):801–3.

44. Meyer BH, Scholtz HE, Schall R, Muller FO, Hundt HK, Maree JS. The effect of fasting on total serum bilirubin concentrations. Br J Clin Pharmacol. 1995;39(2):169–71.

45. McSherry BJ, Lumsden JH, Valli VE, Baird JD. Hyperbilirubinemia in sick cattle. Can J Comp Med. 1984;48(3):237–40.

46. Stockham SL, Scott MA. Urinary system. In: Fundamentals of veterinary clinical pathology. 2nd ed. Ames: Blackwell Publishing; 2008. p. 415–94.

47. Russell KE, Roussel AJ. Evaluation of the ruminant serum chemistry profile. Vet Clin North Am Food Anim Pract. 2007;23(3):403–26.

48. Lefebvre HP, Toutain PL, Serthelon JP, Lassourd V, Gardey L, Braun JP. Pharmacokinetic variables and bioavailability from muscle of creatine kinase in cattle. Am J Vet Res. 1994;55(4):487–93.

49. Bigalke RD. Besnoitiosis and Globidiosis. In: Ristic M, McIntyre I, editors. Diseases of Cattle in Tropics. Volume 6, edn. The Hague: Martinus Nijhoff Publishers; 1981. p. 429–42.

6

Hematological and histopathological effects of swainsonine in mouse

Chenchen Wu, Xiaoxue Liu, Feng Ma and Baoyu Zhao[*]

Abstract

Background: Livestock that consume locoweed exhibit multiple neurological symptoms, including dispirited behavior, staggered gait, trembling, ataxia, impaired reproductive function and cellular vacuolar degeneration of multiple tissues due to toxicity from plant-derived alkaloids such as swainsonine.

Results: Swainsonine was administered to F_0 and F_1 mice by intraperitoneal injection before, during and after pregnancy at the following doses: 0.525 mg/kg BW(I), 0.2625 mg/kg BW(II), 0.175 mg/kg BW(III) and 0 mg/kg BW(IV). Hemosiderin deposits were observed the lamina propria of endometrium in uterus and the red pulp of spleen. Ovary corpus lutea counts in F_0 mice were higher in swainsonine-treated mice compared to control mice. Indirect bilirubin content and reticulocyte numbers were increased in swainsonine-treated F_0 and F_1 generation mice compared to control group ($P < 0.05$). Lactate dehydrogenase, alkaline phosphatase, aspartate aminotransferase and alanine aminotransferase content in F_0-I and F_0-II mice were significantly increased compared with F_0-IV group mice ($P < 0.05$). Red blood cells, hemoglobin and mean corpuscular hemoglobin levels were significantly decreased in F_0 and F_1 mice compared with the control group ($P < 0.05$).

Conclusions: Swainsonine exerts effects on estrus period and reproductive ability, and offspring of dams dosed with swainsonine were affected in-utero or from nursing. Damage to liver, uterus and spleen, as well as hematological changes, are observable before neurological symptoms present.

Keywords: Swainsonine, Locoweed, Hemosiderin deposits, Mouse

Background

Locoweeds are perennial herbaceous plants of the *Astragalus* spp and *Oxytropis* spp. containing the toxic indolizidine alkaloid swainsonine [1]. Locoism causes significant economic losses to the livestock industry on western grasslands in China and the United States [2]. Swainsonine, a trihydroxy indolizidine alkaloid, is the primary toxin in locoweeds [1]. *Astragalus* and *Oxytropis* species that contain swainsonine are found on multiple continents, and have poisoned animals in South America and Asia [3,4]. Early studies demonstrated that natural or experimental long-term ingestion of swainsonine-containing plants causes serious disorders in reproductive functions of livestock (cattle, sheep, horses and goat), including failure to conceive and early embryo loss or abortion, resulting in great economic losses to the livestock industry [5-8]. Therefore, various animal models have

been used to study the toxic effects of swainsonine on reproduction and development, including goat, sheep and cattle. Locoweed poisoning is usually chronic, and the toxic symptoms are observed after a few weeks of locoweed feeding. Mice were fed a small quantity of locoweed for four months, demonstrated that pathological and clinical damage to internal organs and neuronal processes were reversible [9]. In this study, we then selected four groups of mice to treat with either vehicle control or swainsonine (10 each group, F_0-I: 0.525 mg/kg BW; F_0-II: 0.2625 mg/kg BW; F_0-III: 0.175 mg/kg BW and F_0-IV: 0 mg/kg BW). After treatment with swainsonine for two weeks, female mice were mated to untreated male mice, and pups were kept with dams for one month. We sacrificed dams and offspring and observed swainsonine toxicity effects on internal organs via histopathological analysis as well as altered hematological and blood biochemical parameters in both parent and offspring mice.

* Correspondence: zhaobaoyu12005@163.com
College of Animal Veterinary Medicine, Northwest A & F University, Yangling 712100, Shaanxi, People's Republic of China

Results

TLC detection

All extracts were collected using column chromatography, which was placed on the thin layer plate using the capillary sample. Figure 1 show a developed TLC plate. This purple colored spots are swainsonine, the rose red colored spots are the swainsonine analogs as determined by comparison with the swainsonine standard.

Histological effects of swainsonine treatment in F_0 and F_1 mice

Examination of heart, lung and kidney of treated F_0 and F_1 mice revealed no marked changes (**data not shown**).

Histological changes in liver from swainsonine administration are shown in Figure 2 (a-d). Livers of F_0 swainsonine-treated mice displayed few differences compared with their controls, with cellular infiltrates consisting mostly of inflammatory cells, neutrophils and granulocytes in F_0-I, F_0-II and F_0-III mice. No histopathological differences were noted between F_1-I, F_1-II, F_1-III and F_1-IV control mice (Figure 2 (e-h)).

Histological analysis indicated important alterations in the spleen and uterus. As evident in Figure 3 (a-h), dose-related expansion of splenic red pulp was characterized by large numbers of inflammatory cells and lymphocytes, hypertrophy of splenic cells and a considerable number of macrophages and megakaryocytes. Increased extramedullary hemosiderin deposition were also observed in the red pulp of spleen in F_0 and F_1 mice (Figure 3 (a-c)).

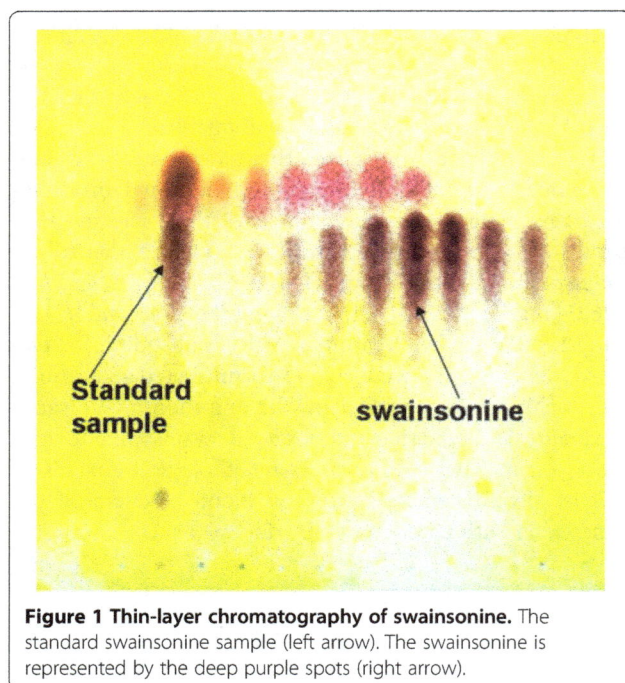

Figure 1 Thin-layer chromatography of swainsonine. The standard swainsonine sample (left arrow). The swainsonine is represented by the deep purple spots (right arrow).

Hemosiderin deposition in the spleen of F_1 mice was not observed (Figure 3 (e-h)).

Histological alterations in uterus of mice exposed to swainsonine were more noticeable, and this effect was independent of dose (Figure 4). Hemosiderin deposits were observed in the lamina propria of endometrium in uterus of F_0 generation mice treated with swainsonine compared with their controls (Figure 4 (a-d)). Focal collection of large numbers of neutrophils were seen in uterus mucosa of F_0 generation mice (Figure 4 (a-c)). However, no noticeable alterations in uterus of F_1 mice were observed (Figure 4 (e-h)).

Histopathological analysis of ovaries in swainsonine-treated mice revealed dose-dependent changes compared with controls (Figure 5 (a-d)). F_0-I and F_0-II mice displayed decreased numbers of primordial and primary follicles compared to F_0-IV controls. F_0-I and F_0-II mice exhibited increased numbers and size of corpus lutea compared with F_0-IV control mice (Figure 5 (a-d)). However, no histopathological changes in the ovary of F_1 mice were observed (Figure 5 (e-h)).

Biochemical marker characterization of swainsonine-treated mice

Indirect bilirubin (IBIL) content of F_0-I, F_0-II and F_0-III mice was significantly increased when compared with F_0-IV controls ($P < 0.05$). Lactate dehydrogenase (LDH), alkaline phosphatase (ALP), aspartate aminotransferase (AST) and alanine aminotransferase (ALT) content of F_0-I and F_0-II mice were significantly increased compared with F_0-IV controls ($P < 0.05$). Furthermore, indirect bilirubin (IBIL) level of F_1-I, F_1-II and F_1-III mice were significantly increased compared with F_1-IV controls ($P < 0.05$). Examination of lactate dehydrogenase (LDH), alkaline phosphatase (ALP), aspartate aminotransferase (AST) and alanine aminotransferase (ALT) content in swainsonine-treated F_1 mice compared with controls revealed no statistically significant differences (Table 1).

Hematological characterization of swainsonine-treated mice

Examination of F_0 dams revealed that WBCs in F_0-I, F_0-II and F_0-III treatment groups were not significantly different from F_0-IV controls ($P > 0.05$). RBCs, and levels of Hb, HCT, PLT, and MCH in F_0-I, F_0-II and F_0-III treatment groups were significantly decreased compared with F_0-IV controls ($P < 0.05$). MCV and reticulocyte levels in F_0-I, F_0-II and F_0-III treatment groups were significantly increased compared with F_0-IV controls ($P < 0.05$). Examination of F_1 mice revealed that reticulocytes in F_1-I, F_1-II and F_1-III treatment groups were significantly increased compared with F_1-IV controls ($p < 0.05$). WBCs counts in F_1-I, F_1-II and F_1-III treatment groups were not significantly different from F_1-IV controls ($P > 0.05$). RBCs, Hb and MCH levels in F_1-I, F_1-II and F_1-III treatment groups

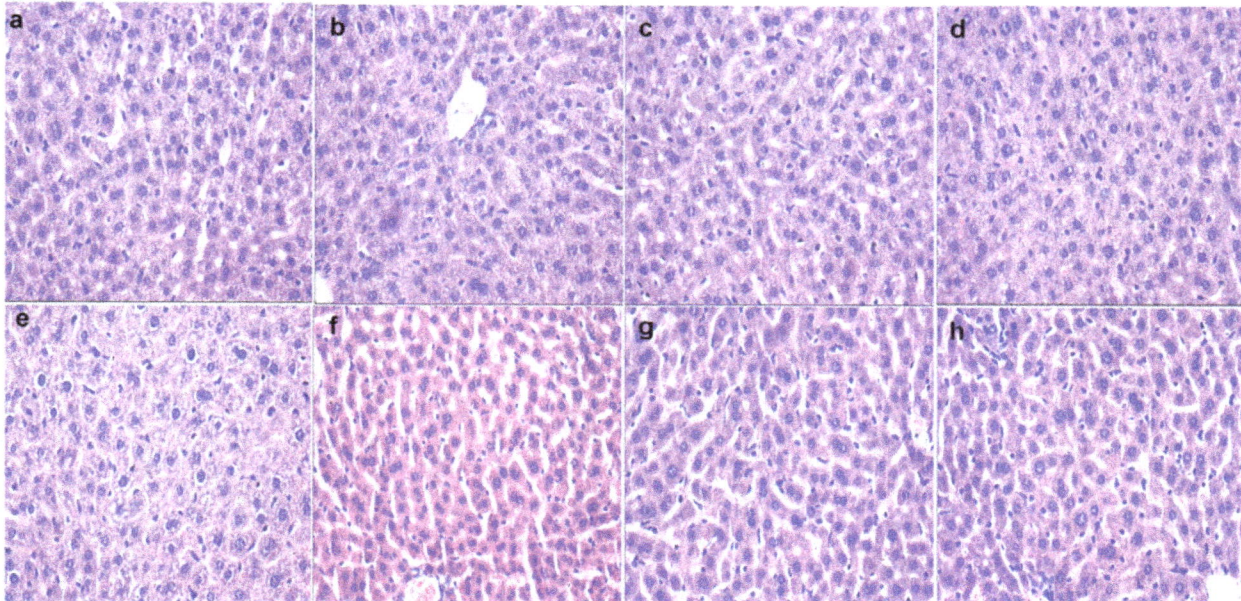

Figure 2 Histological changes in F$_0$ and F$_1$ mice after swainsonine treatment. a-d represent changes in the liver of F$_0$-I, F$_0$-II, F$_0$-III and F$_0$-IV (×400); **e-h** represent changes in the liver of F$_1$-I, F$_1$-II, F$_1$-III and F$_1$-IV (×400).

were significantly decreased compared with F$_1$-IV controls ($P < 0.05$). HCT levels in F$_1$-I group mice were significantly decreased compared with F$_1$-IV control mice ($P < 0.05$), and MCV levels in F$_1$-I and F$_1$-II mice were significantly increased compared with F$_1$-IV control mice ($P < 0.05$) (Table 2).

Discussion

Swainsonine, a trihydroxy indolizidine alkaloid, is the main toxin in locoweed. The structure of the swainsonine cation is similar to the structure of mannose, and it has a higher affinity than mannose for mannosidase [10]. Swainsonine is a well-known inhibitor of lysosomal

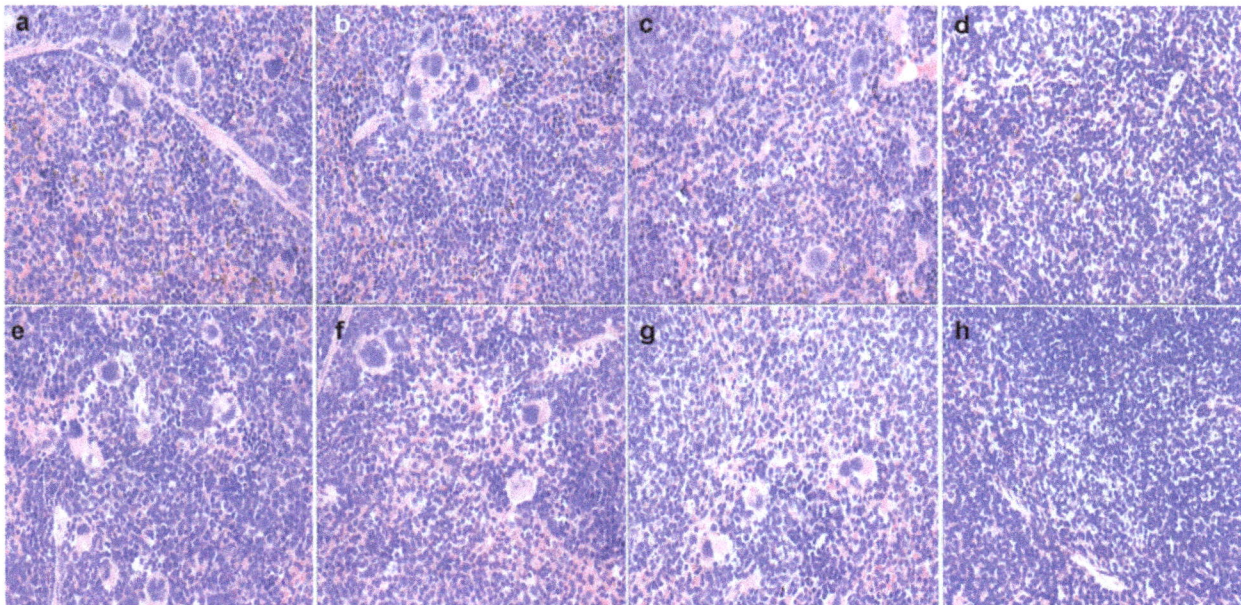

Figure 3 Histological changes in F$_0$ and F$_1$ mice after swainsonine treatment. a-d represent changes in the spleen of F$_0$-I, F$_0$-II, F$_0$-III and F$_0$-IV (×400); **e-h** represent changes in the spleen of F$_1$-I, F$_1$-II, F$_1$-III and F$_1$-IV (×400).

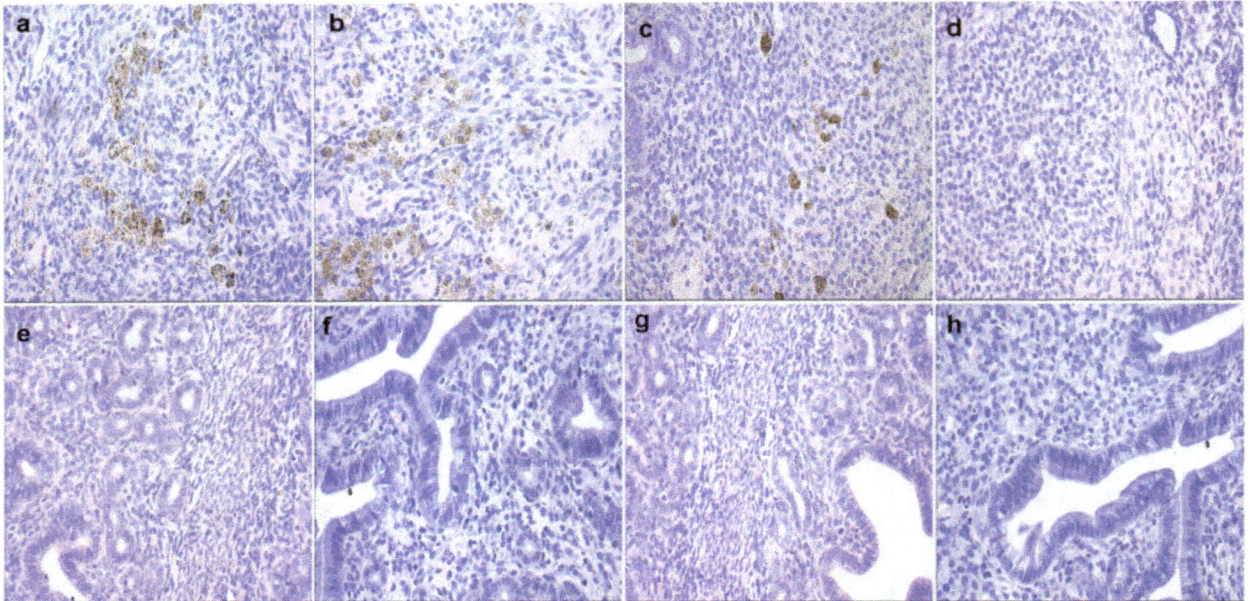

Figure 4 Histological changes in F_0 and F_1 mice after swainsonine treatment. a-d represent changes in the uterus of F_0-I, F_0-II, F_0-III and F_0-IV (×400); **e-h** represent changes in the uterus of F_1-I, F_1-II, F_1-III and F_1-IV (×400).

α-mannosidase and Golgi α-mannosidase II. Swainsonine induces toxicity through inhibition of α-mannosidase and subsequent glycoprotein synthesis. This enzymatic dysfunction causes accumulation of complex oligosaccharides in lysosomes as well as the production of a mixture of mannose and asparagine polysaccharides, resulting in vacuolar degeneration in multiple cells [11]. Clinical symptoms in livestock are characterized by neurological and behavioral disorders, gait abnormalities, difficulty standing, abnormal posture, emaciation, reproductive disorders and cellular vacuolar degeneration of multiple tissues by pathological observation

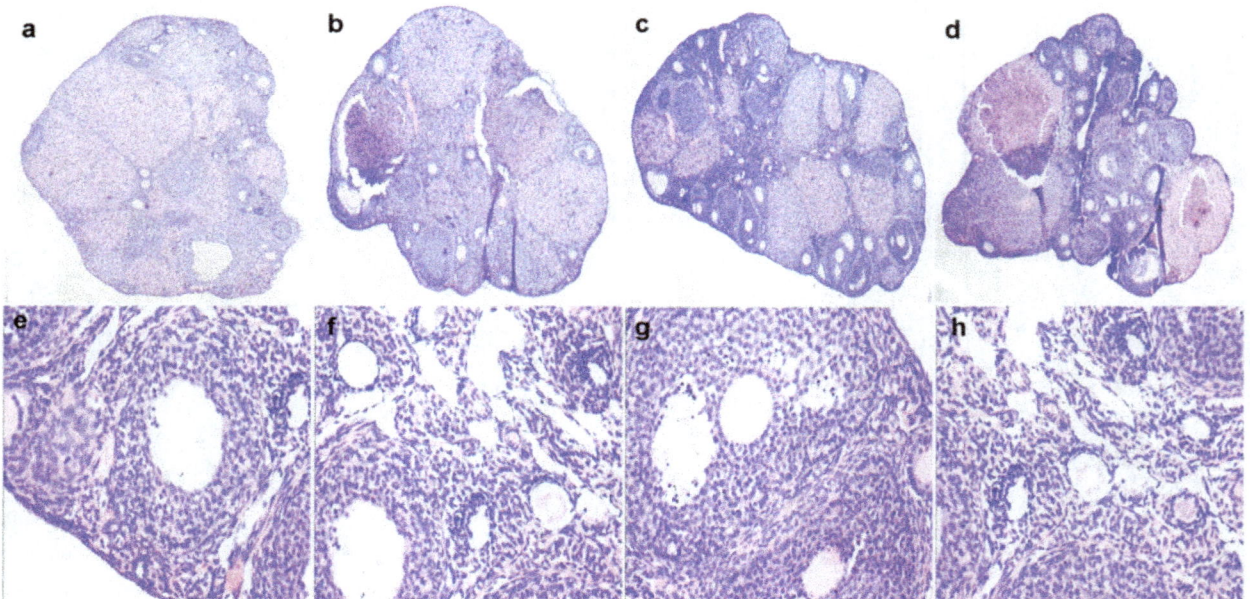

Figure 5 Histological changes in F_0 and F_1 mice after swainsonine treatment. a-d represent changes in the ovary of F_0-I, F_0-II, F_0-III and F_0-IV (×100); **e-h** represent changes in the ovary of F_1-I, F_1-II, F_1-III and F_1-IV (×400).

Table 1 Serum marker assessment in swainsonine-treated mice

	LDHU/L	ALPU/L	ASTU/L	ALTU/L	IBILmg/dL
F0-I	783.9 ± 96.2*	269.84 ± 31.58*	184.32 ± 12.5*	65.87 ± 8.57*	0.43 ± 0.03*
F0-II	718.5 ± 95.7*	221.47 ± 32.85*	178.7 ± 10.8*	59.78 ± 9.55*	0.37 ± 0.05*
F0-III	623.8 ± 99.3	193.58 ± 35.87	120.87 ± 11.8	48.47 ± 8.77	0.029 ± 0.02*
F0-IV	587.2 ± 95.8	188.97 ± 27.31	98.11 ± 9.36	41.05 ± 9.58	0.11 ± 0.011
F1-I	547.54 ± 93.25	214.85 ± 7.5	116.58 ± 9.32	47.32 ± 8.50	0.28 ± 0.03*
F1-II	551.87 ± 90.58	218.55 ± 8.1	111.56 ± 9.65	45.36 ± 8.01	0.20 ± 0.01*
F1-III	569.65 ± 85.79	203.51 ± 7.5	105.8 ± 12.21	42.11 ± 7.59	0.18 ± 0.02*
F1-IV	554.88 ± 80.69	198.65 ± 6.8	92.34 ± 8.65	38.25 ± 7.20	0.095 ± 0.02

The values are the mean ± S.D.
*Significantly different from the control group at same generation ($P < 0.05$).

[12,13]. However, we observed two generations of mice and show organ selective vacuolar degeneration by mice given swainsonine via pathological observation. We found hemosiderin deposition in spleen and enlargement of spleen in F_0 and F_1 mice, and a large amount of hemosiderin deposition in uterus in F_0 mice. When animals are fed a dose of swainsonine arrive to a certain time, the vacuolar degeneration of pathological change will show in the internal organs [9]. Therefore, we think that this experiment period did not arrive to a certain time that vacuolar degeneration found in organ. However, in our previous experiment, we also found hemosiderin deposition in spleen of rat and goat using a different dose of swainsonine [14]. We posited that some tissue bleeding occurred after swainsonine administration and found that hemosiderin deposition leads to damage in some tissues. Whether the presence of hemosiderin deposition can be used as a pathological marker of swainsonine poisoning requires further research.

The experiment results showed that two ways were not significantly different between irrigation and intraperitoneal injection by Liu Tianya [15]. Therefore, we selected the way of intraperitoneal injection for give mice to swainsonine. In this study, we demonstrate that swainsonine exerts hepatotoxicity in F_0 mice. Alterations in liver weight and histopathological changes in liver of swainsonine-treated mice were slight. Liver from swainsonine-treated mice showed cellular infiltrates consisting mostly of inflammatory cells and neutrophil granulocytes. Significant increase of liver weight and significant alterations in levels of AST, ALT and ALP in plasma may indicate hepatic injury in F_0 mice given swainsonine. The elevations of ALT, AST and ALP observed in swainsonine-treated mice may, in part, be due to the hepatic hypertrophic effect of swainsonine and/or may also represent borderline chronic liver toxicity [16,17]. Increased LDH activity levels have been observed in conditions of chemical stress when high levels of energy are required in a short period of time [18]. In the present study, LDH was significantly increased in F_0 mice. However, no significant differences in biochemical markers were found between treatment and control mice F_1 mice. This is consistent with the lack of histopathological changes in liver of F_1 mice.

The present study identifies important histological alterations in the spleen in F_0 and F_1 mice, namely expansion of red pulp with vascular congestion. Furthermore, the endometrium of the uterus displayed notable deposition of hemosiderin granules in a swainsonine-treated dose-dependent manner in F_0 mice. The molecular weight of swainsonine is small enough to penetrate the placental barrier and expose offspring in-utero. A major function of the spleen is to remove aged and damaged

Table 2 Hematological assessment in swainsonine-treated mice

	WBC × 10^9/L	RBC × 10^{12}/L	Hb g/L	HCT %	MCV fL	PLT × 10^9/L	MCH fl	Reticulocytes %
F0-I	7.98 ± 1.12	6.01 ± 1.54*	100.58 ± 21.58*	0.36 ± 0.03*	78.32 ± 6.58*	519.74 ± 53.9*	39.95 ± 7.58*	5.54 ± 0.78*
F0-II	7.21 ± 1.08	6.37 ± 1.23*	108.58 ± 25.46*	0.40 ± 0.03*	76.32 ± 6.68*	523.8 ± 48.5*	40.01 ± 6.52*	4.85 ± 0.85*
F0-III	7.19 ± 1.10	6.58 ± 1.15*	112.87 ± 26.54*	0.41 ± 0.02*	72.58 ± 6.98*	548.9 ± 51.25*	42.11 ± 7.56*	4.56 ± 0.96*
F0-IV	7.85 ± 1.75	8.45 ± 1.12	153.77 ± 20.58	0.53 ± 0.05	54.25 ± 5.44	624.88 ± 58.5	52.10 ± 7.01	2.13 ± 0.58
F1-I	7.89 ± 0.95	6.58 ± 1.12*	121.69 ± 25.41*	0.51 ± 0.025*	69.58 ± 6.32*	588.39 ± 56.21*	40.88 ± 7.85*	4.38 ± 0.29*
F1-II	7.01 ± 0.65	7.05 ± 1.25*	125.6 ± 23.15*	0.59 ± 0.035	65.32 ± 7.32*	605.81 ± 63.5*	42.02 ± 7.96*	4.18 ± 0.74*
F1-III	7.95 ± 0.85	7.55 ± 1.30*	139.85 ± 32.15*	0.60 ± 0.04	60.25 ± 5.91	632.87 ± 65.21	44.32 ± 8.81*	3.66 ± 0.95*
F1-IV	7.75 ± 1.23	8.36 ± 1.05	149.85 ± 23.56	0.62 ± 0.04	58.65 ± 5.64	658.2 ± 63.9	53.53 ± 8.21	2.07 ± 0.66

The values are the mean ± S.D.
*Significantly different from the control group at same generation ($P < 0.05$).

erythrocytes from the blood [19]. Excess hemosiderin deposition in spleen can result in the destruction of macrophages and the release of the contents such as iron, toxic compounds and/or its metabolites into spleen [20]. Toxic effects in both F_1 and F_0 mice include reduction of RBCs, reduction in levels of Hb, HCT, PLT and MCH, as well as an increase in the number of reticulocytes, suggesting the development of anemia [21]. Significant increases in IBIL were observed in F_0 and F_1 mice given swainsonine. The increase of IBIL further indicates that swainsonine could be damaging red blood cells. When organs bleed, red blood cells are phagocytized by macrophages and degraded by lysosomes; Fe^{3+} of hemoglobin from lysed red blood cells can combine with protein to form hemosiderin. Because we observed decreased RBCs, and decreased levels of Hb, MCH and MCV as well as an increase in reticulocytes, we suspect that our dose levels of swainsonine may lead to anemia.

Swainsonine is water-soluble and rapidly distributed to many parts of the body. In previous studies, swainsonine concentrations varied widely in various tissues and organs of sheep that had ingested locoweed [22-24]. In this study, uterus of swainsonine-treated F_0 mice was heavily damaged. This was characterized by the presence of hemosiderin deposits in the lamina propria of endometrium in uterus of F0 mice in this study. In ovary, F_0-I and F_0-II mice displayed decreased numbers of primordial and primary follicles compared to F_0-IV controls. In addition, F_0-I and F_0-II mice displayed increased size and number of corpus lutea compared to F_0-III and F_0-IV. The lesions in ovary and uterus were dose-dependently observed in F_0-I, F_0-II and F_0-III treatment groups. However, F_1 did not display notable histopathological changes in the uterus and ovary. Swainsonine easily accumulates in uterus at high concentrations, which may impair uterus and ovary function and cause toxicity. In the present study, the uterus suffered noticeable damage, which led to a decline in the rate of conception, an increase in the rate of abortion and increases in stillborn births. It is suspected that significant early embryonic loss occurs in cattle and sheep grazing locoweed, and there are documented effects of swainsonine on oocyte maturation, fertilization and subsequent embryonic implantation and development [24]. Increased numbers of corpus lutea in ovary can lead to delayed or halted estrus. The pathological lesions we observed, combined with altered hematological and serum biochemical parameters in swainsonine-treated mice, suggest that exposure to swainsonine may lead to inhibition of reproductive performance under certain doses.

Conclusions

Based on sub-chronic toxicity results, our data establishes effects of swainsonine on reproductive toxicity in a mouse model. In addition, we found that swainsonine can cause hematological changes and lesions in spleen, uterus, ovary and liver. Furthermore, we provide evidence of trans-generational swainsonine toxicity through placental barrier and milk. Spleen, heart, liver, lung, kidney, uterus and ovary were among the organs affected in offspring of dams given swainsonine. Large amounts of hemosiderin deposition in uterus and spleen were observed in the parent generation. We present evidence that hemosiderin deposition may preclude vacuolar degeneration in some tissues of mice given swainsonine. Alterations in hematological and histopathological parameters suggest a link to anemia and decreases in reproduction ability. Our data suggest that anemia and organ-specific hemosiderin deposition followed by destruction of red blood cells are clinical features of swainsonine-treated mice. However, further research is needed to elucidate specific mechanisms of swainsonine toxicity.

Methods
Ethical statement
Female *Rattus norvegicus* mice were supplied by the Animal Center of the Fourth Military Medical University. During the experiment, mice were housed individually in polypropylene cages with laboratory grade pine shavings as bedding. Mice were maintained in a controlled environment with temperature maintained between 19-25°C, relative humidity maintained between 40-70%, >8 air changes/hour, and with a 12:12-h light: dark cycle. The experimental procedures were in accordance with the Ethical Principles (Animal [Scientific Procedures] Act 2012) in Animal Research adopted by the China College of Animal Experimentation and were approved by the College of Veterinary Medicine- Northwest A&F University.

Study design
Extraction of swainsonine from locoweed
The aerial portion of *Oxytropis kansuensis* was collected from the grassland in Tianzhu city, Gansu province in July 2011. The plants were then taxonomically identified by Zhao Bao-Yu, College of Veterinary Medicine, Northwest A and F University, China. The plants were subsequently dried in the shade, finely ground and comminuted.

The extraction and analysis method of swainsonine from *Oxytropis kansuensis* was conducted as previously described [25].

Analysis of swainsonine
Thin-layer chromatography (TLC) detection was performed on silica gel G precoated plates with the developing solvents chloroform:methanol:ammonia:water (70:26:2:2, V/V), chloroform:methanol:ammonia:water (70:26:10:10, V/V), and methanol: ethylacetate: ammonia (4:1:1,V/V) and modified potassium heptaiodobismuthate reagent or

H_2O_2/10% acetic anhydride in EtOH/Ehrlich's reagent was the chromogenic agent.

The extracts were dissolved in methanol, spotted onto the GF254 silica gel G precoated plates. The plates were developed with an ascendant run after saturation with the mobile phase in a s glass chamber for 5–10 min. The plates were dried when the mobile phase was 10 mm from the front edge of the plates. The plates were stained successively with a spray of H_2O_2 (heated for 10 min in an oven at 115°C), a spray of 10% acetic anhydride in dehydrated alcohol (heated at the same temperature until the smell of acetic anhydride disappeared) and finally a spray of Ehrlich's reagent (heated for 15 min at 120°C). The color of the spots in each plate was recorded, and the R_f was determined [25].

Animals to experimental groups
Female mice (N = 40, six weeks old) were divided into four equal groups of 10 mice (10 each group, F_0-I: 0.525 mg/kg BW; F_0-II: 0.2625 mg/kg BW; F_0-III: 0.175 mg/kg BW and F_0-IV: 0 mg/kg BW). All mice were administered swainsonine by intraperitoneal injection 14 days before the mating period followed by re-administration every three days. After this pre-mating period, the treated mice were transferred to the home cage of a male in the same group and cohabited on a 1:1 basis until achievement of successful mating. During the mating period, mice were examined daily for presence of vaginal plugs, and a vaginal plug was considered evidence of successful mating. Pregnant dams continued to receive swainsonine every three days via intraperitoneal injection throughout parturition and the lactation. Upon weaning of four-week-old pups (F_1), the dams (F_0) were sacrificed, and the liver, kidney, heart, spleen, lung, uterus and ovary were collected. In total, F_0 mice were given swainsonine for six to eight weeks in the whole experiment.

Female offspring (F_1) of treated dams were selected from each of the four treatment groups (40 F_1 mice in total, 10 from each F_0 treatment group). The F_1 offspring were not treated with swainsonine, however, the dams continued to be dosed while nursing their F_1 pups. The F_1 offspring were then sacrificed after approximately 1 month of nursing. The liver, kidney, heart, spleen, lung, uterus, and ovary were collected.

All F_0 group mice received intraperitoneal injections of swainsonine once every three days under aseptic conditions. Upon sacrifice, the liver, kidney, heart, spleen, lung, uterus and ovary were trimmed of extraneous fat and weighed immediately.

Histopathological preparation
All tissues were removed and fixed in 10% formaldehyde at room temperature. The tissue samples were then dehydrated and embedded in paraffin according to standard histological procedures. Serial cross-sections of 3 μm were prepared from each organ. The sections were mounted and stained with hematoxylin-eosin.

Hematological assessment
White blood cells (WBCs), red blood corpuscles (RBCs), hemoglobin (Hb), hematocrit (HCT), mean corpuscular volume (MCV), blood platelets (PLTs), mean corpuscular hemoglobin (MCH) and reticulocyte counts were determined by automatic hematological analyzer, MEK-8222 K (TOA Medical Electronics, Kobe, Japan).

Blood biochemical analysis
Blood was collected when mice were sacrificed. Lactate dehydrogenase (LDH), aspartate aminotransferase (AST), alanine aminotransferase (ALT), alkaline phosphatase (ALP) and indirect bilirubin (IBIL) were quantitated using the Beckman Synchron CX7 Delta Chemistry Analyzer (Beckman, USA).

Statistical methods
The statistical software "Statistical Product and Service Solutions" (SPSS V11.3) was used to determine statistically significant differences between treatment groups and the control group. A one-way ANOVA was used to evaluate the homogeneity of the data, and a least squared differences model or Dunnett's multiple comparison test were then used. Values of $p < 0.05$ were considered significant. The data are presented as the group mean values $\pm$ SD (standard deviation).

Competing interests
The authors declare that they have no competing interests.

Authors' contributions
MF carried out the extration of swainsonine from *Oxytropis kansuensis*; ZB participated in the test design and drafted the manuscript; LX raised mice and performed the statistical analysis; WC participated in the design of the study and wrote the manuscript. All authors read and approved the final manuscript.

Acknowledgments
The authors thank Li Xiaoming the research assistant for making pathological, Mr Han from translatinng the manuscript. This study was financed by the grants from the National Natural Science Foundation (No. 31302153) and the origination fee of doctoral research (No. Z111021305), Postdoctoral program (No. K308021401) and the Special Scientific Research Fund of Agriculture Public Welfare industry (No. 201203062).

References
1. Molyneux RJ, James LF. Loco intoxication indolizidine alkaloids of spotted locoweed (Astragalus lentiginosus). Science. 1982;216:190–1.
2. Li JK. The present situation and prospect of the studies on locoweed In China. Agric Sci China. 2003;36:1091–9.
3. Molyneux RJ, Gomez-Sosa E. Presencia del alcaloide indolizidinico swainsonine enAstragalus pehuenches(Leguminosae-Galegueae). Bol Soc Argent Bot. 1991;27:59–64.
4. Molyneux RJ, James LF, Ralphs MH, Pfister JA, Panter KE, Nash RJ. Polyhydroxylated glycosidase inhibitors from poisonous plants of global

distribution: analysis and identification. In: Colegate SM, Dorling PR, editors. Plant-associated toxins, agricultural and phytochemical aspects. Wallingford, UK: CABI; 1994. p. 107–12.

5. Panter KE, James LF, Stegelmeier BL, Ralphs MH, Pfister JA. Locoweeds: effects on reproduction in livestock. J Nat Toxins. 1999;8:53–62.

6. Panter KE, James LF, Mayland HF. Reproductive response of ewes fed alfalfa pellets containing sodium selenate orAstragalus bisulcatusas a selenium source. Vet Hum Toxicol. 1995;37:30–2.

7. Stegelmeier BL, James LF, Panter KE, Molyneux RJ. Serum swainsonine concentration and alpha-mannosidase activity in cattle and sheep ingesting Oxytropis sericea and Astragalus lentiginosus (locoweeds). Am J Vet Res. 1995;56:149–54.

8. James LF, Panter KE, Nielsen DB, Molyneux RJ. The effect of natural toxins on reproduction in livestock. J Anim Sci. 1992;70:1573–9.

9. Chenchen W, Wenlong W, Xiaoxue L. Pathogenesis and preventive treatment for animal disease due to locoweed poisoning. Environ Toxicol Phar. 2014;37:336–47.

10. Galyean ML, Ralphs MH, Reif MN. Effects ofprevious grazing treatment and consumption of locoweed onliver mineral concentrations in beef steers. J Anim Sci. 1996;74:827.

11. Abraham DJ, Rsidebothom BG, Winchester PR. Swainsonine affects the processing of glycoproteins in vivo. FEBS Lett. 1983;163:110–3.

12. Das PC, Roberts JD, White SL. Activation of resident tissue-specific macrophages by swainsonine. Oncol Res. 1995;7(9):425–33.

13. Jacob GS. Glycosylation inhibitors in biology and medicine. Curr Opin Struct Biol. 1995;5(5):605–11.

14. Wang wenlong: Extracts of oxytropis kansuensis induced toxic damage of rats and protective effects of "Jifang E". Northwest A&F University Press 2014; pp.57-59

15. Tianya L, Zongyuan H. Effects of irrigation and intraperitoneal injection on locomotor activity of mice. Editorial Board Acta Academiae Medicinae Wannan. 2010;29(4):241–4.

16. Amacher DE. Serum transaminase elevations as indicators of hepatic injury following the administration of drugs. Regul Toxicol Pharmacol. 1998;27:119–30.

17. Boone L, Meyer D, Cusick P, Ennulat D, Bolliger AP. Selection and interpretation of clinical pathology indicators of hepatic injury in preclinical studies. Vet Clin Pathol. 2005;34:182–8.

18. Kamble N, Velhal V. Cytopathological assessment of uterine cells in rattus norvegicus due to induced sodium fluoride. The bioscan. 2010;5:301–3.

19. Stefanski SA, Elwell MR, Stromberg PC, Boorman GA, Eustis SL, Elwell MR, editors. Pathology of the fischer Rat reference and atlas. San Diego: Academic Press; 1990. p. 369–93.

20. Fujitani T, Tada Y, Yoneyama M. Chlorpropham-induced splenotoxicity and its recovery in rats. Food Chem Toxicol. 2004;42:1469–77.

21. Hui A, Jinyi L, Lujun Y, Shengxue L, Yanhong Z, Huan Y, et al. Acute and subchronic toxicity of hydroxylammonium nitrate in Wistar rats. J Med Colleges PLA. 2008;23:137–47.

22. Tong D, Mu P, Dong Q, Zhao B, Liu W, Zhao J. Immunological evaluation of SW-HSA conjugate on goats. Colloids Surf B Biointerfaces. 2007;58:61–7.

23. Stegelmeier BL, James LF, Panter KE, Molyneux RJ. Tissue and serum swainsonine concentrations in sheep ingesting Astragalus lentiginosus (locoweed). Vet Hum Toxicol. 1995;37:336–9.

24. Stegelmeier BL, James LF, Panter KE, Gardner DR, Ralphs MH, Pfister JA. Tissue swainsonine clearance in sheep chronically poisoned with locoweed (Oxytropis sericea). J Anim Sci. 1998;76:1140–4.

25. Pengbin G, Baoyu Z, Dewen T. Extraction and fractionation and identification of swainsonine on structure from oxytropis glabra. Chin Agric Sci Bull. 2003;19(1):1–5.

7

Suitability of sentinel abattoirs for syndromic surveillance using provincially inspected bovine abattoir condemnation data

Gillian D Alton[1*], David L Pearl[1], Ken G Bateman[1], W Bruce McNab[2] and Olaf Berke[1,3]

Abstract

Background: Sentinel surveillance has previously been used to monitor and identify disease outbreaks in both human and animal contexts. Three approaches for the selection of sentinel sites are proposed and evaluated regarding their ability to capture overall respiratory disease trends using provincial abattoir condemnation data from all abattoirs open throughout the study for use in a sentinel syndromic surveillance system.

Results: All three sentinel selection criteria approaches resulted in the identification of sentinel abattoirs that captured overall temporal trends in condemnation rates similar to those reported by the full set of abattoirs. However, all selection approaches tended to overestimate the condemnation rates of the full dataset by 1.4 to as high as 3.8 times for cows, heifers and steers. Given the results, the selection approach using abattoirs open all weeks had the closest approximation of temporal trends when compared to the full set of abattoirs.

Conclusions: Sentinel abattoirs show promise for integration into a food animal syndromic surveillance system using Ontario provincial abattoir condemnation data. While all selection approaches tended to overestimate the condemnation rates of the full dataset to some degree, the abattoirs open all weeks selection approach appeared to best capture the overall seasonal and temporal trends of the full dataset and would be the most suitable approach for sentinel abattoir selection.

Background

There are various approaches to conduct disease surveillance including sentinel and syndromic surveillance. Sentinel surveillance is a form of surveillance which involves a limited number of recruited participants or organizations, such as farms, veterinarians, abattoirs, healthcare providers or hospitals, which report on certain health events to give an indication of what may be happening in the general population [1]. Sentinel surveillance is a strategy used to sample timely data in a relatively inexpensive manner rather than collect information on the general population, when population-based data collection is unfeasible in a timely or cost-effective manner [2]. Syndromic surveillance involves the amalgamation of signs/symptoms using data from non-traditional data sources [3]; the signs/symptoms are grouped into classifications called 'syndromes' and are used to track disease trends in populations and signal a possible outbreak that warrants further investigation [3].

Sentinel surveillance has been previously used in both human and animal health settings for a variety of disease outcomes. Sentinel surveillance has been used to monitor or identify outbreaks of infectious diseases and to monitor the activity of certain health conditions which can change due to environmental conditions. Though used less often in animal health applications than in human health, sentinel surveillance has been used successfully for surveillance in various applications. For example, following the emergence of Bluetongue virus serotype 8 in Central Europe in 2006, causing a large scale outbreak in 2007 in several countries in Europe, a Bluetongue sentinel surveillance program was established in Belgium in 2010. This surveillance program was intended to demonstrate the absence of Bluetongue virus [4]. This program randomly selected a total of 300 dairy herds, with 30 herds selected from each of the Belgian provinces. The criteria for

* Correspondence: altong@uoguelph.ca
[1]Department of Population Medicine, Ontario Veterinary College, University of Guelph, Guelph, ON N1G 2 W1, Canada
Full list of author information is available at the end of the article

selection of herds was based on dairy herds that were expected to have a minimum of 15 animals present between 4 and 12 months of age at the start of the sentinel program [5]. Other studies have combined both sentinel and syndromic surveillance and utilize data from sentinel veterinarians or veterinary practices [6,7].

Animal health data including abattoir condemnation data have emerged recently as a novel data stream for syndromic surveillance of diseases of animal and public health importance [6,8-13]. Ontario provincial abattoir data have been recently explored as a potential source of information for food animal syndromic surveillance [8-10]. Data from Ontario provincial abattoirs are particularly appealing as they can provide a more regionally specific picture of emerging diseases in Ontario, as the cattle shipped to these abattoirs originate from farms from approximately a 100 km radius [9]. However, there are approximately 100–150 provincial abattoirs in Ontario, many of which are open sporadically and have differing processing capacities, which may bias the results of quantitative methods for disease surveillance. It may be beneficial to conduct enhanced and targeted surveillance at select abattoirs in order to gather more accurate data for syndromic surveillance. In addition, by selecting specific sentinel abattoirs for inclusion in a sentinel syndromic surveillance system, it would allow for more intensive and specialized training of inspectors for syndromic surveillance. Furthermore, if sentinel abattoirs were selected properly, they could help to reduce the cost of surveillance while still being representative of the overall condemnation trends in all Ontario provincial abattoirs. Cost efficiency could result from limiting the number of abattoirs requiring investigation during potential aberrations in condemnation rate, and by reducing the number of abattoirs requiring targeted surveillance and specialized training of inspectors. The criteria used to select sentinel abattoirs require consideration. We proposed three sentinel site selection approaches and compared their ability to detect respiratory disease trends in bovine abattoir condemnation data for use in a sentinel-based syndromic surveillance system.

Pneumonic lung condemnation rates from all Ontario abattoirs processing cattle throughout the 2001–2007 period were compared to those collected from sentinel sites based on three selection approaches: (1) abattoirs processing cattle all weeks of the year; (2) abattoirs processing at least 6500 cattle per year (based on data from abattoirs in the upper 95th percentile in processing capacity); and (3) multi-criteria selection approach of abattoirs that met a predefined set of criteria related to abattoir processing capacity, and animal classes represented.

The goal of the study was to compare abattoir selection approaches for a sentinel surveillance system based on provincially inspected abattoirs in Ontario. Specific

objectives of this study were the following: (1) determine the suitability of sentinel abattoirs for food animal syndromic surveillance using provincial abattoir pneumonic lung condemnation data as an example; and (2) determine which design is most efficient and representative for pneumonic lung condemnation rate in terms of spatial distribution, temporal trends and relative differences between animal classes when compared to data from all the abattoirs over the study period.

Methods

Data source

Pneumonic lung portion condemnation data were obtained from the Food Safety Decision Support System (FSDSS) database maintained by the Ontario Ministry of Agriculture, Food and Rural Affairs (OMAFRA). The database contains information regarding the number and reason for daily organs/body systems condemnations in provincially inspected abattoirs in Ontario. The condemnation category of pneumonic lung was selected for these analyses, as this category represents a major health issue for beef cattle and was among the most frequently reported portion condemnations by provincial inspectors during the study period. Pneumonic lung condemnation refers to bovine lungs which were condemned for lesions indicative of a previous localized and resolved antero-ventral pneumonia infection (personal communication Abdul Rehmtulla, DVM, OMAFRA, Stone Road, Guelph, Ontario).

Data were extracted from the Food Safety Decision Support System (FSDSS) database for cattle animal classes: bulls, calves, cows, heifers, and steers from January 1, 2001 to December 31, 2007. Within the FSDSS database, calves are defined as any animal under 396 lbs dressed weight. All other animal classes are classified at the discretion of the inspector based on age, weight, breed and sex (personal communication Alexandra Reid, DVM, PhD, OMAFRA, Stone Road, Guelph, Ontario). Missing geographical coordinates for abattoirs were approximated using postal codes and/or addresses with the address geocoding software GeoPinpoint Suite 6.4 (DMTI Spatial Inc., Markham, Ontario, Canada). Using the FSDSS database, further variables were created for each month: geographical coordinates of abattoir, year, season, number of weeks an abattoir was operating each year, total number of pneumonic lung condemnations, total number of cattle processed each year, and animal class. Animal class included five categories: bulls, cows, calves, heifers, and steers. Bulls were excluded from subsequent analyses due to missing data and inconsistencies in the use of this classification. The number of weeks an abattoir was operating each year was determined by the total number of weeks in which at least one bovine animal was processed. The total number of animals processed each year was calculated from the total number of condemned cattle plus the number of cattle fit for consumption. The agricultural region where an abattoir was located was classified as: central, eastern, northern, southern or western Ontario using the Ontario Census Agricultural Region boundaries (Statistics Canada, Census Agricultural Regions, Census year 2001). The regional location of each abattoir was determined using the point-in-polygon technique with geographic information system software ArcGIS 9.2 (ESRI, Redlands, California, USA).

This study conducted statistical analyses utilizing a pre-existing government database. As no experimentation or use confidential information for people or animals was used in this study, no ethical approval application was needed.

Descriptive analyses

Monthly bovine pneumonic lung condemnation rates were calculated using data from all abattoirs slaughtering cattle during the study period of January 1, 2001 – December 31, 2007. Condemnation rates were calculated by dividing the total number of pairs of lungs condemned under the pneumonic lung classification each month by the total number of slaughtered bovines for each animal class (e.g., calves, cows, heifers and steers).

During the study period, the number of abattoirs in operation varied from year to year, which was likely due to economic and regulatory changes in the cattle industry. There were a total of 211 provincial abattoirs slaughtering a total of 1,155,535 cattle from 2001–2007. The monthly cattle slaughtered per animal class have been reported in Alton et al. [8]. During the study period there were 36,883 lungs condemned representing approximately 9% of all portion condemnation and among the most frequently reported condemnation in cattle. Further discussion of these data can be found in a previous study by Alton et al. [8]. However, there were only 98 abattoirs that remained in operation for the entire study period and were therefore used to represent the full set of abattoirs in this study. This number is consistent with the current number of abattoirs processing cattle in Ontario in 2014 [14]. There were a total of 33,182 lungs condemned and 856,467 cattle processed during the study period at these 98 abattoirs. Three different design approaches for a sentinel syndromic surveillance system were compared to all data from the full set of 98 abattoirs. The first sentinel selection approach, which we refer to as abattoirs open all weeks, uses data from abattoirs processing cattle 52 weeks per year. The second approach, which we refer to as large abattoirs; uses data from abattoirs in the upper 95th percentile in processing capacity (processing at least 6500 cattle per year). The third approach, which we refer to as multi-criteria approach, uses data from abattoirs that met the following

criteria for each year of the study period: processed at least 499 cattle per year (representing the median total number of cattle processed based on data from all 211 abattoirs open from 2001 – 2007), processed at least 1 bovine carcass 44 weeks or more each year (representing the median number of weeks cattle were processed based on data from all 211 abattoirs open from 2001–2007), and processed cattle representing all animal classes (calves, cows, heifers, and steers).

Data obtained using the three design approaches were summarized graphically using the raw monthly condemnation rates of each animal class. In addition, data were summarized in terms of the number of abattoirs included in each selection approach, percentage of shared abattoirs between each selection approach, and geographical representativeness of each selection approach according to the distribution of abattoirs among census agricultural regions in Ontario.

Statistical analyses

To evaluate the overall condemnation rates within each animal class, a univariable negative binomial model was used to compare monthly pneumonic lung condemnation rates from all sentinel site selection approaches and the full set of abattoirs using a categorical variable for each of the 3 sentinel design approaches. To determine whether the overall seasonal and temporal trends of the full dataset were being captured within each sentinel selection approach, separate multi-level negative binomial regression models were used with a random intercept for abattoir using the xtnbreg command in Stata. This model allows the random effect to follow a beta distribution and for the overdispersion parameter to vary by abattoir. The negative binomial model was used to evaluate the association of monthly condemnation rates of pneumonic lungs for each sentinel selection approach

Table 1 Summary of sentinel abattoirs selection approaches for Ontario provincial abattoirs (2001 – 2007)

Sentinel site selection approach	Selection description	Number of abattoirs
Full dataset	Abattoirs processing at least 1 bovine carcass each year of study period (2001 – 2007)	98
Abattoirs open all weeks	Abattoirs processing at least 1 bovine carcass 52 weeks per year	45
Multi-criteria	Selection of abattoirs meeting the following criteria: processed at least 499 cattle per year, processed at least 1 bovine carcass 44 weeks or more per year, processed cattle representing all animal classes (calves, cows, heifers and steers)	44
Large abattoirs	Abattoirs processing ≥ 6500 cattle per year	7

Table 2 Percentage of shared abattoirs between sentinel selection approaches

Selection approaches	Full dataset[1] (N = 98)	Abattoirs open all weeks[2] (N = 45)	Selection criteria[3] (N = 44)	Large abattoirs[4] (N = 7)
Full dataset[1] (N = 98)	100% (98)	45.9% (45)	44.9% (44)	7.1% (7)
Abattoirs open all weeks[2] (N = 45)	45.9% (45)	100% (45)	71.1% (32)	15.6% (7)
Selection criteria[3] (N = 44)	44.9% (44)	71.1% (32)	100% (44)	6.8% (3)
Large abattoirs[4] (N = 7)	7.1% (7)	15.6% (7)	6.8% (3)	100% (7)

[1]Abattoirs processing at least 1 bovine carcass each year of study period (2001 – 2007).
[2]Abattoirs processing at least 1 bovine carcass 52 weeks per year.
[3]Selection of abattoirs meeting the following criteria: processed at least 499 cattle per year, processed at least 1 bovine carcass 44 weeks or more per year, processed cattle representing all animal classes (calves, cows, heifers and steers).
[4]Abattoirs processing ≥ 6500 cattle per year.

with year, season and animal class. All covariates were evaluated for statistical significance individually and then in a multivariable multi-level negative binomial model. All covariates were forced into the models regardless of univariable significance, due to the identification of these variables as important predictors for pneumonic lung condemnation rates in a previous study [8] and to evaluate overall temporal trends in the data. All statistical models include the log of the number of animals slaughtered for a specific animal class in the offset.

For all regression models, the decision to use a negative binomial model instead of a Poisson regression model was based on evaluating the Akaike Information Criterion (AIC) value of both models and the significance of the over-dispersion term of the negative binomial model. The offset of the negative binomial model was the natural log of the total number of slaughtered cattle for the abattoirs included for each sentinel site selection approach for each animal class and month-year period during the study period. All statistical analyses were conducted using Stata 12 (Stata Corp., College Station, Texas, USA).

Results
Descriptive statistics
Three approaches for sentinel abattoir selection were compared to pneumonic lung condemnation rates for each animal class from the full set of abattoirs (Table 1). Abattoirs for each sentinel selection approach were

chosen from a total of 98 abattoirs processing cattle for the entire study period. The number of abattoirs selected for each sentinel selection approach varied from 7 to 45 (Table 1). In assessing the percentage of overlap of the selected abattoirs among the sentinel site selection approaches, the percentage of shared abattoirs ranged from approximately 7% to 71%, with abattoirs open all weeks and multi-selection criteria approaches having the highest percentage of abattoirs in common (Table 2). All selection approaches led to surveillance systems based on sentinel abattoir condemnation rates representing all census agricultural regions across Ontario with the exception of using the large abattoir criterion, which did not include abattoirs from eastern and northern Ontario (Table 3).

The temporal condemnation rate graphs for all data indicate a gradual decrease in pneumonic lung condemnation rates over time in calves from approximately 100 condemnations per 1000 slaughtered calves in 2001 to approximately 20 condemnations per 1000 slaughtered calves in 2007 (Figure 1). In comparison, pneumonic lung condemnation rates in cows, heifers and steers remained much more stable over the study period (Figures 2, 3 and 4). The overall monthly condemnation rates for the full set of abattoirs compared to the 3 sentinel site selection approaches for each animal class had similar distributions for calves, heifers and steers (Figure 1, 3 and 4), with the exception of the large abattoir selection approach, which tended to have more

Table 3 Distribution of provincial abattoirs 2001 – 2007 among census agricultural regions in Ontario based on three sentinel selection approaches

Selection approach	Number of abattoirs	Central Ontario	Eastern Ontario	Northern Ontario	Southern Ontario	Western Ontario
Full dataset[1]	98	18% (18)	15% (15)	7% (7)	36% (35)	23% (23)
Abattoirs open all weeks[2]	45	18% (8)	13% (6)	7% (3)	38% (17)	24% (11)
Multi-criteria[3]	44	9% (4)	18% (8)	5% (2)	39% (17)	30% (13)
Large abattoirs[4]	7	29% (2)	0% (0)	0% (0)	43% (3)	29% (2)

[1]Abattoirs processing at least 1 bovine carcass each year of study period (2001 – 2007).
[2]Abattoirs processing at least 1 bovine carcass 52 weeks per year.
[3]Selection of abattoirs meeting the following criteria: processed at least 499 cattle per year, processed at least 1 bovine carcass 44 weeks or more per year, processed cattle representing all animal classes (calves, cows, heifers and steers).
[4]Abattoirs processing ≥ 6500 cattle per year.

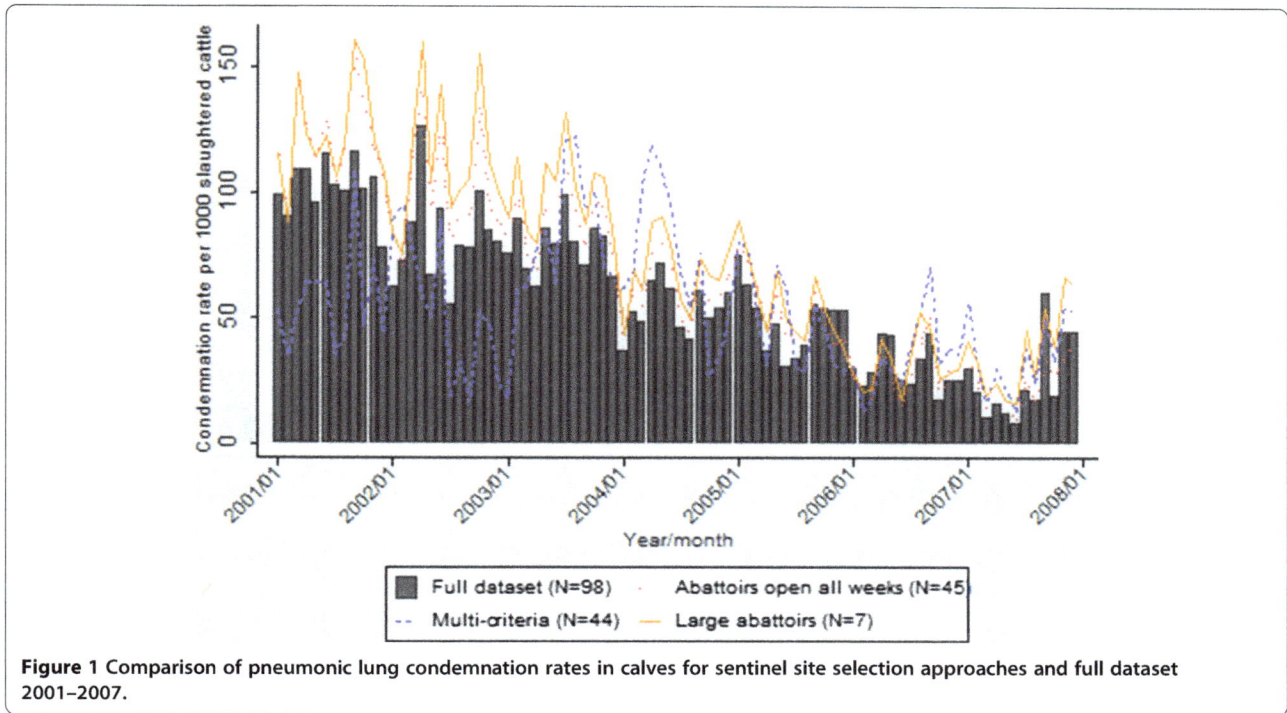

Figure 1 Comparison of pneumonic lung condemnation rates in calves for sentinel site selection approaches and full dataset 2001–2007.

variability when compared to the other selection approaches and full set of abattoirs.

Based on descriptive plots for calves (Figure 1), the multi-criteria selection approach did not show a good fit with the full dataset, with alternating trends of either overestimating or underestimating the condemnation rate of the full dataset. However, the other two alternative selection approaches tended to approximate the overall secular trends of the full dataset, but generally overestimated the condemnation rates of the full dataset

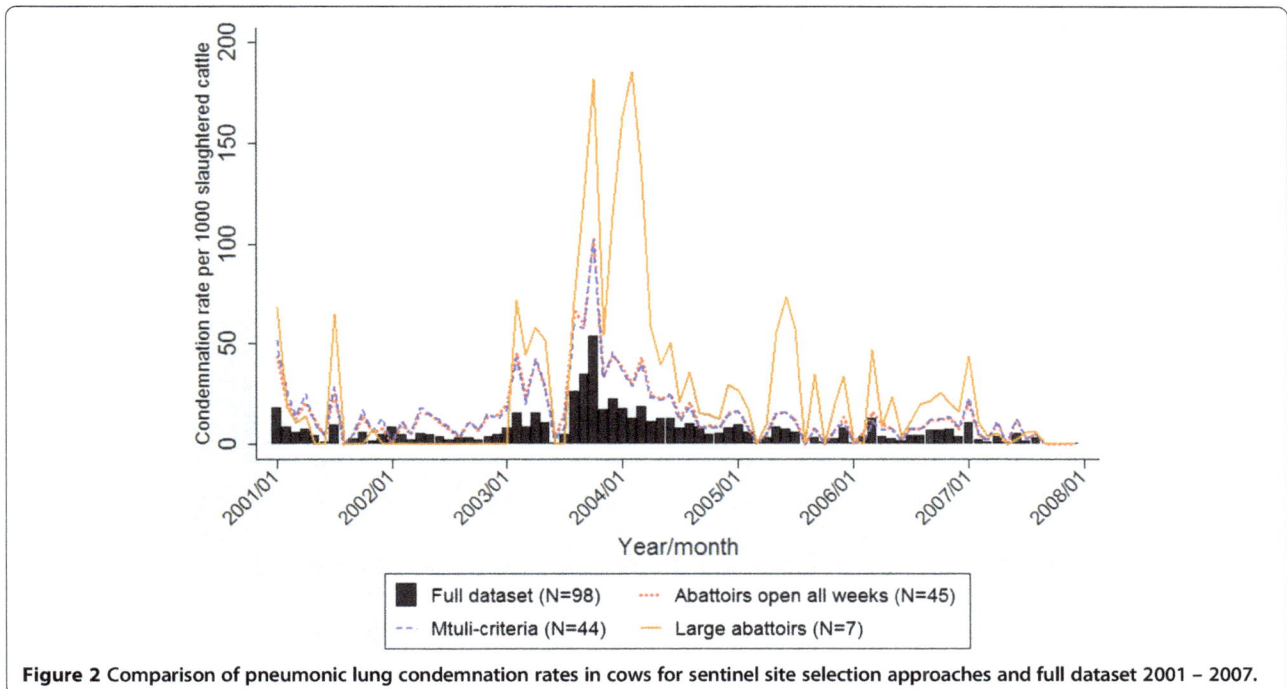

Figure 2 Comparison of pneumonic lung condemnation rates in cows for sentinel site selection approaches and full dataset 2001 – 2007.

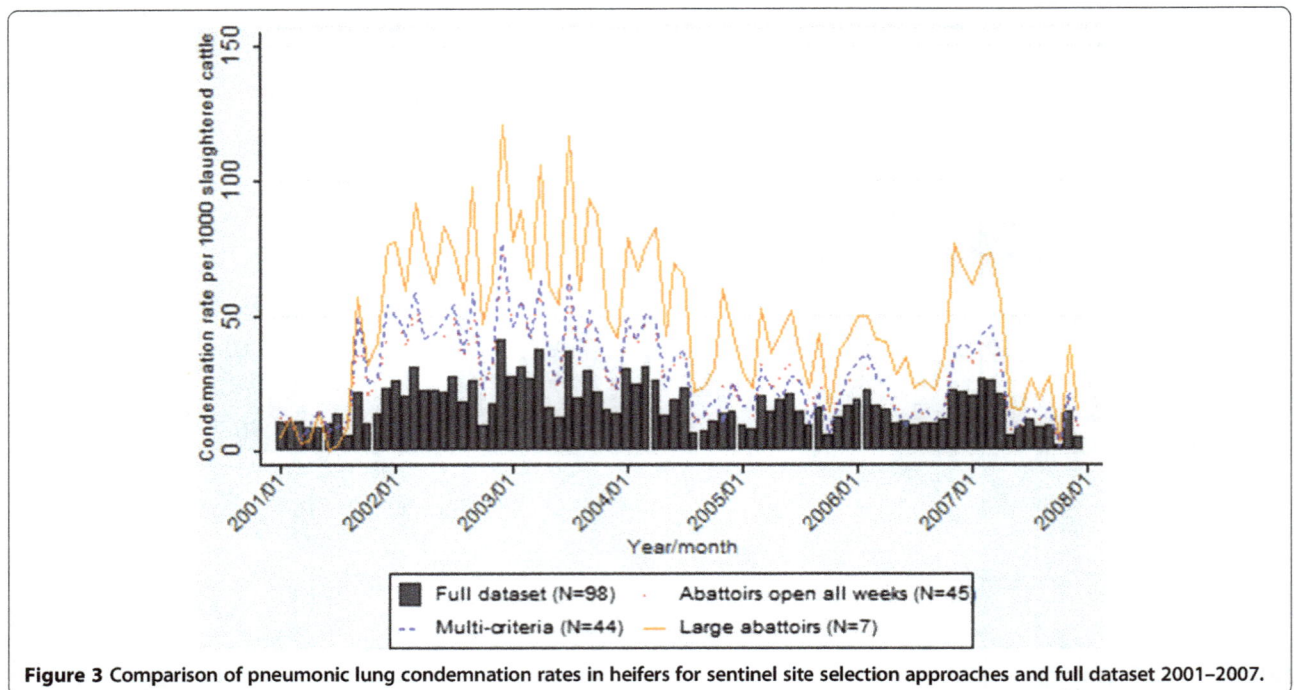

Figure 3 Comparison of pneumonic lung condemnation rates in heifers for sentinel site selection approaches and full dataset 2001–2007.

throughout the study period. Based on the descriptive plots for cows, heifers and steers (Figures 2, 3 and 4), all three design approaches tended to overestimate the condemnation rate relative to the full set of data, however, the large abattoir selection approach had the largest overestimation in all animal classes.

Negative binomial models

We used a negative binomial regression model to compare the monthly pneumonic lung condemnation rates from the 3 sentinel surveillance system selection approaches for each animal class to the full dataset. The model involving calves (Table 4a) found a difference

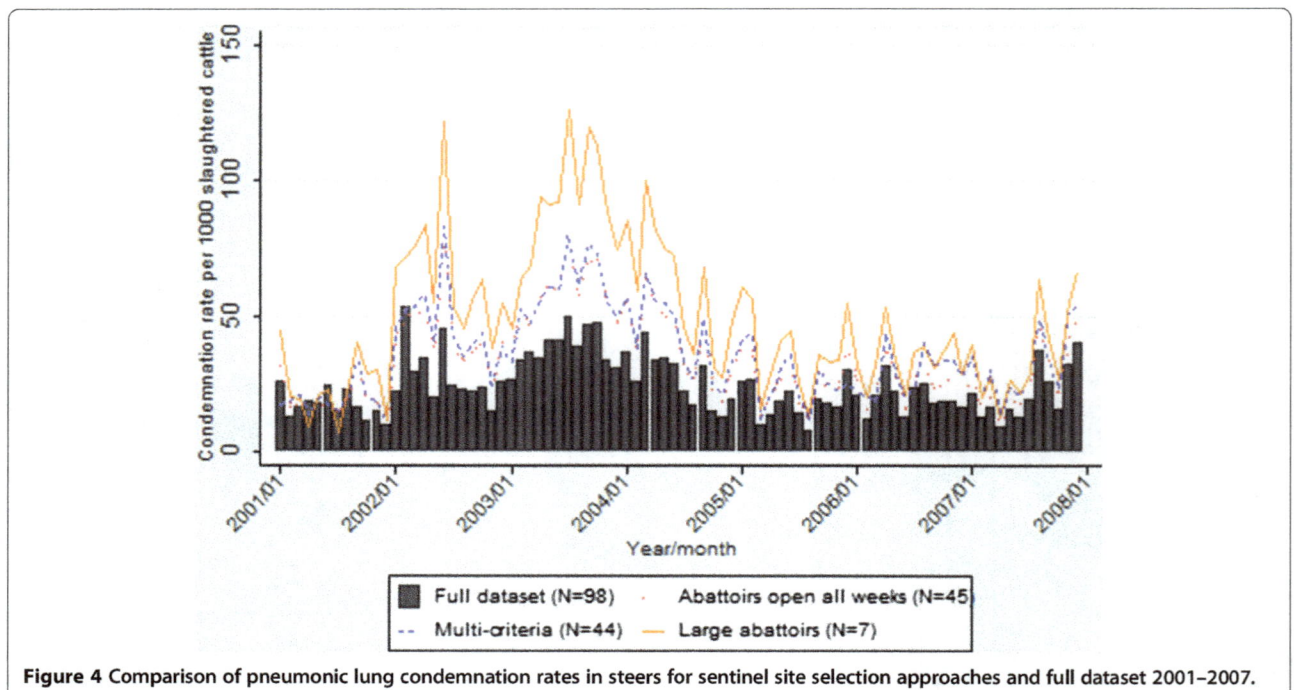

Figure 4 Comparison of pneumonic lung condemnation rates in steers for sentinel site selection approaches and full dataset 2001–2007.

Table 4 Negative binomial regression models comparing monthly pneumonic lung condemnation rates for all abattoirs for each animal class with three methods of sentinel abattoir selection

Sentinel selection method	IRR	95% CI	P-value
a) Calves			
Full dataset[1]	—	—	—
Abattoirs open all weeks[2]	1.12	0.95 – 1.32	0.16
Multi-criteria[3]	0.90	0.76 – 1.06	0.21
Large abattoirs[4]	1.25	1.06 – 1.47	0.01
b) Cows			
Full dataset[1]	—	—	—
Abattoirs open all weeks[2]	2.08	1.49 – 2.91	<0.01
Multi-criteria[3]	2.06	1.47 – 2.89	<0.01
Large abattoirs[4]	3.83	2.73 – 5.38	<0.01
c) Heifers			
Full dataset[1]	—	—	—
Abattoirs open all weeks[2]	1.61	1.35 – 1.94	<0.01
Multi-criteria[3]	1.70	1.42 – 2.04	<0.01
Large abattoirs[4]	2.86	2.38 – 3.43	<0.01
d) Steers			
Full dataset[1]	—	—	—
Abattoirs open all weeks[2]	1.39	1.20 – 1.61	<0.01
Multi-criteria[3]	1.48	1.28 – 1.72	<0.01
Large abattoirs[4]	2.02	1.74 – 2.34	<0.01

[1]Abattoirs processing at least 1 bovine carcass each year of study period (2001 – 2007).
[2]Abattoirs processing at least 1 bovine carcass 52 weeks per year.
[3]Selection of abattoirs meeting the following criteria: processed at least 499 cattle per year, processed at least 1 bovine carcass 44 weeks or more per year, processed cattle representing all animal classes (calves, cows, heifers and steers).
[4]Abattoirs processing ≥ 6500 cattle per year.

between the large abattoir selection approach and the full set of data. In comparison, negative binomial modelling of cow data (Table 4b) found that all 3 design approaches overestimated the condemnation rate by a factor of 2 to 4 times, when compared to the full dataset. Similarly, relative to the full dataset, all the sentinel selection approaches overestimated the condemnation rates for heifers (Table 4c) and steers (Table 4d).

There were similar seasonal and temporal trends noted among all sentinel site selection approaches and the full set of abattoirs (Table 5a – d). However, the abattoirs open all weeks sentinel selection approach tended to have coefficients and trends which best resembled the seasonal and temporal trends of the full dataset. Abattoirs open all weeks also tended to have the closest approximation of coefficients when compared to the full dataset for the animal class variable.

Discussion

Three sentinel site selection approaches for a sentinel syndromic surveillance system using abattoir condemnation data were proposed and compared to the full set of provincially inspected abattoirs in Ontario from 2001–2007. While pneumonic lung condemnation data were used as an exemplar in this study, the process of sentinel abattoir selection could be extended to other disease categories as well. While all selection approaches tended to overestimate the condemnation rates of the full dataset to some degree, the abattoirs open all weeks selection approach appeared to best capture the overall seasonal and temporal trends of the full dataset and would be the most suitable approach for sentinel abattoir selection. This selection approach utilizes data from 45 abattoirs. It may be advantageous to conduct enhanced surveillance at carefully selected sentinel abattoirs rather than at the approximately 100 abattoirs slaughtering cattle in Ontario [14]. This allows for more intensive and specialized training of inspectors for syndromic surveillance. Furthermore, if sentinel abattoirs were selected properly, sentinel abattoirs could help to reduce the cost of surveillance while still being representative of Ontario provincial abattoirs.

While there was not one design approach that perfectly fit the full dataset in all analyses, the results of the descriptive and quantitative analyses found a fairly good fit between abattoirs open all weeks and the full dataset. This sentinel selection approach utilizes less than half of the abattoirs from the full set of abattoirs. By collecting data from fewer abattoirs, the cost of data collection and analysis is reduced. This approach also allows for the use of targeted training of inspectors to reduce any presence of inspector bias on the data, which appeared to be a possible issue with these data based on previous studies [9,10]. The multi-criteria sentinel selection approach also utilizes data from approximately the same number of abattoirs as the abattoirs open all weeks, however, this approach had larger amount of overestimation for heifers and steers than abattoirs open all weeks and did not approximate the overall seasonal, secular and animal class condemnation trends of the full dataset as well as the abattoirs open all weeks. This suggests that the number of abattoirs selected is not necessarily as important as the criteria used to select the abattoirs. While the abattoirs open all weeks sentinel selection approach drastically reduced the number of abattoirs needed to conduct syndromic surveillance involving provincial abattoir condemnation data compared to the full dataset, it is uncertain whether this reduction is sufficient and manageable to conduct intensive and targeted surveillance. Further research is needed to determine if there are other sentinel selection approaches that could reduce this number of abattoirs even further.

Table 5 Multivariable multilevel negative binomial regression model examining seasonal and annual variability in monthly pneumonic lung condemnations for three sentinel selection approaches

Model	IRR	95% CI	P-value
a) Full dataset[1]			
Winter	—	——	—
Spring	0.97	0.85 – 1.11	0.61
Summer	0.90	0.78 – 1.03	0.12
Fall	0.89	0.78 – 1.03	0.11
2001	—	—	—
2002	0.93	0.79 – 1.08	0.34
2003	0.99	0.85 – 1.16	0.93
2004	0.53	0.44 – 0.63	<0.01
2005	0.45	0.38 – 0.54	<0.01
2006	0.39	0.32 – 0.47	<0.01
2007	0.32	0.26 – 0.40	<0.01
Calves	—	—	—
Cows	1.05	0.87 – 1.27	0.60
Heifers	0.68	0.57 – 0.80	<0.01
Steers	0.75	0.66 – 0.85	<0.01
b) Abattoirs open all weeks[2]			
Winter	—	—	—
Spring	1.01	0.88 – 1.16	0.93
Summer	0.92	0.80 – 1.05	0.22
Fall	0.91	0.79 – 1.05	0.22
2001	—	—	—
2002	0.94	0.80 – 1.11	0.50
2003	1.03	0.88 – 1.21	0.68
2004	0.57	0.48 – 0.68	<0.01
2005	0.46	0.38 – 0.55	<0.01
2006	0.40	0.38 – 0.49	<0.01
2007	0.34	0.28 – 0.42	<0.01
Calves	—	—	—
Cows	1.03	0.84 – 1.26	0.75
Heifers	0.73	0.62 – 0.87	<0.01
Steers	0.75	0.66 – 0.86	<0.01
c) Multi-criteria[3]			
Winter	—	—	—
Spring	1.08	0.92 – 1.28	0.33
Summer	0.95	0.80 – 1.12	0.51
Fall	0.92	0.78- 1.09	0.35
2001	—	—	—
2002	1.03	0.84 – 1.27	0.76
2003	1.30	1.11 – 1.63	<0.01
2004	1.04	0.85 – 1.28	0.72
2005	0.67	0.54 – 0.84	<0.01

Table 5 Multivariable multilevel negative binomial regression model examining seasonal and annual variability in monthly pneumonic lung condemnations for three sentinel selection approaches (Continued)

Model	IRR	95% CI	P-value
2006	0.67	0.49 – 0.79	<0.01
2007	0.62	0.62 – 0.96	<0.01
Calves	—	—	—
Cows	0.77	0.62 – 0.96	0.02
Heifers	0.62	0.51 – 0.75	<0.01
Steers	0.71	0.61 – 0.82	<0.01
d) Large abattoirs[4]			
Winter	—	—	—
Spring	0.97	0.82 – 1.15	0.74
Summer	0.92	0.77 – 1.09	0.32
Fall	0.99	0.84 – 1.18	0.94
2001	—	—	—
2002	1.38	1.11 – 1.72	<0.01
2003	1.56	1.26 – 1.93	<0.01
2004	0.97	0.77 – 1.22	0.78
2005	0.75	0.59 – 0.94	0.01
2006	0.64	0.50 – 0.82	<0.01
2007	0.64	0.50 – 0.82	<0.01
Calves	—	—	—
Cows	1.22	0.92 – 1.62	0.16
Heifers	1.02	0.83 – 1.25	0.86
Steers	0.87	0.74 – 1.03	0.10

[1]Abattoirs processing at least 1 bovine carcass each year of study period (2001 – 2007).
[2]Abattoirs processing at least 1 bovine carcass 52 weeks per year.
[3]Selection of abattoirs meeting the following criteria: processed at least 499 cattle per year, processed at least 1 bovine carcass 44 weeks or more per year, processed cattle representing all animal classes (calves, cows, heifers and steers).
[4]Abattoirs processing ≥ 6500 cattle per year.

Geographical representativeness is also an important consideration when establishing sentinel selection criteria. While the sentinel selection approaches based on abattoirs that are open all weeks and multi-criteria are geographically representative, the large abattoir selection approach is geographically over-representative of abattoirs in central and southern Ontario and has no representation of abattoirs in northern and eastern Ontario. This could pose an issue for syndromic surveillance, as abattoirs generally receive animals from relatively local farms [9], and a lack of representation from abattoirs in these regions could lead to the inability to identify emerging health issues in these under-represented areas. The distribution of abattoirs among regions is almost identical for abattoirs open all weeks selection approach and the full dataset. In addition, region has been shown to be an important variable associated with partial and whole carcass condemnations [8,9] and excluding certain regions could bias the results of spatio-temporal cluster detection methods for syndromic surveillance involving these data.

While the number of abattoirs processing cattle varied over the study period, these fluctuations are likely due to the large economic and regulatory changes in the cattle industry during the study period. If the number of abattoirs fluctuates greatly over time, the process of sentinel selection would have to be repeated on a regular basis and could pose inefficiency issues for the surveillance system. To address this issue in our study, we opted to select only the abattoirs that were open during the study period to represent the full dataset. However, in recent years that number of abattoirs processing cattle has remained fairly consistent and this is not expected to be an issue for sentinel selection in Ontario provincial abattoirs.

This study found bovine provincial abattoir condemnation data to be suitable for sentinel surveillance assuming it is a cost-effective option. However, this study did not investigate outbreak detection, as there were no documented animal health outbreaks in cattle during the study period. Consequently, further research is needed to assess the effectiveness of sentinel selection approaches for detecting emerging health issues using documented or simulated outbreak data of both respiratory diseases as well as other disease syndromes important to both animal health and food safety.

Conclusions

Sentinel abattoirs show promise for integration into a food animal syndromic surveillance system using Ontario provincial abattoir condemnation data. The selection of the sentinel abattoirs is extremely important in order to maintain representativeness of the disease trends in the entire population. The information extracted from surveillance systems varied by its respective selection approach and for each animal class. While all selection approaches tended to overestimate the condemnation rates of the full dataset to some degree, the abattoirs open all weeks selection approach appeared to best capture the overall seasonal and temporal respiratory condemnation trends of the full dataset and would be most suitable approach for sentinel abattoir selection involving these data. However, should the purpose of the surveillance system be to measure the overall condemnation rates, the overestimation of all sentinel abattoir selection approaches would give inaccurate results. Further studies should examine the performance of the proposed sentinel selection approaches using simulated data that include disease outbreaks for both respiratory diseases as well as other condemnation syndromes relevant to animal health and food safety.

Competing interests
The authors declare that they have no competing interests.

Authors' contributions
GDA performed the statistical analysis and drafted the manuscript. WBM was involved in the acquisition of data, and the drafting and revision of the manuscript for intellectual content. DLP and OB were involved in the conception and design, analysis and interpretation of data, and revising manuscript critically for important intellectual content. KGB was involved in the interpretation of data, and the revising of the manuscript critically for important intellectual content. All authors read and approved the final manuscript.

Acknowledgements
The authors would also like to acknowledge the following organizations for their support for infrastructure, data retrieval and funding for this project: Canada Foundation for Innovation (CFI), the Ontario Research Fund, the Ontario Graduate Scholarship, and Ontario Ministry of Agriculture & Food (OMAF).

Author details
[1]Department of Population Medicine, Ontario Veterinary College, University of Guelph, Guelph, ON N1G 2 W1, Canada. [2]Ontario Ministry of Agriculture & Food, Guelph, ON N1G 4Y2, Canada. [3]Department of Mathematics and Statistics, University of Guelph, Guelph, ON N1G 2 W1, Canada.

References
1. Salman MD. Animal Disease Surveillance and Survey Systems: methods and Applications. Ames, Iowa: Iowa State Press; 2003.
2. Lee LM, Teutsch SM, Thacker SB, St. Louis ME. Principles and Practice of Public Health Surveillance. 3rd ed. New York: Oxford University Press; 2010.
3. Lawson AB, Kleinman K. Spatial and Syndromic Surveillance for Public Health. Chichester, West Sussex: J. Wiley; 2005.
4. Vangeel I, De Leeuw I, Meroc E, Vandenbussche F, Riocreux F, Hooyberghs J, et al. Bluetongue sentinel surveillance program and cross-sectional serological survey in cattle in Belgium in 2010–2011. Prev Vet Med. 2012;106:235–43.
5. Amezcua M, Pearl D, Friendship R, McNab W. Evaluation of a veterinary-based syndromic surveillance system implemented for swine. CJVR. 2010;74:241–50.
6. Dórea F, Sanchez J, Revie CW. Veterinary syndromic surveillance: current initiatives and potential for development. Prev Vet Med. 2011;101:1–17.
7. Alton GD, Pearl DL, Bateman KG, McNab WB, Berke O. Suitability of portion condemnations at Ontario provincially-inspected abbatoirs for food animal syndromic surveillance. BMC Vet Res. 2012;8:88.
8. Alton GD, Pearl DL, Bateman KG, McNab WB, Berke O. Factors associated with whole carcass condemnation rates in provincially-inspected abattoirs in Ontario 2001–2007: implications for food animal syndromic surveillance. BMC Vet Res. 2010;6:42.
9. Thomas-Bachli AL, Pearl DL, Friendship RM, Berke O. Suitability and limitations of portion-specific abattoir data as part of an early warning system for emerging diseases of swine in Ontario. BMC Vet Res. 2012;6:3.
10. Weber WD. Development of an animal monitoring system based on slaughter condemnation data. Miami: Proceedings of the Eighth International Society for Disease Surveillance Conference; 2009. 3–4 December.
11. O'Sullivan T, Friendship RM, Pearl DL, McEwen B, Dewey CE. Identifying an outbreak of a novel swine disease using test requests for porcine reproductive and respiratory syndrome as a syndromic surveillance tool. BMC Vet Res. 2012;8:192.
12. Palmer S, Sully M, Fozdar F. Farmers, animal disease reporting and the effect of trust: a study of West Australian sheep and cattle farmers. Rural Society. 2009;19:32–48.
13. Provincially Licensed Meat Plants. [http://www.omafra.gov.on.ca/english/food/inspection/maps/TblBeef.htm]

8

Development of intestinal microflora and occurrence of diarrhoea in sucking foals: effects of *Bacillus cereus* var. *toyoi* supplementation

Jenny John[1,4], Kathrin Roediger[2], Wieland Schroedl[3], Nada Aldaher[3] and Ingrid Vervuert[1*]

Abstract

Background: Almost all foals develop transient diarrhoea within the first weeks of life. Studies indicated different viral, bacterial, and parasitic causes, such as rotavirus, *Clostridium perfringens*, *Escherichia coli,* and *Cryptosporidium* are discussed. But little is known about the development of intestinal microflora in foals. The present study investigated whether the supplementation with *Bacillus cereus* var. *toyoi* would modify the developing intestinal microflora and consequently reduce diarrhoea in foals. From birth, the foals were randomly assigned to three treatment groups: placebo (10 mL isotonic NaCl, $n = 8$), low dosage (LD; 5×10^8 cfu *B. cereus* var. *toyoi*, $n = 7$) and high dosage (HD; 2×10^9 cfu *B. cereus* var. *toyoi*, $n = 10$). Treatment groups were supplemented orally once a day for 58 days. Faeces scoring and sampling were performed within the first 24 h after birth and on day 9, 16, 23, 30, 44, 58 of the foal's life and also on the first day of diarrhoea. Culture-plate methods were used to analyse the bacterial microflora.

Results: Eighty-eight per cent of the foals developed diarrhoea (placebo 7/8, LD 5/7, HD 10/10) during the first 58 days of life. *Bacillus cereus* var. *toyoi* supplementation had no effect on bacterial microflora. *Clostridium perfringens* and enterobacteria were equally prevalent in foals with diarrhoea and those who were not afflicted.

Conclusions: We conclude that the supplementation of *B. cereus* var. *toyoi* had no effect on the occurrence of diarrhoea and health status in the foals.

Keywords: Microflora, Foal, Diarrhoea, Probiotic, *Bacillus cereus* var. *toyoi*

Background

Diarrhoea is a common problem in neonatal foals. Almost all foals develop transient diarrhoea within the first weeks of life [1,2]. Studies have reported different viral, bacterial, and parasitic causes [3–6]. Between the days 5 and 15 of a foal's life, when the dam's first post partum oestrus is expected, diarrhoea in foals is observed frequently [3]. The diarrhoea is termed 'foal heat diarrhoea'. Although commonly there is no reduction in behaviour of the foals, some of them suffer from diarrhoea more than 20 days within the first 2 months of life and develop not as good as foals with shorter diarrhoea periods. The establishment of intestinal microflora and maturation of the gastrointestinal mucosa are some reasons proposed for diarrhoea in this period of life [2].

However, little is known about the development of the intestinal microflora during this period. During and following birth, neonates are exposed to a variety of microorganisms originally from the dam or environment. On the day of birth, aerobes, facultative anaerobes, and strict anaerobes were already detected in the faeces of the foals [7]. Before foals are fed solid food, cellulolytic bacteria have already colonized the digestive tract [7]. Because the intestinal microflora is a crucial line of resistance against colonization by exogenous microbes, it is highly relevant in the prevention of tissue invasion by pathogens [8].

Probiotic bacteria were defined by a joint FAO, WHO [9] as 'live microorganism which when administered in adequate amounts confer a health benefit on the host'. Some probiotics are known to have a positive effect on the intestinal microflora. For example, Yuyama et al. [10] reported that supplementation with probiotics led to an earlier recovery from foal heat diarrhoea, probably by enhancing establishment of the normal intestinal

* Correspondence: ingrid.vervuert@vetmed.uni-leipzig.de
[1]Institute of Animal Nutrition, Nutrition Diseases and Dietetics, Faculty of Veterinary Medicine, University of Leipzig, Leipzig, Germany
Full list of author information is available at the end of the article

microflora. However, other studies that showed that supplementation with probiotics in foals increased the occurrence and duration of diarrhoea compared to placebo-treated foals [11], and Weese and Rousseau [12] reported that probiotic administration was significantly associated with development of signs of depression, anorexia, and colic in foals.

The aim of the study was to investigate the effects of oral probiotic supplementation on the growing intestinal microflora in equine neonates. Previous studies have shown positive effects of *Bacillus cereus* var. *toyoi* on intestinal health in calves, piglets, poultry, broiler chickens, and growing rabbits [13–16]. Baum et al. [17] observed trophic effects of *Bacillus cereus* var. toyoi on the small intestinal mucosa of pigs as demonstrated by longer villi, thicker mucosa and more mature, i.e. acidic mucins. Vilà et al. [15] showed that feeding of *Bacillus cereus* var. *toyoi* reduced the prevalence of pathogens such as Salmonella in poultry and improved the performance variables of broiler chickens. We hypothesized that oral supplementation with *B. cereus* var. *toyoi* from birth until 2 months of the foal's life would modify the intestinal microflora and mucosa, and therefore lead to a reduction of diarrhoea in foals.

Results

During the observation period, haematolgy parameters like erythrocytes, haematocrit or leukocytes were in the reference range obtained for foals (data not shown, treatment p > 0.05). 24 h after birth serum IgG levels were always higher than the lowest critical threshold of 8 g/L. Serum IgG levels of the foals were in median between 17.1 g/l and 25.6 g/l (treatment p > 0.05). During the observation period, serum IgG levels decreased down to 60 − 70% of initial value at day 58 (time p < 0.05, treatment p > 0.05). Diarrhoea occurred in up to 90% of the foals for at least one 1 day between days 8 and 16 of life. In particular, during transition period between orange-brown milk faeces and more adult-like greenish faeces a loose consistency (faeces score: 6–9) was observed in 92% of the foals. Despite this, foals remained bright and alert and continued to nurse.

Supplementation with *B. cereus* var. *toyoi* had no significant effect on dry matter content of the faeces of the foals. Furthermore, supplementation with *B. cereus* var. *toyoi* had no significant effect on blood parameters and there was no change in the incidence of diarrhoea in foals in the first 58 days of life (Table 1).

Lactobacilli in the foals faeces increased on days 1 to 9 of foals life. Maximum level was 4.50×10^7 cfu/g (LD, Table 2). Declining counts of Lactobacilli were noticed until day 58 where Lactobacilli counts almost reached the levels of the mares (measured at the time of birth).

Table 1 Number of foals with diarrhoea, duration of diarrhoea (days) and faecal score in placebo (*n* = 8), low dosage (*n* = 7), and high dosage (*n* = 10) during period of oral supplementation with *Bacillus cereus* var. *toyoi* (days 1 to 58 of life), data expressed as numbers, median, 25 and 75% quartile

Item	Placebo	Low dosage	High dosage	P-value
Number of foals with diarrhoea (n)				
	7/8	5/7	10/10	>0.05
Duration of diarrhoea (days)				
25% quartile	2	2	2.8	0.7072
Median	2.5	10	3.5	
75% quartile	5.3	11	4.8	
Faecal score				
25% quartile	3	2	2	0.132
Median	3	3	3	
75% quartile	3	6	5	

Supplementation with *B. cereus* var. *toyoi* had no significant effect on lactobacilli counts in faeces of the foals.

Both frequency of detection (Table 3) and bacteria counts of enterococci (data not shown) in the faeces of the foals increased in the first 9 days of life and then declined until day 58. Enterococci were found in 15.2% of the mares samples (measured at the time of birth). Supplementation with *B. cereus* var. *toyoi* had no significant effect on enterococci counts in faeces of the foals.

Bacteroides spp. were detected in the faeces of three foals respectively in one to three samples between days 9 and 30 of life. Two out of three foals had days of diarrhoea above-the-average. Four out of six samples with *Bacteroides spp.* were samples from diarrhoea. No *Bacteroides spp.* were found in the mares samples (data not shown).

Enterobacteria were not detected in faeces of the foals at every time point during the treatment period (days 1 to 58 of life, Table 4). Enterobacteria were found in 30% (10 of 33) of the mare samples (measured at the time of birth), at a maximum of 6.00×10^5 cfu/g (data not shown). Enterobacteria were equally prevalent in foals with diarrhoea and in foals those not afflicted (data not shown). No significant treatment effect was observed for enterobacteria.

In the first faeces of the foals after meconium, *Clostridium perfringens* was detectable in 50–71% of the samples (Table 5). In the placebo group, *C. perfringens* was detectable in 100% of the foals on day 3. Among all groups, the maximum count was 6.00×10^6 cfu/g on day 3. *C. perfringens* was found in 75% of the mare samples (measured at the time of birth) and ranged from 1.00×10^3 to 2.50×10^5 cfu/g (data not shown). *Clostridium perfringens* was equally prevalent in foals with or without

Table 2 Lactobacilli in faeces (cfu/g) of the foals from days 1 to 58 of life in placebo, low dosage (LD), and high dosage (HD) groups and for all foals, data expressed as numbers, median, 25 and 75% quartile, time p = 0.002, treatment p = 0.522

Group	Measure	Day of foal's life							
		1	3	9	16	23	30	44	58
Placebo	25% quartile	2.8×10^4	2.7×10^6	3.2×10^6	2.1×10^6	2.9×10^5	5.0×10^5	4.3×10^5	4.1×10^4
	Median	3.4×10^4	1.7×10^7	2.5×10^7	2.0×10^7	1.4×10^6	1.0×10^6	1.9×10^6	2.2×10^5
	75% quartile	4.0×10^5	8.3×10^7	4.0×10^7	3.0×10^7	5.0×10^6	2.5×10^6	2.6×10^6	3.3×10^5
LD	25% quartile	1.9×10^4	n.d.	8.2×10^6	3.6×10^6	2.5×10^5	2.8×10^5	3.4×10^5	2.7×10^5
	Median	4.0×10^5	n.d.	4.5×10^7	5.5×10^6	5.4×10^5	3.9×10^5	4.0×10^5	6.0×10^5
	75% quartile	2.0×10^6	n.d.	6.7×10^7	1.9×10^7	2.9×10^6	4.2×10^5	5.4×10^5	9.7×10^5
HD	25% quartile	7.0×10^3	2.3×10^6	4.7×10^6	4.2×10^6	2.7×10^5	3.1×10^5	1.4×10^5	1.5×10^5
	Median	2.5×10^4	3.7×10^6	2.1×10^7	1.5×10^7	1.6×10^6	2.7×10^6	4.3×10^5	4.9×10^5
	75% quartile	2.3×10^6	3.8×10^7	4.6×10^7	4.6×10^7	1.3×10^7	7.1×10^6	7.3×10^5	4.4×10^6
Total	25% quartile	1.6×10^4	2.3×10^6	3.5×10^6	3.2×10^6	1.9×10^5	2.5×10^5	2.7×10^5	1.9×10^5
	Median	3.4×10^4	3.7×10^6	2.3×10^7	1.7×10^6	1.3×10^6	6.0×10^5	5.0×10^5	3.2×10^5
	75% quartile	2.2×10^6	4.5×10^7	5.0×10^7	2.8×10^7	5.0×10^6	2.9×10^6	1.2×10^6	1.0×10^6

n.d.: non-determinable, total: over all treatments.

diarrhoea (data not shown). Supplementation with *B. cereus* var. *toyoi* had no significant effect on *C. perfringens*.

Occasionally yeasts were found in samples of the mares (2 out of 24 samples) and the foals (17 out of 191 samples, data not shown).

Discussion

The present study was performed on a studfarm under typical field conditions. To minimize effects related to husbandry, feeding, and season, our study took place at one thoroughbred farm, within one foaling period from February to May. According to Lahrssen and Zentek [18] such a study design is important when working with a limited number of animals. Probiotic dosing and treatment period were in accordance with studies by Jeroch et al. [19], Jadamus et al. [20], and Vilà et al. [15].

Unfortunately some foals were treated with antibiotics during a severe period of illness which may have an impact on the subsequent microbial profile in faeces.

Bacterial microflora in faeces was used as an indication of the effects of *B. cereus* var. *toyoi* on the intestinal

Table 3 Detection rate (> 10^3 cfu/g,%) of enterococci in faeces of the foals from days 1 to 58 of life in placebo, low dosage (LD), and high dosage (HD) groups and for all foals, data expressed in %, treatment p > 0.05

Group	Day of foal's life							
	1	3	9	16	23	30	44	58
Placebo	66,7%	100.0%	85.7%	50.0%	50.0%	25.0%	25.0%	12.5%
LD	57.1%	n.d.	85.7%	85.7%	42.9%	42.9%	42.9%	14.3%
HD	60.0%	83.3%	100.0%	60.0%	40.0%	40.0%	40.0%	30.0%
Total	61.1%	90.0%	91.7%	64.0%	44.0%	36.0%	36.0%	20.0%

n.d.: non-determinable, total: over all treatments.

health of foals. Although faeces might have some limitations for describing the gut ecosystem, by comparing microflora and the digestion process in the colon with faeces in fistulated horses Julliand and Goachet [21] showed that the faecal ecosystem is an appropriate marker of intestinal changes appearing in the colon ecosystem.

Culture-plate methods were used to access bacterial microflora in the faeces of the foals to establish basic knowledge. For following studies culture-dependent methods should be extended by PCR methods to improve knowledge about diversity of genes.

In our study, diarrhoea did not lead to changes in normal foal behaviour. Foals remained bright and alert and continued to nurse. Clinical parameters including heart and respiratory rate, body temperature, and body weight were in the proper physiological range. We conclude that diarrhoea in foals between days 6 and 16 of the foal's life is not primarily pathogen related. During this period, we observed diarrhoea when orange-brownish faeces changed to green, soft faeces. These changes in faeces colour might mark the transition from only digestion of milk to increasing digestion of solid nutrients like crude fibre. In that context, hemicellulose and cellulose could be responsible for a higher water-binding capacity and a reduction of intestinal passage. As a result, adsorptive and secretory intestinal processes are influenced and free water in the colon could simulate lower dry matter content in faeces of the foals. Another reason for the reduction of dry matter content in faeces could be osmotically-acting metabolites of bacterial digestion of crude fibre.

Meconium has been reported to be free of bacteria [22] and no bacterial PCR products were obtained from

Table 4 Detection rate (> 10^3 cfu/g,%) of enterobacteria in faeces of the from days 1 to 58 of life in placebo, low dosage (LD), and high dosage (HD) groups and for all foals, data expressed in %, treatment p > 0.05

Group	Day of foal's life							
	1	3	9	16	23	30	44	58
Placebo	0%	25.0%	14.3%	25.0%	25.0%	37.5%	37.5%	50.0%
LD	28.6%	n.d.	42.9%	42.9%	42.9%	57.1%	28.6%	57.1%
HD	20.0%	16.7%	60.0%	40.0%	40.0%	30.0%	40.0%	20.0%
Total	16.7%	20.0%	36.0%	36.0%	40.0%	40.0%	36.0%	40.0%

n.d.: non-determinable, total: over all treatments.

meconium samples [11], which confirmed that the gastrointestinal tract of a foetus is sterile [23]. In mares, bacterial flora remained largely stable from 14 days before until 42 days after foaling, whereas the presence of bacterial species and intensity of bacterial growth changed over time in foals [2]. These results were confirmed in our study, as aerobic and anaerobic bacteria (data not shown), but also lactobacilli, enterococci and *C. perfringens* counts in the faeces of the foals increased after birth until day 3 or day 9. Foals start to consume forages and concentrates very early in life. As a result, the intestinal microflora is adapting rapidly to improve digestion of the feed. In foals, there may be great genetic selective pressure for early colonisation of microflora to avoid acidic stomach conditions and to occupy a more distal region (post-gastric) than would be the case in calves or lambs [24]. By day 58 of a foal's life, aerobic and anaerobic bacteria, enterobacteria, lactobacilli, and enterococci had decreased to the levels in the faeces of mares (measured at the time of birth). These changes seemed to be related to the stabilisation of microflora by increasing fibre intake and digestion processes within the first 2 months of the foal's life.

Bacillus cereus var. *toyoi* did not have any effects on the health status of the foals. There is a great diversity of bacteriophages, bacteria, fungi, and protozoa that might have an unselective entry to the gastrointestinal tract of the foals. Therefore, even if probiotic bacteria survive the acidic conditions after day 2 of life, they will experience heavy competition within the very rapidly developing intestinal microflora of foals.

Probiotic supplementation with *Lactobacillus pentosus* WE7 was significantly associated with development of signs of depression, anorexia, and colic in foals [12]. Also, supplementation with *Lactobacillus rhamnosus* and *Enterococcus faecium* led to increased diarrhoea in foals [11]. In contrast, we found that supplementation with *B. cereus* var. *toyoi* had no effect on the growth and health parameters in foals kept under high-quality standard husbandry.

Conclusions

Supplementation with *B. cereus* var. *toyoi* had no effect on health status or the intestinal microflora in suckling foals. Diarrhoea occurred in up to 90% of the foals for at least one 1 day between days 8 and 16 of life. Despite this, foals remained bright and alert and continued to nurse. Diarrhoea might be a part of the normal physiological development of the intestinal microflora. Competition with diverse, rapidly colonizing intestinal microflora seems to suppress *B. cereus* var. *toyoi* and its possible effects.

Methods
Animals
The project (V54-19c20/15-V/04) was approved by the Ethics Committee for Animal Rights Protection of the District government in Darmstadt, in accordance with German legislation for animal rights and welfare.

A total of 25 mares and their foals with one thoroughbred stud were included in the study. The mares had been stabled at least 2 months before foaling at the stud farm. Mares were kept in separate stalls with straw beddings and were turned out daily on sand paddocks for several hours every day. They were fed ad libitum haylage or hay and 2–3 kg of concentrates per day. Mares had free access to fresh water at all times. Foals were born between February and May 2011. Twenty-two foals first came into contact with the mares' udder within the first hour of life, and 1 foal required 90 min. (In the other two mares, foaling was not observed.) Mares were dewormed with ivermectin immediately after foaling and 2–3 months post partum. After foaling, mares were fed ad libitum hay, 4–5 kg of alfalfa hay, and 2–3 kg of a complement feed per day (Equilac Zuchtstutenfutter Spezial Etzean; Additional file 1: Table S1). Passive transfer of antibodies was controlled with SNAP Foal IgG Test (Idexx Laboratories, Westbrook, Maine, USA). Twenty-four of the 25 foals had immunoglobulin levels of > 800 mg/dL at 12 h of age.

Table 5 Detection rate (> 10^3 cfu/g,%) of *Clostridium perfringens* in faeces of the foals from days 1 to 58 of life in placebo, low dosage (LD), and high dosage (HD) groups and for all, foals, data expressed in %, treatment p > 0.05

Group	Day of foal's life							
	1	3	9	16	23	30	44	58
Placebo	50.0%	100%	42.9%	25.0%	12.5%	0%	0%	0%
LD	71.4%	n.d.	71.4%	71.4%	28.6%	14.3%	14.3%	28.6%
HD	60.0%	66.7%	90.0%	60.0%	10.0%	0%	0%	0%
Total	61.1%	80.0%	70.8%	52.0%	16.0%	4.0%	4.0%	8.0%

n.d.: non-determinable, total: over all treatments.

Feeding

In the first weeks of life foals had access to the mare's feed. From day 2 of the foal's life, the mare and foal were turned out on sand paddocks twice a day for 1–2 h. From day 7 to 14, two mares and foals had access to pasture twice a day for 2 to 4 h. At this time, no additional alfalfa hay was fed to the mares. From 4 to 8 weeks, groups of mares and foals were turned out on pasture and foals were fed complement feed for foals (1.7–2.5 kg per foal; Fohlenfutter Spezial Etzean; Additional file 1: Table S1) in a separate area. Once or twice a week foals were given 50 mL of a mineral mixture (Meganutril junior; Additional file 1: Table S1).

Deworming and treatments

All foals received pyrantel in week 2 of life, ivermectin in week 8, and pyrantel in month 4. Five foals were treated for an omphalic inflammation with cefquinome or trimethoprim-sulfadimethoxine at day 2–4 or at day 24–26 of foals life, two foals were treated for congenital neuromyodysplasia with oxytetracycline at day 2–4 of foals life and three foals were treated because of high-grade diarrhoea with cefquinome or trimethoprim-sulfadimethoxine at day 24–26 of foals life.

Probiotic and administration protocol

Bacillus cereus var. *toyoi* was provided as an odourless, white to greyish-brown dry powder supplemented with 1.0×10^{10} viable spores of *B. cereus* var. *toyoi* per gram. The viability was confirmed at the beginning of the study by use of the microbiological spread plate method.

Foals were randomly allocated to three groups and received their respective placebo or supplement once a day orally for 58 days, starting on the first day of life. Eight foals were given 10 mL of isotonic saline solution (placebo), seven foals received 5.0×10^{8} cfu of *B. cereus* var. *toyoi* (low dosage, LD), and ten foals were given 2.0×10^{9} cfu of *B. cereus* var. *toyoi* (high dosage, HD).

Examinations and faeces samples

Behaviour, appetite, heart and respiratory rates, rectal temperature, and body weights were monitored during the treatment period (day 1 to 58 of life) and monthly from age 3 to 5 months. Blood work was done four times in month 1 and at the end of month 2. The time schedule of the study is given in Table 6.

Within the first day of life, on days 9, 16, 23, 30, 44, and 58, and on the first day of diarrhoea faecal samples were taken from the rectum or by the use of a collection bag. Faeces were visually classified by a faeces score (Table 7), and faeces dry matter content was determined after oven-drying (103°C) to constant mass.

Table 6 Time schedule of the study

Measure	Day of foal's life												Month of foal's life		
	1	4	6	9*	10	12	14	16	23	30	44	58	3	4	5
Health status	X	X	X	X	X	X	X	X	X	X	X	X	X	X	X
Body weight	X		X					X	X	X	X	X	X	X	X
Faeces	X		X					X	X	X	X	X			
Blood	X		X					X		X		X			

*Additional measurements and sampling were done on the first day of diarrhoea.

Mares' faeces were taken from the rectum immediately after foaling. Faeces samples were frozen at –18°C until analysis.

Haematology and serum chemistry analysis

Serum and EDTA blood was subjected to haematology and serum chemistry determination. The parameters of red blood count and differential leukocyte count were determined photometric, optical or calculated using an ADVIA®120 haematology system (Fa. Bayer Vital GmbH, Fernwald, Germany).

Serum-IgG was determined quantitatively with a competitive ELISA as previously described by Schroedl et al. [25]. Thereby serum-IgG in the samples and equine IgG conjugated to peroxidase (purity according to SDS-PAGE > 90%) competed for antibodies against equine IgG. After washing and the addition of a chromogenic substrate quantity of peroxidase was optically measurable at 405 nm (reference wavelength 492 nm). Equine reference serum was used as standard. Out of the measuring data IgG concentration was calculated with Table Curve 2D v4 (Systat Software Inc, Chicago, USA). Limit of detection with a serum dilution factor of 4000 was 0.15 g/l. The level of specificity was at 100%.

Table 7 Faeces score

Score	Faeces quality
0	Orange-brownish first faeces after meconium
1	Dry balled
2	Soft balled, formed
3	Not formed, soft
4	Pasty
5	Mushy
6	Inhomogeneous: structured and watery part
7	Mucous like
8	Green diarrhoea
9	Yellow diarrhoea

Bacterial analysis

Faecal specimens (0.5 g in 4.5 mL phosphate buffered saline) were serially diluted in phosphate buffered saline for quantitative bacterial investigations. Dilutions were tested for total aerobic cell numbers developing on sheep blood agar (Oxoid, Germany), gram negative cell numbers on Gassner agar (SIFIN, Berlin), Enterococci on Citrate azide tween carbonate agar (CATC agar, SIFIN, Berlin), total anaerobe cell numbers on sheep blood agar (OXOID, Germany), Lactobacilli on deMan, Rogosa and Sharpe Lactobacillus agar (MRSA agar, SIFIN, Berlin), Bacteroides spp. on sheep blood agar supplemented with vitamin K, Clostridium perfringens on sheep blood agar containing polymyxin B and neomycin, and yeasts and fungi on Sabouraud agar (SIFIN, Berlin). The total aerobic cell numbers, gram negative cell numbers and enterococci were cultured aerobically at 37 _C for 24 h. The anaerobic bacteria were cultured at 37 _C for 48 h in anaerobic chamber (MACS anaerobic workstation, Don Whitley Scientific limited, England). Yeasts and fungi were cultured aerobically at 37 _C for 5 days. The different isolated strains were identified based on their characteristic colony- and micromorphology and by their biochemical characteristics according to Bisping and Amtsberg [26] and finally analyzed with the use of matrix-assisted laser desorption/ionization time of flight (MALDI-TOF) as described by Shehata et al. [27].

Statistical analysis

Data are expressed as median, 25% quartile, and 75% quartile. Data analysis was performed by the Statistica software program (StatSoft, Hamburg, Germany). The Shapiro-Wilk test was used to assess data for normality. Data were not normally distributed. Non-parametric tests (Kruskal-Wallis ANOVA) were used to compare the effects of time and diet. Pearson's chi-squared test was used to compare the frequency of foals with diarrhoea between treatments.

Statistical significance was accepted at $P < 0.05$.

Additional file

> **Additional file 1: Table S1.** Nutrient composition of the feedstuffs provided to the foals and mares during experimental period (expressed in %).

Abbreviations

B. cereus var. *toyoi*: Bacillus cereus var. toyoi; *C. perfringens*: Clostridium perfringens; HD: High dosage (5.0 × 10^8 cfu of *B. cereus* var. *toyoi*); LD: Low dosage (2.0 × 10^9 cfu of *B. cereus* var. *toyoi*).

Competing interests

Rubinum Animal Health supplied *Bacillus cereus* var. *toyoi*, the probiotic used in this study. Rubinum Animal Health played no role in the study design or in the collection, analysis, and interpretation of data, nor in the decision to submit the manuscript for publication. None of the authors has any financial or personal relationships that could inappropriately influence or bias the content of the paper.

Authors' contributions

JJ has made substantial contributions to acquisition, analysis and interpretation of data, helped to perform the statistical analysis and drafted the manuscript. KR has made contributions to conception of the study and helped to acquire data. WS has revised the manuscript critically for important intellectual content and has given final approval of the version to be published. NA carried out the bacterial analysis. IV conceived the study, and participated in its design and coordination, performed the statistical analysis and helped to draft the manuscript. All authors read and approved the final manuscript.

Acknowledgements

The authors are grateful to the team at Etzean Stud. We wish to thank Jana Tietke for her technical assistance. We acknowledge support from the German Research Foundation (DFG) and the Leipzig University within the programme of Open Access Publishing.

Author details

[1]Institute of Animal Nutrition, Nutrition Diseases and Dietetics, Faculty of Veterinary Medicine, University of Leipzig, Leipzig, Germany. [2]Pferdeklinik Großostheim, Großostheim, Germany. [3]Institute of Bacteriology and Mycology, Faculty of Veterinary Medicine, University of Leipzig, Leipzig, Germany. [4]Present address: Tierklinik Teisendorf, Teisendorf, Germany.

References

1. Masri MD, Merritt AM, Gronwall R, Burrows CF. Faecal composition in foal heat diarrhoea. Equine Vet J. 1986;18:301–6.
2. Kuhl J, Winterhoff N, Wulf M, Schweigert FJ, Schwendenwein I, Bruckmaier RM, et al. Changes in faecal bacteria and metabolic parameters in foals during the first six weeks of life. Vet Microbiol. 2011;151:321–8.
3. Magdesian KG. Neonatal foal diarrhea. Vet Clin North Am Equine Pract. 2005;21:295–312.
4. Knottenbelt DC, Holdstock N, Madigan JE. Diarrhö. In: Knottenbelt DC, editor. Neonatologie der Pferde. 1st ed. München: Elsevier, Urban & Fischer, München; 2007. p. 265–88.
5. Dunkel B. Infectious foal diarrhoea: pathophysiology, prevalence and diagnosis. Equine Vet Educ. 2004;16(2):94–101.
6. Velde K, Kolm G. Entzündlich und funktionell bedingte Störungen des Darms. In: Fey K, Kolm G, editors. Fohlenmedizin. 1st ed. Stuttgart: Enke; 2011. p. 327–37.
7. Julliand V, De Vaux A, Villard L, Richard Y. Preliminary studies on the bacterial flora of faeces taken from foals, from birth to twelve weeks: effects of the oral administration of a commercial colostrum replacer. Pferdeheilkunde. 1996;12:209–12.
8. Sadet-Bourgeteau S, Julliand V. Equine microbial gastro-intestinal health. In: Ellis AD, Longland AC, Coenen M, Miraglia N, editors. The Impact of Nutrition on the Health and Welfare of Horses, EAAP Publications, vol. 128. Cirencester: Wageningen Academic Publishers; 2010. p. 161–82.
9. FAO, WHO. Report of a joint FAO/WHO expert consultation on evaluation of health and nutritional properties of probiotics in food including powder milk with live lactic acid bacteria. In: Health and Nutritional Properties of Probiotics in Food Including Powder Milk with Live Lactic Acid Bacteria. 2001. ftp://ftp.fao.org/docrep/fao/009/a0512e/a0512e00.pdf.
10. Yuyama T, Yusa S, Takai S, Tsubaki S, Kado Y, Morotomi M. Evaluation of a host-specific *Lactobacillus* probiotic in neonatal foals. Int J Appl Res Vet Med. 2004;2:26–33.
11. Günther E, Ströbel C, Romanowski K, Urubschurov V, Büsing K, Souffrant W, et al. Effects of probiotic strains of *Enterococcus faecium* and *Lactobacillus rhamnosus* on diarrhoea patterns and the faecal microbiome of sucking foals. In: Szymeczko R, Iben C, Burlikowska K, Sitkowska B, editors. Proceedings of the16th Congress of the European Society of Veterinary and Comparative Nutrition: 13–15 September 2012; Bydgoszcz. Multiskop Sp: Z o.o; 2012. p. 79.
12. Weese JS, Rousseau J. Evaluation of *Lactobacillus pentosus* WE7 for prevention of diarrhea in neonatal foals. J Am Vet Med Assoc. 2005;226:2031–4.
13. Erhard MH, Leuzinger K, Stangassinger M. Untersuchungen zur prophylaktischen Wirkung der Verfütterung eines Probiotikums und von

erregerspezifischen Kolostrum- und Dotterantikörpern bei neugeborenen Kälbern. J Anim Physiol Anim Nutr. 2000;84:85–94.

14. Jadamus A, Vahjen W, Simon O. Growth behavior of a spore forming probiotic strain in the gastrointestinal tract of broiler chicken and piglets. Arch Anim Nutr. 2001;54:1–17.

15. Vilà B, Fontgibell A, Badiola I, Esteve-Garcia E, Jiménez G, Castillo M, et al. Reduction of Salmonella enterica var. enteritidis colonization and invasion by Bacillus cereus var. toyoi inclusion in poultry feeds. Poult Sci. 2009;88:975–9.

16. Matusevicius P, Bartkeviciute Z, Cernauskenie J, Kozlowski K, Jeroch H. Effect of probiotic preparation "Toyocerin" and phytogenic preparation "Cuxarom Spicemaster" in growing rabbits. Eur Poult Sci. 2011;75(1):67–71.

17. Baum B, Liebler-Tenorio EM, Enß ML, Pohlenz JF, Breves G. Saccharomyces boulardii and Bacillus cereus var. toyoi influence the morphology and the mucins of the intestine of pigs. Z Gastroenterol. 2002;40:277–84.

18. Lahrssen M, Zentek J. Wirksamkeit von probiotischen Mikroorganismen als Futterzusatzstoff: Leitlinien zur Prüfung der Wirksamkeit bei den Tierkategorien Hund, Katze und Pferd. Tierarztl Wochenschr. 2002;109(1):22–5.

19. Jeroch H, Strobel E, Zachmann R. Untersuchungen zur Wirksamkeit des Probiotikums Bacillus cereus toyoi in der Putenmast. Vetarinarija Ir Zootechnika. 2004;28(50):57–60.

20. Jadamus A, Vahjen W, Schäfer K, Simon O. Influence of the probiotic strain Bacillus cereus var. toyoi on the development of enterobacterial growth and on selected parameters of bacterial metabolism in digesta samples of piglets. J Anim Physiol Nutr. 2002;86:42–54.

21. Julliand V, Goachet AG. Fecal microflora as a marker of cecal or colonic microflora in horses. In: Proceedings of the19th Equine Science Symposium: 31 May- 3 June. Tucson; 2005. p. 140–1.

22. Sakaitani Y, Yuki N, Nakajima F, Nakanishi S, Tanaka H, Tanaka R, et al. Colonization of intestinal microflora in newborn foals. J Intestinal Microbiol. 1999;13:9–14.

23. Mackie RI, Sghir A, Gaskins HR. Developmental microbial ecology of the neonatal gastrointestinal tract. Am J Clin Nutr. 1999;69:1035S–45.

24. Egan CE, Snelling TJ, Mc-Ewan NR. The onset of ciliate populations in newborn foals. Acta Protozool. 2010;49:145–7.

25. Schroedl W, Jaekel L, Krueger M. C-reactive protein and antibacterial activity in blood plasma of colostrum-fed calves and the effect of lactulose. J Dairy Sci. 2003;8:3313–20.

26. Bisping W, Amtsberg G. Colour Atlas for the Diagnosis of Bacterial Pathogens in Animals. Verlag Berlin: Paul Parey; 1988.

27. Shehata A, Schrödl W, Neuhaus J, Krüger M. Antagonistic effect of different bacteria on Clostridium botulinum types A, B, D and E in vitro. Vet Rec. 2013;172:47.

9

Establishment of a mouse model to express bovine *CD14* short hairpin RNA

Xiangping Li[1,3]*, Shihai Huang[2], Yanping Ren[1,3], Meng Wang[1,3], Chao Kang[2], Liangliang Xie[1,3] and Deshun Shi[1,3]*

Abstract

Background: Cluster of differentiation 14 (CD14) functions as a co-receptor for Toll-like receptor (TLR)-4 and myeloid differentiation factor (MD)-2 in detecting bacterial lipopolysaccharide. Together, these complexes promote the phagocytosis and digestion of Gram-negative bacteria, and initiate immune responses. To date, much of our understanding of CD14 function during Gram-negative bacterial inflammation comes from studies on mouse knockout models and cell transfection. To identify the effect of *CD14* knockdown in this process in large livestock animals, we established a mouse model expressing bovine *CD14* short hairpin (sh) RNA. shRNA fragments targeting bovine *CD14* were screened by co-transfection in HEK 293 cells, and the most effective *CD14* shRNA fragment was cloned into the eukaryotic expression vector pSilencer4.1-CD14 shRNA-IRES (internal ribosome entry site) and transferred into mouse zygotes by pronuclear microinjection to obtain transgenic mice. Expression of the enhanced green fluorescent protein (EGFP) reporter and genes related to the TLR4 signaling pathway was detected by immunohistochemistry (IHC) and quantitative polymerase chain reaction (PCR), respectively.

Results: One effective shRNA fragment (shRNA-674) targeting bovine *CD14* was obtained, the sequence of which was shown to be conserved between cows, buffalos, sheep, and humans. Thirty-seven founder pups were obtained by pronuclear microinjection, of which three were positive for the transgene. In the F_1 generation, 11 of 33 mice (33%) were positive for the transgene as detected by PCR. IHC analysis detected exogenous EGFP expression in the liver, kidney, and spleen of transgenic F_1 mice, indicating that they were chimeric. The expression of endogenous *CD14* mRNA in the heart, liver, spleen, lung, and kidney of transgenic F_1 mice was decreased 8-, 3-, 19.5-, 6-, and 11-fold, respectively. The expression patterns of endogenous *MD-2*, *TLR4*, interleukin-6 and tumor necrosis factor-α genes in transgenic mice also varied.

Conclusions: This study confirms that transgenic mice expressing bovine *CD14* shRNA can be generated by pronuclear microinjection, and demonstrates inhibited endogenous mouse *CD14* expression that alters gene expression related to the TLR4 signaling pathway.

Keywords: Bovine *CD14*, shRNA, Mouse model, TLR4, Gene expression

Background

CD14 is a 55 kDa glycoprotein expressed mainly on the surface of monocytes, macrophages, and granulocytes [1], which plays a crucial role in the inflammatory response to lipopolysaccharide (LPS) [2-4]. Currently, LPS-induced cellular activation is thought to occur through signal complexes comprised of CD14 and either myeloid differentiation factor (MD)-2 or Toll-like receptor (TLR) 4 [5-7]. LPS binding to these complexes facilitates activation of the TLR4/nuclear factor (NF)-κB inflammatory pathway, ultimately leading to the production of proatherogenic cytokines including tumor necrosis factor alpha (TNF-α), interleukin-6 (IL-6), and IL-1 [8-11].

Strategies aimed at inhibiting the expression of TLR4 complex genes have been used to analyze their contribution to inflammatory reactions [12-14]. In addition to inhibiting TLR4 expression, many CD14-deficient mice have also been established by *CD14* knockout strategies [15-17]. When infected by live Gram-negative bacteria or LPS, CD14-deficient mice demonstrate reduced bacteremia and

* Correspondence: xiangpingli@163.com; ardsshi@163.com
[1]State Key Laboratory of Subtropical Bioresource Conservation and Utilization at Guangxi University, Nanning, Guangxi, China
[3]Guangxi High Education Key Laboratory for Animal Reproduction and Biotechnology, Guangxi University, Nanning 530004, China
Full list of author information is available at the end of the article

systemic inflammation [18]. Thus, inhibiting signals through CD14 may limit the release of a broad range of inflammatory mediators, and prevent rapid bacterial dissemination following infection by Gram-negative bacteria [1,19-22].

Numerous approaches using monoclonal antibodies, small molecule antagonists, and RNA interference have demonstrated that inhibiting LPS signals through lipopolysaccharide-binding protein, CD14, MD-2, and TLR4 reduce the release of inflammatory cytokines [20,23-26]. For instance, small interfering (si) RNA targeting CD14 in the mouse cell line RAW264.7 was found to inhibit the release of TNF-α, macrophage inflammatory protein-2, IL-6, and the production of nitric oxide following exposure to LPS [27]. Thus far, most of our understanding about the role of CD14 during Gram-negative bacterial inflammation comes from studies of mouse knockout models or mouse and human immune cells. However, because of the serious harm caused by bacterial infections such as mastitis and Brucella in large livestock animals and huge resultant losses to the breeding industry, it is essential to establish knockout models of such animals to investigate the CD14 role in LPS-induced inflammation. This would also be of benefit in the development of a practical and effective measure to prevent bacterial infection in livestock. Based on our previous discovery of the effect of CD14 down-regulation in buffalo monocytes/macrophages [28], the present study aimed to establish a transgenic mouse model to express bovine CD14 short hairpin (sh) RNA, and to determine the effect of endogenous mouse CD14 down-regulation on gene expression of the mouse TLR4 signaling pathway.

Results
Screening of shRNA sequences targeting bovine CD14
Given the importance of CD14 in LPS signaling, we first sought to screen shRNA sequences for their ability to inhibit bovine CD14 expression in vitro. Using ABI siRNA online software (http://www.ambion.com), three different sites of the bovine CD14 mRNA sequence (GenBank Accession No. NM_174008.1) were used to design three CD14 shRNA sequences (shRNA-279, –326, and –674). CD14 shRNA lentiviral expression vectors with human U6 promoters were constructed (pSicoR-CD14 shRNA-279/326/674), and lentiviral particles were produced using the calcium-phosphate method, with titers reaching 1×10^7 (data not shown). Lentiviral particles expressing bovine CD14 shRNA were used to infect HEK 293 cells expressing CD14 at a multiplicity of infection (MOI) of 100, using a non-infected cell line as blank control, the scrambled shRNA as negative control. The infected cells were harvested 72 h after infection and total RNA was extracted for quantitative reverse-transcription polymerase chain reaction (qRT-PCR) analyses. As expected, cells infected with the shRNA-negative control showed no reduction in CD14 expression (Figure 1A). Compared

with scrambled shRNA-1864, shRNA-279 and shRNA-326 fragments were also unable to reduce bovine CD14 expression. However, the shRNA-674 fragment significantly inhibited CD14 mRNA expression in vitro ($p < 0.01$) (Figure 1A). shRNA-674 nucleotides were highly conserved between cows, sheep, buffalos, and humans, indicating that this shRNA fragment could potentially be used in related research of multiple species.

To confirm if the shRNA-674 fragment also reduced expression of the CD14 protein, we performed western blot analysis. At two different MOIs, the intracellular expression of shRNA-674 completely abolished CD14 protein expression (Figure 1B), which was consistent with RT-PCR analysis.

shRNA transgenic mice demonstrated reduced CD14 expression
We next determined the effects of the shRNA-674 fragment on CD14 expression in vivo. To avoid the biological safety problems of lentiviruses, the shRNA-674 fragment was inserted into the eukaryotic shRNA expression vector pSilencer™4.1-CMV neo. Internal ribosome entry site (IRES) elements were then ligated with the vector to construct the pSilencer4.1-CD14 shRNA-674-IRES plasmid (Figure 1). This plasmid was linearized with Nhe I digestion and microinjected into the pronucleus of fertilized eggs from FVB mice to create CD14 shRNA transgenic mice. After transferring two-cell stage embryos into pseudo-pregnant females, a total of 37 founder pups were obtained. Transgene integration in F_0 offspring was analyzed by amplifying EGFP and neo genes that were both amplified in three founder mice (8.1%): one male (11[#]) and two females (22[#], 32[#]) that were regarded as transgenic. Within the F_1 generation (wild-type mouse with transgenic F_0 mouse cross), 33 mice were born, of which 11 were found to be transgenic (33.3%; data not shown). In the 11 transgenic F1 mice, 3 was offspring of 11[#] F0 mouse, 5 and 3 were offspring of 22[#] and 32[#] mouse respectively. Three of the 33 F_1 mice were selected for Southern blot analysis to confirm the PCR data. Two (lane2, 4, offspring of 22[#], 32[#] respectively) were transgenic while the third was not (lane3, offspring of 11[#]) (Figure 1E). These findings were consistent with PCR results (data not shown).

To further characterize the transgene insertion, organs of F_1 transgenic mice (offspring of 22[#]) were analyzed for eGFP expression by confocal microscopy. This protein was shown to be expressed in the liver, kidney, and spleen tissue of all transgenic mice, with the highest expression detected in the spleen. However, eGFP expression was absent from heart and lung tissues. The expression pattern was similar in both male and female mice (Figure 2). Together these data demonstrated that the transgenic mice were chimeric.

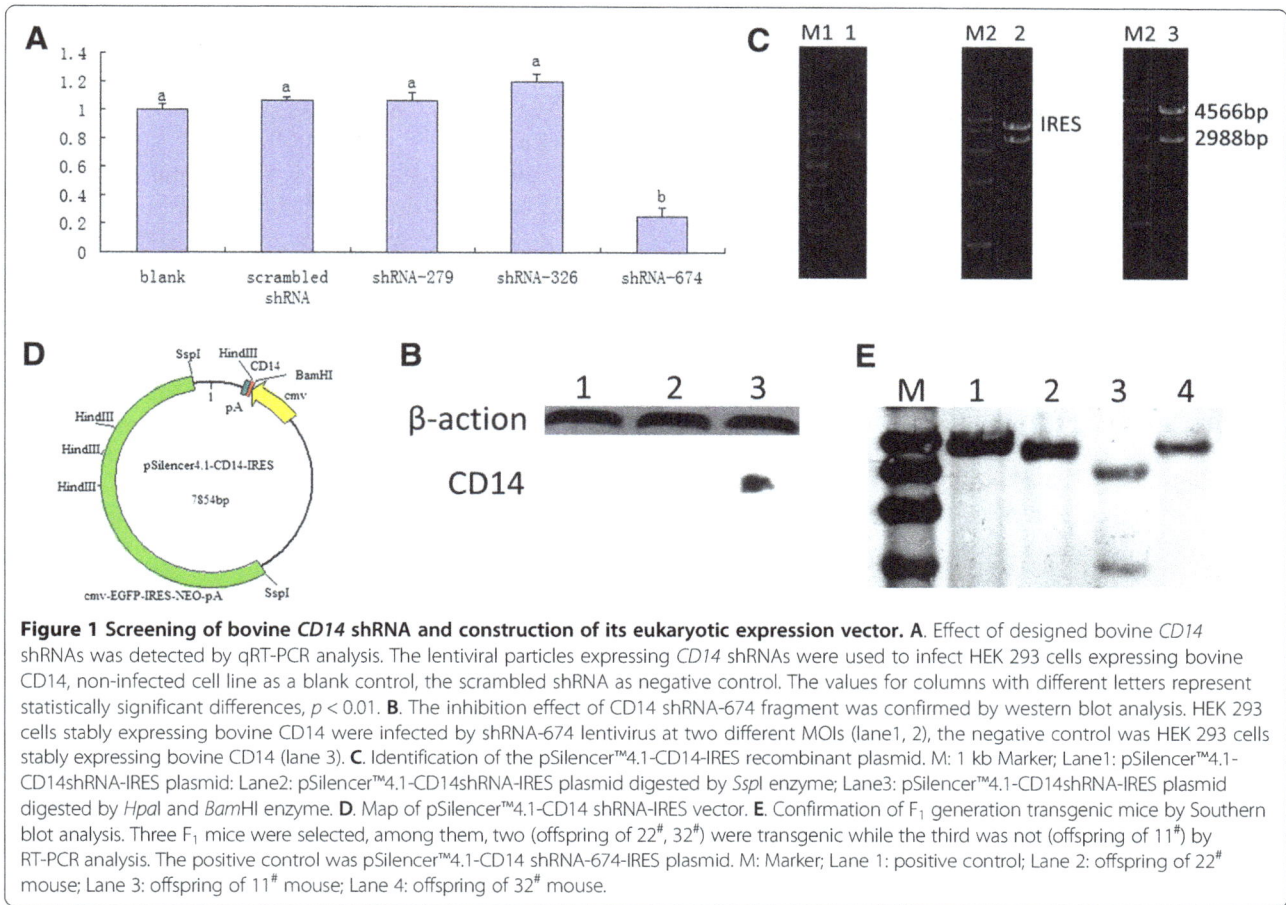

Figure 1 Screening of bovine *CD14* shRNA and construction of its eukaryotic expression vector. A. Effect of designed bovine *CD14* shRNAs was detected by qRT-PCR analysis. The lentiviral particles expressing *CD14* shRNAs were used to infect HEK 293 cells expressing bovine CD14, non-infected cell line as a blank control, the scrambled shRNA as negative control. The values for columns with different letters represent statistically significant differences, $p < 0.01$. **B**. The inhibition effect of CD14 shRNA-674 fragment was confirmed by western blot analysis. HEK 293 cells stably expressing bovine CD14 were infected by shRNA-674 lentivirus at two different MOIs (lane1, 2), the negative control was HEK 293 cells stably expressing bovine CD14 (lane 3). **C**. Identification of the pSilencer™4.1-CD14-IRES recombinant plasmid. M: 1 kb Marker; Lane1: pSilencer™4.1-CD14shRNA-IRES plasmid: Lane2: pSilencer™4.1-CD14shRNA-IRES plasmid digested by *Ssp*I enzyme; Lane3: pSilencer™4.1-CD14shRNA-IRES plasmid digested by *Hpa*I and *Bam*HI enzyme. **D**. Map of pSilencer™4.1-CD14 shRNA-IRES vector. **E**. Confirmation of F_1 generation transgenic mice by Southern blot analysis. Three F_1 mice were selected, among them, two (offspring of 22[#], 32[#]) were transgenic while the third was not (offspring of 11[#]) by RT-PCR analysis. The positive control was pSilencer™4.1-CD14 shRNA-674-IRES plasmid. M: Marker; Lane 1: positive control; Lane 2: offspring of 22[#] mouse; Lane 3: offspring of 11[#] mouse; Lane 4: offspring of 32[#] mouse.

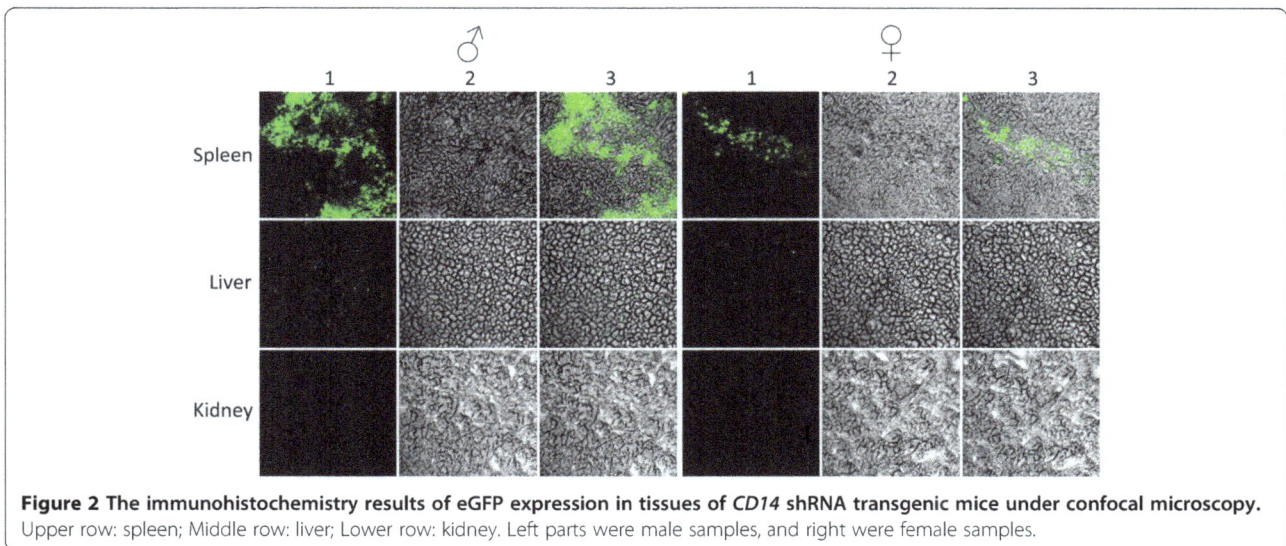

Figure 2 The immunohistochemistry results of eGFP expression in tissues of *CD14* shRNA transgenic mice under confocal microscopy. Upper row: spleen; Middle row: liver; Lower row: kidney. Left parts were male samples, and right were female samples.

To explore if the transferred shRNA fragment affected the expression of endogenous *CD14* mRNA *in vivo*, we used qRT-PCR to analyze the relative expression of *CD14* expression in tissues of F_1 transgenic mice (offspring of $22^{\#}$). Compared with non-transgenic mouse RNA samples, the expression of endogenous *CD14* mRNA in the heart, liver, spleen, lung, and kidney tissues of transgenic mice was reduced 8-, 3-, 19.5-, 6-, and 11 fold, respectively (Figure 3). Thus, the expression of endogenous *CD14* mRNA was inhibited in transgenic mice.

We next examined the expression pattern of genes in the TLR4 signaling pathway. *TLR4* demonstrated a significantly increased expression level in the heart and liver of *CD14* shRNA transgenic mice compared with wild-type mice ($p < 0.05$), although there were no significant differences in expression in the spleen, lung, or kidney between transgenic and wild-type mice. *MD-2*, *TNF-α*, and *IL-6* transcripts showed similar expression patterns, except for the kidney, with significantly increased expression in the heart, liver, and lung ($p < 0.05$), and significantly lower expression in the spleen ($p < 0.05$) compared with wild-type mice. Exogenous *neo* expression showed the same pattern as that of *MD-2* and *IL-6* (Figure 3) but with greater differences between transgenic and wild-type mice. Together, these results revealed the successful generation of a mouse model expressing bovine *CD14* shRNA, and indicated that

the inhibition of exogenous *CD14* expression altered the expression levels of genes in the TLR4 signaling pathway *in vivo*.

Discussion

Several studies have previously demonstrated that CD14 plays a crucial role in the inflammatory response to LPS [2-4]. In the CD14-dependent signaling pathway, CD14 binds to LPS and facilitates activation of the TLR4/NF-κB inflammatory pathway [28]. Upstream inhibition of the bacterial LPS/TLR4/CD14-mediated inflammation pathway has been proven to be an effective therapeutic approach for attenuating dysfunctional immune activation [20,29]. However, very few studies have investigated the role of *CD14* in LPS-induced inflammation in large livestock animals such as sheep, cows, and buffalos. Nevertheless, this is of particular importance because of the multiple reproductive and veterinary problems associated with these species, and the need to develop a practical and effective measure to prevent bacterial infections in livestock.

We previously found that knockdown of endogenous *CD14* had clear regulatory effects on the signal transduction of TLR4 after stimulation with LPS in buffalo monocyte/macrophages *in vitro* [28]. To determine if *CD14* knockdown had similar effects in large livestock animals *in vivo*, it is first necessary to establish a mouse

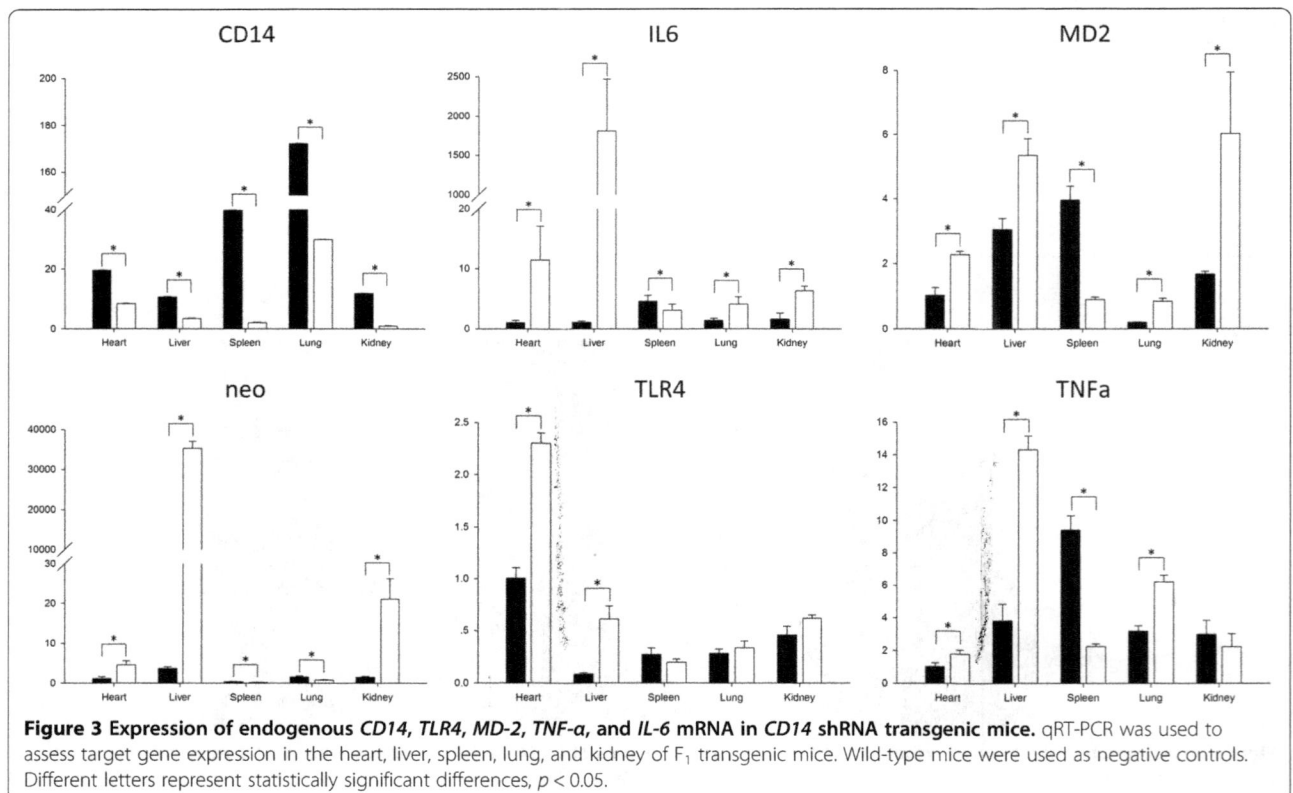

Figure 3 Expression of endogenous *CD14*, *TLR4*, *MD-2*, *TNF-α*, and *IL-6* mRNA in *CD14* shRNA transgenic mice. qRT-PCR was used to assess target gene expression in the heart, liver, spleen, lung, and kidney of F_1 transgenic mice. Wild-type mice were used as negative controls. Different letters represent statistically significant differences, $p < 0.05$.

model expressing bovine *CD14* shRNA. This model would provide basic data about *CD14* knockdown on animal development, gene expression in the CD14-dependent signaling pathway, and most importantly on toxicity experiments. Future work could then build on these data and establish a larger animal model with the aim of developing novel therapeutic interventions to inflammatory diseases caused by Gram-negative bacteria.

Conclusions

We successfully generated a mouse model expressing bovine *CD14* shRNA by pronuclear microinjection. Moreover, we showed that the inhibited expression of exogenous *CD14* shRNA altered the expression levels of some genes in the TLR4 signaling pathway in transgenic mice.

Methods

All experiments and protocols were performed in strict accordance with the Guiding Principles for the Care and Use of Research Animals from the Guangxi University Committee on Animal Research and Bioethics, the committee explicitly approved the animal study.

Reagents and antibodies

All chemicals used in this study were purchased from Sigma-Aldrich (St. Louis, MO), unless otherwise stated. TCM-199 powder was purchased from Gibco BRL (Paisley, Scotland, UK), and Dulbecco's modified Eagle's medium was purchased from Hyclone (Logan, UT). The pSilencer4.1 vector (Life technology, USA), the pEF-EGFP-IRES-neo-SV40-polyA vector, and the pSicoR-GFP vector were generated or maintained by our laboratory. The anti-buffalo CD14 primary antibody was kindly provided by Dr. Wang Fengyang (Hainan University, Haikou, China).

Bovine *CD14* cloning and expression vector construction

The bovine *CD14* coding sequence fragment (1,340 bp) was cloned by RT-PCR, confirmed by sequencing, and used to construct the pDsRed1-N1-bovine CD14 fusion vector by inserting the CD14 fragment into the *SalI* and

SacII sites. This plasmid was then transfected into HEK 293 cells using Lipofectamine® LTX reagent according to the manufacturer's instructions, and cell lines that stably expressed bovine *CD14* were selected using G418 selection.

shRNA design and synthesis

Using ABI siRNA online software (http://www.life technologies.com/cn/zh/home/life-science/rnai/synthetic-rnai-analysis/ambion-silencer-select-sirnas/silencer-select-sirna.html?ICID=search-am16704), three different regions of the bovine *CD14* mRNA sequence (GenBank Accession No. NM_174008.1) were used to design *CD14* shRNA sequences, which were synthesized by Nanjing GenScript Co. (Nanjing, China). A universal shRNA scramble control (NC) sequence was also purchased (Cat. No. 1864, Open Biosystem, Huntsville, AL). The 71 bp oligonucleotide sequence of each shRNA fragment followed the same pattern: 5′-*Xho* I-CCGG-shRNA (sense strand)-TTGAA GAGA (loop structure)-shRNA (antisense strand)-TTTT TT-*Not* I-3′ (Table 1). shRNA lentiviral expression vectors were constructed by inserting the synthesized shRNA fragments into the pSicoR-GFP vector (Addgene, USA) after digestion with *Xho* I and *Not* I. These vectors are referred to as pSicoR-GFP-CD14 shRNA (279/326/674) and scrambled shRNA-1864. The constructed shRNA lentiviral vectors were confirmed by restriction enzyme digestion and sequencing.

Lentivirus packaging and titer determination

Lentiviral particles were produced as previously described [30]. The pSicoR-GFP CD14 shRNA vector was co-transfected into 293 T cells with vesicularstomatitis virusG (VSVG) and NRF plasmids using the calcium-phosphate method [30]. Supernatant was harvested 48–72 h after transfection, centrifuged at 2,000 rpm for 10 min at 4°C to remove cellular debris, and filtered through a 0.45 μm membrane. Viral titers were determined using a serial dilution method in 293 T cells [30].

Table 1 The designed shRNA sequences of the bovine CD14 gene

Name	Duplexes of DNA coding specific shRNA (5′-3′)
shRNA-674	S 5 ′-GCCTAGACCTGTCTGACAATTTCAAGAGAATTGTCAGACAGGTCTAGGC-3′
	AS 5′-CGGATCTGGACAGACTGTTAAAGTTCTCTTAACAGTCTGTCCAGATCCG-3′
shRNA-279	S 5′-GCCTGGAACAGTTTCTCAAGGTTCAAGAGACCTTGAGAAACTGTTCCAGGC-3′
	AS 5′-CGGACCTTGTCAAAGAGTTCCAAGTTCTCTGGAACTCTTTGACAAGGTCCG-3′
shRNA-326	S 5′-GCTGACACAATCAAGGCTCTGTTCAAGAGACAGAGCCTTGATTGTGTCAGC-3′
	AS 5′-CGACTGTGTTAGTTCCGAGACAAGTTCTCTGTCTGGCAACTAACACAGTCG-3′
Scrambled shRNA-1864	S 5′-CTCGAGCCGGCCTAAGGTTAAGTCGCCCTCGCTCG AGCGAGGGCGACTTAACCTTAGGTTTTTTGGCGGCCGC-3′
	AS 5′-GCGGCCGCCAAAAAACCTAAGGTTAAGTCGCCCTC GCTCGAGCGAGGGCGACTTAACCTTAGGCCGGCTCGAG-3′

Screening of shRNA sequences targeting bovine *CD14*

shRNA sequences were screened by infecting HEK293 cells expressing bovine *CD14* with lentiviral particles containing different *CD14* shRNAs. Cells were harvested 72 h after infection and total RNA was extracted using Trizol reagent. The inhibition effects of each shRNA sequence on CD14 were quantified using qRT-PCR and western blot analysis.

For qRT-PCR analysis, total RNA was extracted with Trizol (Invitrogen, USA), digested with DNaseI (Tiangen, Beijing) to remove contaminating genomic DNA, then reverse transcribed into cDNA using AMV reverse transcriptase (Takara, Dalian) according to the manufacturer's instructions. cDNA was diluted to 100 ng/μL for subsequent TaqMan quantitative PCR analysis (ABI 7500) using the probes and primers listed in Table 2. PCR conditions were: 94°C for 30 s, followed by 40 cycles of 94°C for 15 s and 60°C for 30 s. Duplicate PCR experiments were performed for each transcript. The comparative Ct method was used for the relative quantification of target gene expression levels (ABI Prism Sequence Detection System). The histone H2a gene was used for normalization. Within the log-linear phase region of the amplification curve, fold-changes in the relative mRNA expression of the target gene were determined using the formula $2^{-\Delta\Delta CT}$.

Western blot analysis was performed using standard protocols. The primary antibody was a rabbit anti-bovine CD14 polyclonal (1:200) (a gift from Dr. Fengyang Wang), and the secondary antibody was horseradish peroxidase-conjugated goat anti-rabbit IgG (Tiangen Biotech, Beijing, China; 1:1,000). Bovine CD14 shRNA-674 lentivirus was used to infect HEK 293 cells stably expressing bovine CD14 at two different MOIs, 50 and 100 respectively. The cells were harvested at 72 h after infection, HEK 293 cells stably expressing bovine CD14 were used as negative controls.

Construction of CD14 shRNA-674 eukaryotic expression vector

The pSilencer™4.1-CMV neo and pSicoR-CD14 shRNA-674 plasmids were first digested with *Bam*HI and *Hin*dIII, respectively, then the CD14 shRNA-674 fragment was inserted into the pSilencer™4.1-CMV neo backbone to construct the pSilencer™4.1-CD14 shRNA plasmid. The IRES fragment was amplified by PCR using pEF-EGFP-IRES-neo-SV40-polyA vector as template and primer sequences listed in Table 2. It was then ligated with pSilencer™4.1-CD14 shRNA-674 to construct the pSilencer™4.1-CD14 shRNA-674-IRES plasmid. Plasmid

Table 2 The primers used in the paper

Gene	Primer sequences	Fragment length (bp)
Histone H2a	Forward: 5'-AACAAGCTGCTGGGCAAAGT-3'	80
	Reverse: 5'-TTATGGTGGCTCTCCGTCTTCT-3'	
	Probe: 5'-CCCAACATCCAGGCCGTGCTG-3'	
CD14	Forward: 5'-CCGTTCAGTGGTAATGGTTGC-3'	100
	Reverse: 5'-TGGTGTCGGCTCCCTTGAG-3'	
	Probe: 5'-CCGCCCGCCACTGATCTTCCCACCTCTT-3'	
EGFP	Forward: 5'- ACGTAAACGGCCACAAGTTC -3'	440
	Reverse: 5'- GATCTTGAAGTTCACCTTGATGC -3'	
Neo	Forward: 5'- AGAGGCTATTCGGCTATGAC -3'	211
	Reverse: 5'-GCTTCAGTGACAACGTCGAG -3'	
IRES	Forward: 5'-CGGAATATTATAACTTCGTATAATGTATGCTATACGAAGTTATCTTCCGACATTGATTATTGAC-3'	4300
	Reverse: 5'-CGGAATATTATAACTTCGTATAGCATACATTATACGAAGTTATGATCCAGACATGATAAGATAC-3'	
TLR4	Forward: 5'-CTGCCTGAGAACCGAGAGTTG-3'	300
	Reverse: 5'-GCTCCATGCACTGGTAACTAATGT-3'	
IL-6	Forward: 5'- ATCAGAACACTGATCCAGATCC-3'	300
	Reverse: 5'-CAAGGTTTCTCAGGATGAGG-3'	
TNF-α	Forward: 5'-GCTCCAGAAGTTGCTTGTGC-3'	300
	Reverse: 5'-AACCAGAGGGCTGTTGATGG-3'	
MD2	Forward: GAGTTGCCGAAGCGTAAG	213
	Reverse: GCGGTGAATGATGGTGAA	
β-actin	Forward: 5'-GCCCTGGCACCCAGCACAAT-3'	150
	Reverse: 5'-GGAGGGGCCGGACTCATCGT-3'	

construction was confirmed by enzyme digestion and cell transfection experiments.

Generation and detection of transgenic mice

The pSilencer™4.1-CD14 shRNA-674-IRES cassette was digested with *Nhe* I (Takara, Dalian, China) and purified by gel extraction (Qiagen, USA). The purified fragment was then microinjected into the pronucleus of 200 fertilized FVB mice eggs, which were implanted into pseudopregnant FVB females. All mice were housed at the transgenic mouse facility of Cyagen Biosciences Inc. (Guangzhou, China).

DNA purified from the tails of F_0 offspring mice was used to screen for transgene integration by the PCR amplification of *EGFP* and *neo* (Table 2). Transgenic F_0 mice were crossed with wild-type mice to obtain an F_1 generation that was also screened using PCR amplification as above. Three of the 33 F_1 mice were selected for Southern blot analysis to confirm PCR data using the DIG High Prime DNA Labeling and Detection Starter kit II (Roche, USA). The probe was complemented with the neo fragment by digesting the pSilencer4.1-CD14shRNA-IRES plasmid with *Nco* I and *Eag* I. The positive control was pSilencer™4.1-CD14 shRNA-674-IRES plasmid.

Transgene expression analysis

The expression of eGFP in tissues of F_1 transgenic mice was assayed by confocal microscopy (LSM 510, Zeiss, Oberkochen, Germany). Briefly, 10-μm-thick cryostat sections from snap frozen tissues were prepared and fixed with 4% paraformaldehyde. Specimens were visualized using an Olympus BX61 microscope, and digital pictures were acquired with a CCD camera.

The relative expression of *CD14*, *MD-2*, *TLR4*, *IL-6*, *TNF-α*, and *neo* mRNA in the heart, liver, spleen, lung, and kidney of F_1 transgenic mice was assessed by SYBR® Green qRT-PCR; tissues of wild-type mice were used as a negative control. ACTB and histone H2a were used as internal control genes (Table 2), and non-transcribed RNA samples served as an RT-minus control. The expression level of each target gene was calculated using the $2^{-\Delta\Delta CT}$ formula as above.

Statistical analysis

qRT-PCR mRNA expression data were analyzed using SPSS16.0 and Excel 2003 to statistically process multiple samples. Single-factor analysis of variance and the q-test were used for pairwise comparisons. A *P*-value of less than 0.05 was considered to be significant.

Abbreviations

CD14: Cluster of differentiation antigen 14; LPS: Lipopolysaccaride; TLR: Toll-like receptor; IL-6: Interleukin-6; TNF-α: Tumor necrosis factor-α; NF-KB: Nuclear factor kappaB; shRNA: Short hair RNA; MOI: Multiplicity of infection.

Competing interests
The authors declare that they have no competing interests.

Authors' contributions
XPL drafted the manuscript and participated in all study design. SHH participated in gene expression assays and virus package. YPR constructed the CD14 shRNA-674 eukaryotic expression vector and participated in some gene expression assays. MW analyzed the trangenic mouse. CK cloned the bovine CD14 gene and screened the shRNAs. LLX participated in mouse breeding. DSS conceived the study and helped draft the manuscript. All authors read and approved the final manuscript.

Acknowledgements
This work was supported by the National Transgenic Project (2009ZX08007-009B), Guangxi Natural Science funding (2012GXNSFCB053002), funding from the State Key Laboratory of Subtropical Bioresource Conservation and Utilization (KSL-CUSAb-2012-02) and State Education Ministry's Scientific Research Foundation for the Returned Overseas Chinese Scholars.

Author details
[1]State Key Laboratory of Subtropical Bioresource Conservation and Utilization at Guangxi University, Nanning, Guangxi, China. [2]College of Life Science and Technology, Guangxi University, Nanning, Guangxi, China. [3]Guangxi High Education Key Laboratory for Animal Reproduction and Biotechnology, Guangxi University, Nanning 530004, China.

References
1. Ziegler-Heitbrock HW, Ulevitch RJ. CD14: cell surface receptor and differentiation marker. Immunol Today. 1993;14:121–5.
2. Le Roy D, Di Padova F, Adachi Y, Glauser MP, Calandra T, Heumann D. Critical role of lipopolysaccharide-binding protein and CD14 in immune responses against gram-negative bacteria. J Immunol. 2001;167:2759–65.
3. Song G, Li X, Shen Y, Qian L, Kong X, Chen M, et al. Transplantation of iPSc Restores Cardiac Function by Promoting Angiogenesis and Ameliorating Cardiac Remodeling in a Post-infarcted Swine Model. Cell Biochem Biophys. 2014; [Epub ahead of print].
4. Li XQ, Pryds A, Carlsen J, Larsen M. Multifocal central serous chorioretinopathy with photoreceptor-retinal pigment epithelium diastasis in heritable pulmonary arterial hypertension. Retinal Cases Brief Rep. 2015;9:83–7.
5. Thorgersen EB, Hellerud BC, Nielsen EW, Barratt-Due A, Fure H, Lindstad JK, et al. CD14 inhibition efficiently attenuates early inflammatory and hemostatic responses in Escherichia coli sepsis in pigs. FASEB J. 2010;24:712–22.
6. Li X, Cai J, Zhuang Z, Liu J, Xia B, Hu G, et al. Investigation of the action mechanisms of poly-ADP-ribosylation in hexavalent chromium induced cell damage. Zhonghua Yu Fang Yi Xue Za Zhi. 2014;48:720–5.
7. Zuo H, Liao D, Lin L, Zhang R, Li X. Resveratrol attenuates hypoxia-reperfusion injury induced rat myocardium microvascular endothelial cell dysfunction through upregulating PI3K/Akt/SW pathways]. Zhonghua Xin Xue Guan Bing Za Zhi. 2014;42:670–4.
8. Miyake K. Innate immune sensing of pathogens and danger signals by cell surface Toll-like receptors. Semin Immunol. 2007;19:3–10.
9. Miyake K. Innate recognition of lipopolysaccharide by CD14 and toll-like receptor 4-MD-2: unique roles for MD-2. Int Immunopharmacol. 2003;3:119–28.
10. Miyake K. Innate recognition of lipopolysaccharide by Toll-like receptor 4-MD-2. Trends Microbiol. 2004;12:186–92.
11. Takeuchi O, Akira S. Pattern recognition receptors and inflammation. Cell. 2010;140:805–20.
12. Chen S, Lee LF, Fisher TS, Jessen B, Elliott MW, Evering W, et al. Combination of 4-1BB agonist and PD-1 antagonist promotes anti-tumor effector/memory CD8 T cells in a poorly immunogenic tumor model. Cancer Immunol Res. 2015;3:149–60.
13. Xu Z, Huang CX, Li Y, Wang PZ, Ren GL, Chen CS, et al. Toll-like receptor 4 siRNA attenuates LPS-induced secretion of inflammatory cytokines and chemokines by macrophages. J Infect. 2007;55:e1–9.

14. Mancek-Keber M, Gradisar H, Pestana MI, de Tejada GM, Jerala R. Free Thiol Group of MD-2 as the Target for Inhibition of the Lipopolysaccharide-induced Cell Activation. J Biol Chem. 2009;284:19493–500.

15. Qian L, Zhao H, Li X, Yin J, Tang W, Chen P, et al. Pirenzepine Inhibits Myopia in Guinea Pig Model by Regulating the Balance of MMP-2 and TIMP-2 Expression and Increased Tyrosine Hydroxylase Levels. Cell Biochem Biophys 2014. [Epub ahead of print].

16. Haziot A, Ferrero E, Kontgen F, Hijiya N, Yamamoto S, Silver J, et al. Resistance to endotoxin shock and reduced dissemination of gram-negative bacteria in CD14-deficient mice. Immunity. 1996;4:407–14.

17. Roncon-Albuquerque R, Moreira-Rodrigues M, Faria B, Ferreira AP, Cerqueira C, Lourenco AP, et al. Attenuation of the cardiovascular and metabolic complications of obesity in CD14 knockout mice. Life Sci. 2008;83:502–10.

18. Haziot A, Rong GW, Lin XY, Silver J, Goyert SM. Recombinant soluble CD14 prevents mortality in mice treated with endotoxin (lipopolysaccharide). J Immunol. 1995;154:6529–32.

19. Li XX, Guan HJ, Liu JP, Guo YP, Yang Y, Niu YY, et al. Association of selenoprotein S gene polymorphism with ischemic stroke in a Chinese case–control study. Blood Coagul Fibrinolysis. 2015;26:131–5.

20. Nagaoka I, Hirota S, Niyonsaba F, Hirata M, Adachi Y, Tamura H, et al. Cathelicidin family of antibacterial peptides CAP18 and CAP11 inhibit the expression of TNF-alpha by blocking the binding of LPS to CD14 (+) cells. J Immunol. 2001;167:3329–38.

21. Li X, Lu C, Dai J, Dong S, Chen Y, Hu N, et al. Novel multiferroicity in GdMnO3 thin films with self-assembled nano-twinned domains. Sci Rep. 2014;4:7019. doi:10.1038/srep07019.

22. Hou Y, Wang Y, Zhao J, Li X, Cui J, Ding J, et al. Smart soup, a traditional chinese medicine formula, ameliorates amyloid pathology and related cognitive deficits. PLoS One. 2014;9:e111215.

23. Mookherjee N, Wilson HL, Doria S, Popowych Y, Falsafi R, Yu JJ, et al. Bovine and human cathelicidin cationic host defense peptides similarly suppress transcriptional responses to bacterial lipopolysaccharide. J Leukocyte Biol. 2006;80:1563–74.

24. Nemchinov LG, Paape MJ, Sohn EJ, Bannerman DD, Zarlenga DS, Hammond RW. Bovine CD14 receptor produced in plants reduces severity of intramammary bacterial infection. Faseb J. 2006;20:1345–51.

25. Song YX, Dou H, Gong W, Liu XQ, Yu ZG, Li EG, et al. Bis-N-norgliovictin, a small-molecule compound from marine fungus, inhibits LPS-induced inflammation in macrophages and improves survival in sepsis. Eur J Pharmacol. 2013;705:49–60.

26. Shao Y, Cheng Z, Li X, Chernaya V, Wang H, Yang XF. Immunosuppressive/anti-inflammatory cytokines directly and indirectly inhibit endothelial dysfunction- a novel mechanism for maintaining vascular function. J Hematol Oncol. 2014;7:80.

27. Li X, Kolomeisky AB. Theoretical analysis of microtubule dynamics at all times. J Phys Chem B. 2014;118:13777–84.

28. Li X, Li M, Huang S, Qiao S, Qin Z, Kang C, et al. The effect of buffalo CD14 shRNA on the gene expression of TLR4 signal pathway in buffalo monocyte/macrophages. Cell Mol Biol Lett. 2014;19:623–37.

29. Verbon A, Dekkers PE, ten Hove T, Hack CE, Pribble JP, Turner T, et al. IC14, an anti-CD14 antibody, inhibits endotoxin-mediated symptoms and inflammatory responses in humans. J Immunol. 2001;166:3599–605.

30. Li X, Hou L, Liu M, Lin X, Li Y, Li S: Primary effects of extracellular enzyme activity and microbial community on carbon and nitrogen mineralization in estuarine and tidal wetlands. Applied microbiology and biotechnology 2014. [Epub ahead of print].

10

Natural *Besnoitia besnoiti* infections in cattle: chronology of disease progression

Nicole S Gollnick[1*], Julia C Scharr[2], Gereon Schares[3] and Martin C Langenmayer[4]

Abstract

Background: Bovine besnoitiosis is an emerging protozoan disease in cattle. Neither vaccines nor chemotherapeutic drugs are currently available for prevention and treatment of *Besnoitia besnoiti* infections. Therefore the implementation of appropriate disease management strategies is of utmost importance. The aim of this longitudinal study was to complement current knowledge on the chronology of disease progression. This was realized by correlating clinical findings in early stages of naturally acquired bovine besnoitiosis with results of real-time PCR of skin biopsies and of two western immunoblots and an immunofluorescent antibody test (IFAT).
Animals for this study were obtained by i) closely monitoring a cow-calf operation with a high prevalence of bovine besnoitiosis for cases of acute disease, and by ii) conducting a 12-week cohabitation experiment on pasture with five healthy heifers, a healthy bull and five *B. besnoiti* infected cows. A control group of six healthy heifers was kept at a minimal distance of 20 m. Further, the spectrum of potential insect vectors was determined.

Results: Infected cattle were followed up to a maximum of 221 days after first detection of *B. besnoiti* antibodies. Two severely affected cows developed visible and palpable alterations of skin, a decrease in body condition despite good feed intake, and chronic bovine besnoitiosis-associated laminitis leading to non-healing sole ulcers. The cows also had high reciprocal IFAT titers and high loads of parasite DNA in skin samples. Two heifers developed a mild clinical course characterized by few parasitic cysts visible in the scleral *conjunctivae* and *vestibula vaginae*. Both heifers became infected during the time of high insect activity of the species *Musca domestica*, *Musca autumnalis*, *Haematobia irritans*, and *Stomoxys calcitrans*. When a third heifer became subclinically infected, low insect activity was recorded. None of the six control heifers contracted a *B. besnoiti* infection.

Conclusions: In chronic besnoitiosis, the severe clinical course apparently corresponded with high reciprocal IFAT titers and high loads of parasite DNA in skin, whereas mild and subclinical cases displayed lower values. Bovine besnoitiosis-associated laminitis represents an important complication in severe chronic disease which severely impairs animal welfare.

Keywords: *Besnoitia besnoiti*, Bovine besnoitiosis, Cattle, Natural infection, Acute disease, Chronic disease, Laminitis

Background

Bovine besnoitiosis is caused by the apicomplexan parasite *Besnoitia besnoiti* [1]. Severe acute disease is characterized by fever, subcutaneous edema, conjunctivitis, nasal discharge, salivation, lameness, and depression [2-6]. In the chronic stage of bovine besnoitiosis, the parasite forms cysts in connective tissues, especially the dermis and the non-intestinal mucosa [5-8]. Of special diagnostic value are the superficially located cysts in the scleral *conjunctivae*, mucous membranes lining the nasal cavity and the *vestibulum vaginae* [9-11]. These pin-head sized, white protuberances are pathognomonic for bovine besnoitiosis [5]. In severe cases of the disease, the massive parasitism of the dermis also leads to visible and palpable changes of the skin. It becomes uneven and thicker, and disturbance of local blood perfusion may lead to alopecia and skin necrosis [5,8]. To date, vaccines and chemotherapeutical drugs for prevention and treatment of the disease are not available [6,12].

Cattle are considered to be intermediate hosts while the definitive host is still unknown [13,14]. Therefore, the complete life cycle of *B. besnoiti* remains yet to be elucidated. However, it has been established by experiments

* Correspondence: nicole.gollnick@web.de
[1]Clinic for Ruminants with Ambulatory and Herd Health Services at the Centre for Clinical Veterinary Medicine, Veterinary Faculty, Ludwig-Maximilians-Universitaet Muenchen, Sonnenstrasse 16, 85764 Oberschleissheim, Germany
Full list of author information is available at the end of the article

that hematophagous insects are able to transmit the parasite between cattle [2]. Further, the close contact of infected and healthy animals has been suggested to play a pivotal role in disease transmission [2,12].

Clinical and pathophysiological aspects of chronic bovine besnoitiosis are well described in the literature, as a number of such cases of naturally or experimentally acquired disease in cattle has been reported over the past century [8,10,11,15-25]. But especially studying the early stages of naturally acquired bovine besnoitiosis has proved to be difficult. This may be either due to the limitation of access to individual animals in extensive management systems where acute cases may go undetected or simply due to subclinical course of infections [2,25,26].

As bovine besnoitiosis is spreading within Europe, the demand for more scientific investigations is increasing [12,27]. Thus far, longitudinal studies focusing on early stages of naturally acquired bovine besnoitiosis combining the results of clinical examinations and current state-of-the-art laboratory tests are lacking [5]. Therefore, the objective of the present study was to augment current knowledge concerning the chronology of disease progression.

Animals for this study were obtained by i) closely monitoring a German cattle herd with a high prevalence of bovine besnoitiosis for cases of acute disease (Herd-BbGer1) [28], and by ii) conducting a cohabitation experiment involving healthy and B. besnoiti infected cattle. Clinical examinations were correlated with the results on antibody development and the detectability of B. besnoiti DNA over time in one of the parasite's target organs, the skin.

Methods

Ethical statement

Permission for this study was granted by the responsible authorities (Animal ethics committee; Regional government of Upper Bavaria). The experiment was registered under TV Az. 55.2-54-2531-83-09. After completion of the cohabitation period, all animals remained on the premises for fattening or breeding purposes until submitted to slaughter or necropsy.

Animals and experimental design

The study consisted of a 12-week cohabitation period (August 18, 2009, until November 9, 2009) and a five-month follow-up period. Six healthy Simmental heifers (Study animals [SA] 2, 5, 7, 10, 11, and 12) were randomly assigned to a paddock (control) group. Five healthy Simmental heifers (SA 3, 4, 6, 8, and 9) and a healthy Simmental bull (SA 1) were kept on a 2,500 m^2 pasture together with three clinically infected non-pregnant Limousin cows (SA 13, 15, and 16) with a well documented history of chronic bovine besnoitiosis. These cows showed typical parasitic cysts in the scleral

conjunctivae and vestibula vaginae, alterations of skin, and had tested positive in IFAT, immunoblot, histology and PCR (Additional file 1). Further, two pregnant Limousin cows (SA 20 and 22) in the acute stage of disease were added to the pasture group on trial day [td] 3 and 51, respectively. Both animals came from subsets of Herd-BbGer1 with B. besnoiti seroprevalence of 92.5% and 82.8%, respectively (data not shown). The minimal distance between both groups was 20 m. The age range of Simmental and Limousin cattle was 11 to 20 months and three to eight years, respectively. All cattle tested negative for Neospora caninum antibodies by an immunofluorescent antibody test (IFAT) and by immunoblots as previously described [29,30]. During a two-week quarantine period, claws of all Simmental cattle were trimmed and thorough clinical examinations were conducted daily.

Throughout the 12-week cohabitation period, social and reproductive behavior of study animals was recorded daily. This included heat detection in non-pregnant animals on pasture during the morning hours before, during, and after clinical examinations, and in the evening after feeding time. Mating activity of the bull was recorded. The non-pregnant females on pasture were treated regularly with 150 μg Cloprostenol i.m., a synthetic PGF2α analog (Dalmazin®, FATRO S.p.A., Ozzano Emilia, Italy) to induce estrus. For ovarian cyst treatment, 100 μg Lecirelin i.m., a synthetic GnRH analog was used (Dalmarelin®, FATRO S.p.A., Ozzano Emilia, Italy). In accordance with animal welfare regulations (see Ethical statement), it was required to treat animals showing signs of acute bovine besnoitiosis with 0.5 mg/kg of Meloxicam s.c. (Metacam®, Boehringer Ingelheim, Vetmedica GmbH, Ingelheim/Rhein, Germany). This treatment was repeated every 48 hours until clinical signs of disease subsided. Cattle with a lameness score of ≥ 3 underwent functional claw trimming and appropriate treatment. Deep claw ulcers were treated under intravenous regional analgesia using 20 ml of Procain-Hydrochlorid 2% (Procasel 2%®, Selectavet, Weyarn/Holzolling, Germany).

Clinical examinations and samplings

Clinical examinations and samplings were performed in the morning while cattle were restrained in a cattle chute (paddock group) or in headlocks at the feed bunk (pasture group). See Table 1 for further details about the examination protocols 'daily exam' and 'status exam'. Scores 1 (mild), 2 (moderate), and 3 (severe) were assigned to classify the degree of alterations. The body condition score (BCS) was determined according to Edmonson et al. [31]. For grading gait disturbances, the five-point scoring system described by Sprecher et al. (1997) was used [32]: Normal gait (1), mild (2), moderate

Table 1 Clinical examination protocols

Examination of	Daily exam protocol[a]	Status exam protocol[b,c]
Temperament	●	●
Posture	●	●
Gait	●	●
Temperature	●	●
Body condition		●
Cardiovascular system	●	●
Respiratory tract	●	●
Digestive tract	●	●
Musculosceletal system	●	●
Female reproductive system		●
Skin		●
Palpable lymph nodes[d]		●
Abdominal cavity by rectal exploration		●
Scleral *conjunctivae*		●
Mucous membrane of *vestibulum vaginae*		●

[a]Used daily (except Mondays and Thursdays) for *Besnoitia besnoiti* negative Simmental cattle.
[b]Used Mondays and Thursdays for *B. besnoiti* negative Simmental cattle.
[c]Used daily for Simmentals after developing signs of clinical besnoitiosis until the end of the cohabitation experiment. Used daily for study animal 20, and for study animal 22 on trial days 51, 52, 56, 63, 70, and 80. Used on all animals examined during the five-month follow-up period.
[d]*Lymphonodi [Inn.] mandibulares, Inn. parotidei, Inn. retropharyngei mediales, Inn. cervicales superficiales, Inn. subiliaci, Inn. ileofemorales.*

(3), moderate to severe (4), and severe lameness (5). The number of cysts in the mucous membrane of the *vestibulum vaginae* and the mean number of cysts in the scleral *conjunctivae* were estimated and the result were assigned to the following categories: 1: 1–5 cysts; 2: 6–10 cysts; 3: 11–20 cysts; 4: 21–30 cysts; 5: >30 cysts.

Blood and skin biopsy sampling

On td 0, blood samples were collected from all Simmentals and SA 13, 15, and 16. Further, skin biopsies for PCR (except SA 13, 15, and 16) and histological examinations were taken under local anesthesia with 8-mm punch biopsy devices at the femoral regions of the hind legs [33,34]. Thereafter, skin biopsies for PCR were taken on Mondays and Thursdays over the 12-week cohabitation period from healthy Simmental cattle. In case a *B. besnoiti* infection had been observed in an individual animal, blood samples were taken every day and skin samples were obtained at least every other day at the femoral region or, less often, laterally at the neck during 21 days after initial signs of acute disease. Thereafter, blood and skin samples were again taken twice a week. With regards to SA 20, the sampling regime for acutely infected cattle was applied. Due to its uncooperative behavior, SA 22 was only sampled on days 51, 52, 56, 63, 70, and 80. During regular herd visits in the five-month follow-up period, complete samplings were performed on SA 4, 6, 8, 20, and 22 every two to three weeks.

Serology and real-time PCR examinations

An immunofluorescent antibody test (IFAT) and two western immunoblots (one with tachyzoite and the second with bradyzoite antigen) were performed to define the serological status of the animals. The combination of results of these three serological tests is referred to as "serological reference system" later on. Thus, a blood sample was regarded as seropositive if it revealed a positive result in at least two of the three tests applied. In IFAT, a serum was regarded as positive if the reciprocal IFAT titer was ≥ 200. In the immunoblot, a positive serological reaction was recorded if ≥ 4 of 10 bands selected per antigen (tachyzoite, bradyzoite) were recognized [29]. Previously published real-time PCR results for the detection of a *B. besnoiti* infection were included for data interpretation [34]. For calculation of mean cycle threshold [ct]-values and statistical analysis, negative real-time PCR results were counted with a ct-value of 45.0.

Examinations by light microscopy

Immediately after collection of blood into tubes precoated with EDTA, a blood smear was performed on a glass slide. Smears were stained with a Pappenheim stain (Haema Schnellfaerbung, LT-SYS® Labor + Technik Eberhard Lehmann GmbH, Berlin, Germany) and examined for *B. besnoiti* tachyzoites. At necropsy of SA 20 and 22, samples of the claws were fixed in paraformaldehyde 4% for 24 to 48 hours, decalcified for one week and subsequently embedded in plastic [35]. Sections of 2 μm thickness were routinely stained with hematoxylin and eosin (HE) and according to Giemsa.

Insects: collection, DNA extraction and real-time PCR

Insects alighting on or flying in the vicinity of the trunk, neck and head of the pasture group cattle restrained in headlocks were caught using a Japan insect hand net on td 24 at 1 and 2 pm, and on td 32 at 11 am. Insects were stored in 96.5% ethanol. Using a dissecting microscope, insect classification was conducted based on morphological characteristics at the Institute for Parasitology and Tropical Veterinary Medicine, Berlin, Germany. Using a vacuum evaporator (Alpha-RVC, Martin Christ Gefriertrocknungsanlagen GmbH, Osterode am Harz, Germany), insects were dried for 60 min at 37°C. DNA extraction was performed using the ZR Insect/Tissue DNA Kit-25™ (ZYMO Research Corporation, Irvine, CA, USA) following the manufacturer's procedure with a variation in bead beater process time (15 min instead of 10 min). Every 11th sample, a negative processing control (empty tube), was included during DNA extraction.

All DNAs were tested by real-time PCR using the Bb-RT2 assay as previously described [36].

Definitions

Acute, subacute, and chronic bovine besnoitiosis are characterized by a number of specific and non-specific clinical signs reviewed by [5,6]. In our study we chose specific clinical features for assigning a study animal to a respective disease stage: Animals in the acute stage of bovine besnoitiosis had to show fever (body temperature > 39.0°C) or at least two of the following clinical signs/diagnoses: depression, conjunctivitis, subcutaneous edema, lymphadenitis, lameness. Cattle were classified as chronically infected by *B. besnoiti* when first parasitic cysts were visible in the scleral *conjunctivae* or mucous membranes. The time period between the acute and chronic stage is referred to as subacute stage of disease. The assumed time period of infection is defined as the period of 11–14 days prior to the onset of clinical signs and was based on previous studies [2].

Results

New infections by *B. besnoiti*

Only Simmental heifers SA 4, 6, and 8 kept in direct contact with clinically affected cattle became *B. besnoiti* infected. SA 1 (bull), 3, and 9, kept under the same conditions and the six control females remained free of *B. besnoiti* infection (Figure 1). Overall, five female cattle were followed for at least 152 days (SA 8) to a maximum of 221 days (SA 20) after first detection of *B. besnoiti* antibodies. SA 4, 6, 20, and 22 became clinically infected. In case of SA 8, only routine laboratory tests revealed an infection with *B. besnoiti*. Skin samples tested *B. besnoiti* DNA positive on td 70 (cycle threshold [ct]-value: 39.1) and SA 8 seroconverted on td 73 (Figure 2) [34]. *B. besnoiti* tachyzoites could not be demonstrated in blood smears of SA 8.

Duration of the acute and subacute stages and the beginning of the chronic stage varied between study animals. To compare diagnostic characteristics between cattle, the time course of infection was adjusted to the day of seroconversion (based on the reference system). For the correlation of clinical findings with laboratory results, periods of time were defined at which SA 4, 6, and 20 were most likely in a particular stage of clinical disease: Acute disease: +/− 3 *dps*; subacute disease: 7 to 18 *dps*; chronic disease: 32 to 152 *dps*. For better comparability of results, these periods of time were also applied to SA 8 and SA 22. In cases where more than two test values were available for the respected clinical periods, the mean of real-time PCR ct-values and the mean of reciprocal IFAT titers were determined for each animal (Table 2).

Acute stage of bovine besnoitiosis

The period of acute bovine besnoitiosis of SA 4 and 6 lasted for 12 and 13 days, respectively (Figure 3). *B. besnoiti* DNA could be demonstrated in skin samples of SA 4 and 6, one and four days after the beginning of the acute phase, respectively (SA 4: ct-value: 38.7; SA 6: ct-value: 35.0) (Figure 2) [34]. Limousin cow SA 20, tested positive for *B. besnoiti* DNA in skin samples on the day of admission (ct-value: 30.3) and seroconversion was noted one day later (Figures 2 and 3) [34]. Clinical findings during the acute stage for SA 4, 6 and 20 are shown in Figures 3 and 4.

On the day of admission (td 51), SA 22 had a body temperature of 38.7°C. The Limousin cow was severely depressed, had mucopurulent nasal discharge and showed mild to moderate conjunctival hyperemia and moderate injection of episcleral and conjunctival vessels. The animal walked reluctantly with a very stiff gait on td 51 and 52. Further, *B. besnoiti* DNA could be detected in skin samples (ct-value: 31.5) and the animal had already seroconverted (Figure 2) [34]. According to our definition, SA 22 entered the study on the last day of acute disease. Hereafter, for comparability with other study animals, td 51 will be referred to as day of seroconversion for SA 22.

Disorders of the cardiovascular, respiratory, and digestive systems were not observed in all four clinically affected cattle.

Examinations of blood smears for SA 4, 6, 20, and 22 prepared on days of acute disease did not reveal free or intracellular tachyzoites in peripheral blood. Further serological and real-time PCR results are detailed in Table 2.

Subacute stage of bovine besnoitiosis

Subacute disease, i.e. the phase between the end of acute disease and the macroscopic observation of first tissue cysts, lasted 15, 24, 18, and 10 days for SA 4, 6, 20, and 22, respectively (Figure 2). No abnormal clinical findings were recorded in SA 4 and 6 during the subacute period. In SA 20 and 22, the only alteration noted was a rough and dull hair coat (SA 20: 2, 9, 15, 16 and 19 *dps*; SA 22: 8 *dps*). Good ruminal fill and no decrease in BCS was recorded for SA 4, 6, 20, and 22 (Figure 5).

Serological and real-time PCR results are detailed in Table 2.

Chronic stage of bovine besnoitiosis

Chronic besnoitiosis led to macroscopical changes of the scleral *conjunctivae* and *vestibula vaginae* in all clinically affected animals. Further, in severely affected cattle SA 20 and 22, effects on body condition, skin and claw health were noted. Serological and real-time PCR results are detailed in Table 2.

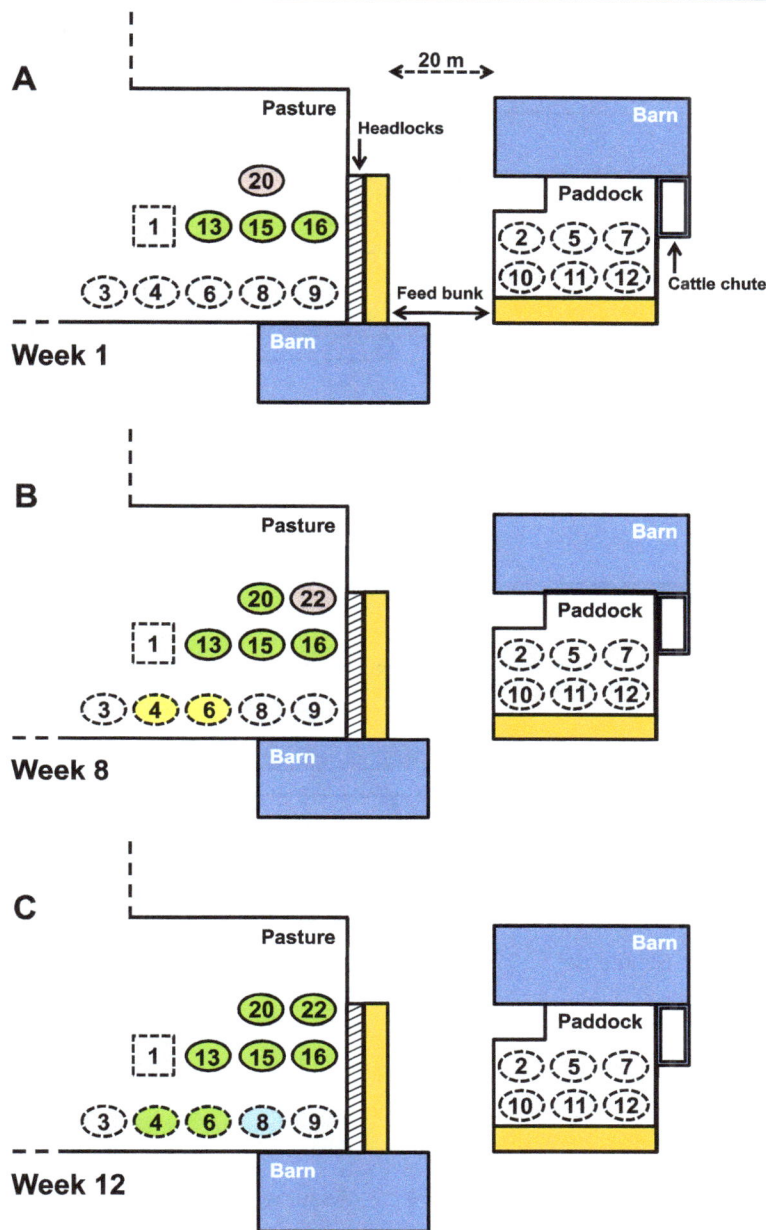

Figure 1 Experimental design and results of cohabitation trial. Sixteen female adult cattle (O) and one breeding bull (□) of the breeds Limousin (—) and German Simmental (– – –) were enrolled in the 12-week cohabitation trial. Pink, yellow, green, and blue indicate animals in the acute, subacute, chronic, and subclinical stage of bovine besnoitiosis, respectively. **A)** Five healthy, non-pregnant Simmental heifers (Study animals [SA] 3, 4, 6, 8, and 9), and a healthy Simmental bull (SA 1) were kept together with three chronically *Besnoitia besnoiti* infected, non-pregnant Limousin cows (SA 13, 15, and 16) on a 2,500 m² pasture. A control group of six healthy, non-pregnant Simmental heifers (SA 2, 5, 7, 10, 11, and 12) were confined at a minimal distance of 20 m in a 200 m² paddock area. On trial day [td] 3, the acutely *B. besnoiti* infected, pregnant Limousin cow SA 20 was introduced into the pasture group. **B)** The acutely *B. besnoiti* infected, pregnant Limousin cow SA 22 was introduced on td 51. By this time SA 20 had entered the chronic stage, and SA 4 and 6 were in the subacute stage of disease. **C)** In the final week of the trial, SA 4, 6, and 22 had reached the chronic stage of bovine besnoitiosis and SA 8 was identified as subclinically infected.

Clinical changes of mucous membranes and skin

First parasitic cysts in the scleral *conjunctivae* were detected macroscopically 19 and 32 *dps* in SA 4 and 6, respectively. In the *vestibulum vaginae,* parasitic cysts appeared 180 and 135 *dps* for SA 4 and 6, respectively. Throughout the study, the skin of both animals remained clinically unaffected (Figure 5).

In SA 20 first, very minute parasitic cysts were observed in the scleral *conjunctivae* of both eyes 23 *dps*

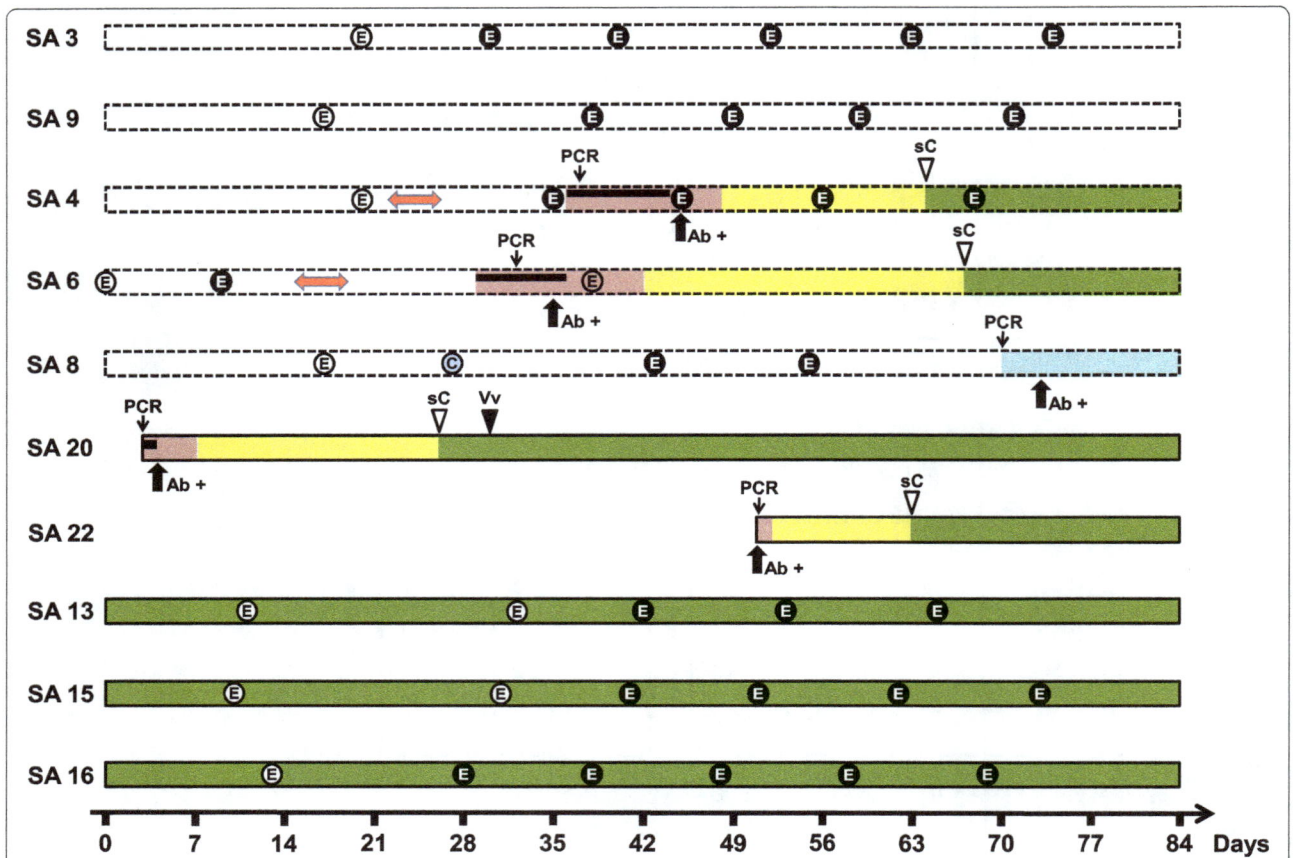

Figure 2 Chronology of events during the 12-week cohabitation period. Clinical, serological, and PCR findings in female animals of the pasture group are shown. The acutely *Besnoitia besnoiti* (Bb)-infected Limousin cows SA 20 and 22 were introduced into the experiment on trial days 3 and 51, respectively. Simmental heifers SA 4, 6, and 8 became infected with *B. besnoiti* during the experimental period. In the reference system used, a blood sample was regarded as seropositive if it revealed a positive result in at least two of the three tests applied: IFAT, tachyzoite and bradyzoite immunoblot.

(Figure 6A) and first parasitic cysts became visible in the mucous membrane of the *vestibulum vaginae* 26 *dps.* The number of visible parasitic cysts in the scleral *conjunctivae* and *vestibulum vaginae* exceeded 30

(Category 5) within 28 *dps* and 42 *dps*, respectively (Figure 5). Palpable indurations of 3–5 mm in diameter in the skin of the teat basis were detected for the first time 23 *dps* (Figure 5). Open skin lesions on the teats were

Table 2 Serology and real-time PCR results based on stage of bovine besnoitiosis[a]

Animal data		SA 4	SA 6	SA 8	SA 20	SA 22
Animal ID		SA 4	SA 6	SA 8	SA 20	SA 22
Breed		S	S	S	L	L
Age (months)		20	19	13	53	49
Pregnancy status		np	np	np	p	p
Study entry (td)		1	1	1	3	51
Acute disease						
Start/End (dps)[b]		−9/2	−6/6	subclinical	unknown/4	unknown/0
Ct (+/− 3 dps)[c]	Lowest/highest/mean (# sample)	32.5/36.7/33.9 (4)	30.4/36.0/33.8 (7)	39.1/ND/ND (1)	29.5/31.4/30.3 (5)	31.5/ND/ND (1)
IFAT (+/− 3 dps)	Lowest/highest/mean (# sample)	100 /400/260 (5)	50/400/229 (7)	50/800/ND (2)	800/1600/1280 (5)	400/400/ND (2)
Subacute disease						
Start/End (dps)		3/18	7/31	subclinical	5/22	1/11
Ct (7–18 dps)[c]	Lowest/highest/mean (# sample)	34.5/45.0/ND (2)	33.6/35.3/ND (2)	45.0/45.0/45.0 (3)	28.0/32.9/ND (2)	31.6/ND/ND (1)
IFAT (7–18 dps)[d]	Lowest/highest/mean (# sample)	800/1600/1120 (5)	400/1600/867 (6)	800/800/800 (3)	1600/1600/ND (2)	1600/ND/ND (1)
Chronic disease						
Start (dps)		19	32	subclinical	23	12
Ct (32–152 dps)[c]	Lowest/highest/mean (# sample)	45.0 /45.0/45.0 (4)	23.2/37.6/27.6 (5)	27.4/45.0/41.5 (9)	15.5/18.8/16.9 (4)	11.6/19.5/15.3 (3)
IFAT (32–152 dps)	Lowest/highest/mean (# sample)	1600/3200/2200 (8)	800/3200/1829 (7)	800/1600/1244 (9)	1600/6400/3556 (9)	6400/6400/6400 (5)

[a] Abbreviations: SA = study animal; S = Simmental; L = Limousin; np = not pregnant; p = pregnant; td = trial day; dps = days post seroconversion; ND = not determined; PCR = polymerase chain reaction; IFAT = immunofluorescent antibody test; Ct = Cycle threshold in BbRT2 PCR [30].

[b] Data on the date of seroconversion are previously published [29].

[c] For determination of mean ct-values, negative real-time PCR results were depicted at cycle threshold [Ct] = 45.0.

[d] For SA 22 only laboratory results between 7 to 11 dps were regarded.

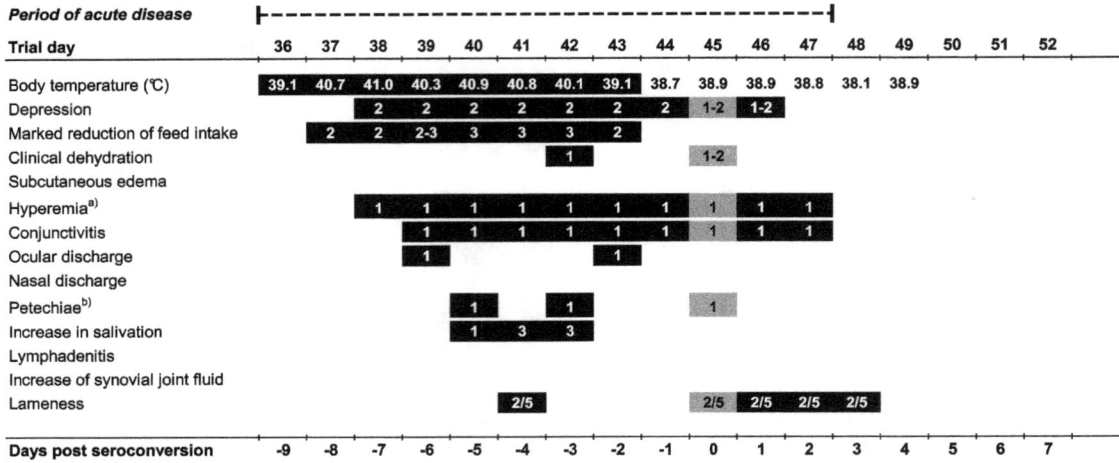

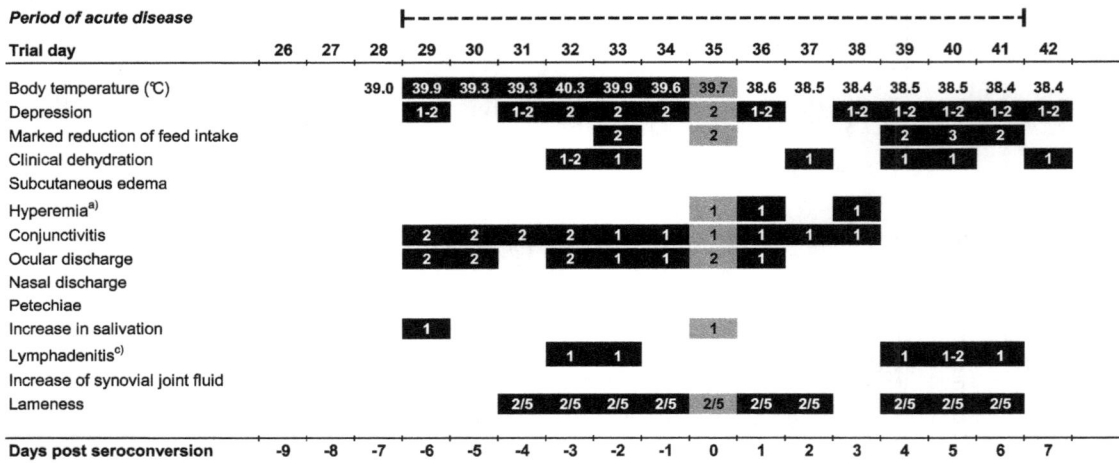

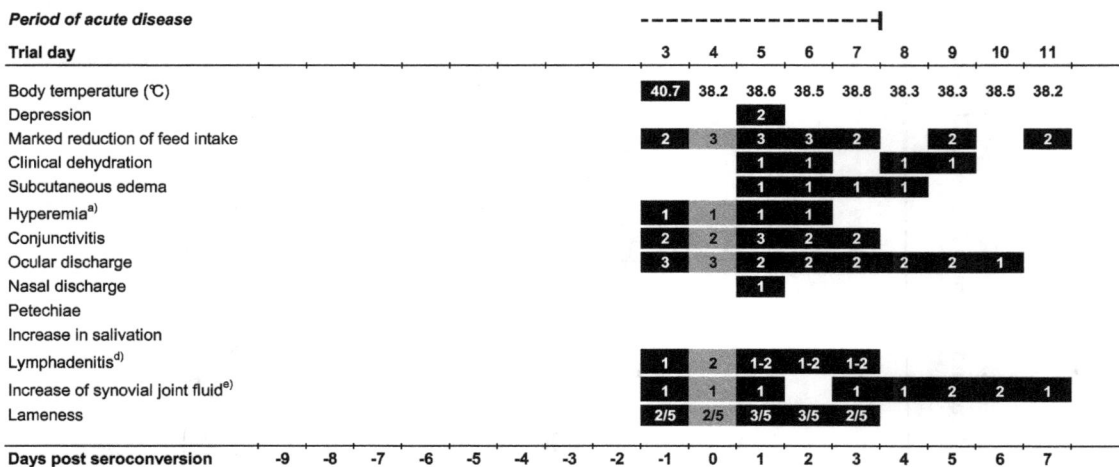

Figure 3 (See legend on next page.)

(See figure on previous page.)
Figure 3 Clinical findings in acute bovine besnoitiosis in study animals [SA] 4, 6, and 20. The exact period of acute disease was determined retrospectively after serology results confirmed an infection with *Besnoitia besnoiti*. The acute stage is defined as the period in which an animal had a body temperature of > 39.0°C or showed at least two of the following clinical signs/diagnoses: depression, conjunctivitis, subcutaneous edema, lymphadenitis, lameness. A black bar indicates on which day an animal showed specific clinical alterations during the acute stage of disease. The day of seroconversion is marked by dark grey. The scores 1 (mild), 2 (moderate), and 3 (severe) indicate the severity of alteration from physiological values. For lameness evaluations a five-point scoring system was utilized: Normal gait (1), mild (2), moderate (3), moderate to severe (4), and severe lameness (5) [28]. [a]Hyperemia of unpigmented skin and mucous membranes; [b]*Petechiae* in the nasal and oral mucous membranes; [c]Lymphadenitis of *Lnn. cervicales superficiales*; [d]Lymphadenitis of *Lnn. cervicales superficiales* and *Lnn. subiliaci*; [e]Increase of synovial joint fluid in the stifle, carpal and tarsal joints.

recorded 32 *dps* (Figure 6E). Intradermal knots especially at the teat basis increased in size (up to 1 cm in diameter by 116 *dps*) and open skin lesions as well as encrusted epidermal areas were noted throughout the follow-up period (Figure 6F). The skin of the proximal part of the hind legs was first recorded to be slightly, yet notably uneven 25 *dps* (Figure 6H). These skin alterations became more prominent with time and by 166 *dps* intradermal indurations were palpable and clearly visible on the eyelids, neck, proximal hind legs (Figure 6J), and the distal limbs. The skin of the proximal hind legs was noted to be hypotricheic (Figure 6J) and partial alopecia was found on the distal limbs.

In SA 22, first parasitic cysts were noted in the scleral conjunctivae and *vestibulum vaginae* 13 and 84 days after the end of the acute stage, respectively. First palpable changes were recorded for the teat skin 30 *dps* and for the skin of the upper hind legs and neck 120 *dps* (Figure 5).

Effects on body condition

During the chronic stage, ruminal fill was recorded as "good" at all status examinations for SA 4, 6, 20 and 22. Weight gain was recorded for SA 4 and 6, while SA 20 and 22 lost body condition (Figure 5).

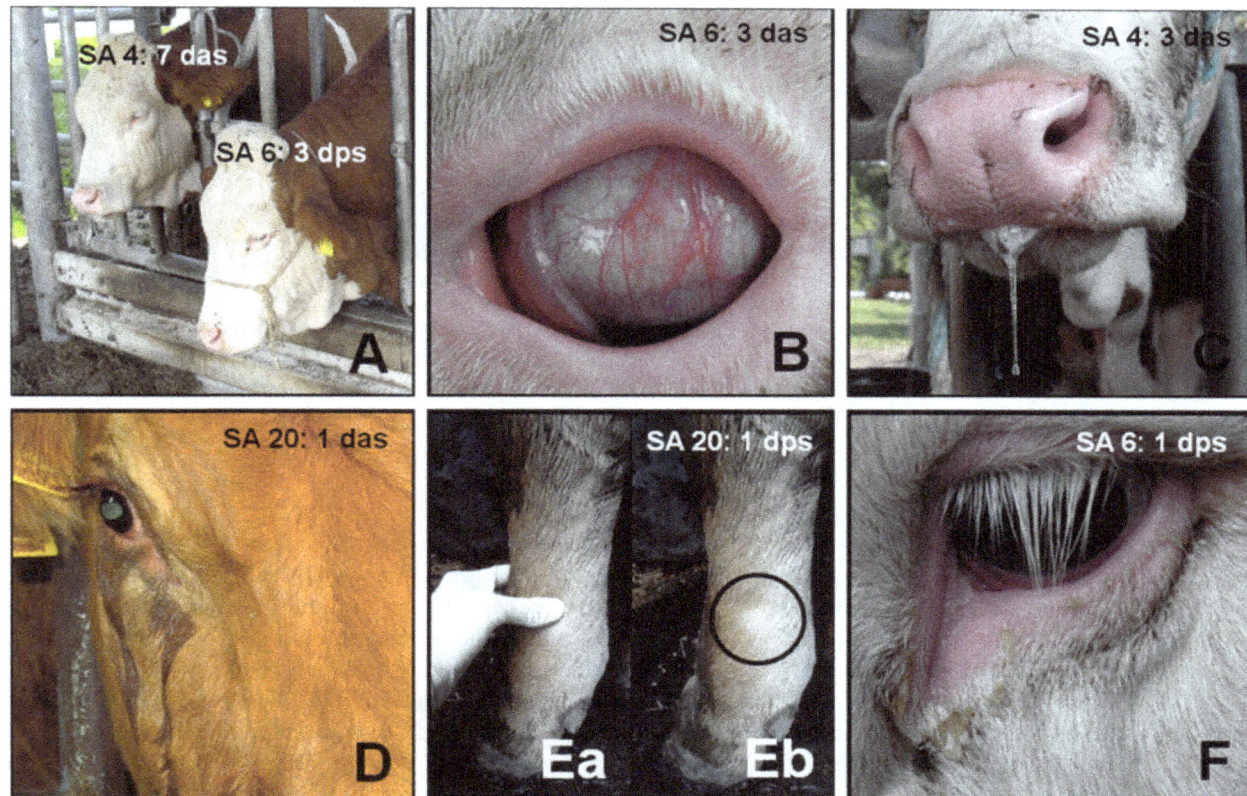

Figure 4 Study animals [SA] 4, 6, and 20 in acute stage of bovine besnoitiosis. Animal ID and day when picture was taken are provided in the figure (*das* = days ante seroconversion, *dps* = days post seroconversion). **A)** Depression and inappetence. **B)** Injected scleral vessels and considerable dehydration (sunken eye bulb). **C)** Increase of salivation. **D)** Serous ocular discharge. **E)** Pitting edema on distal left front limb. Note the indentation after applying pressure to the metacarpal skin (Eb: Black circle). **F)** Mild purulent ocular discharge.

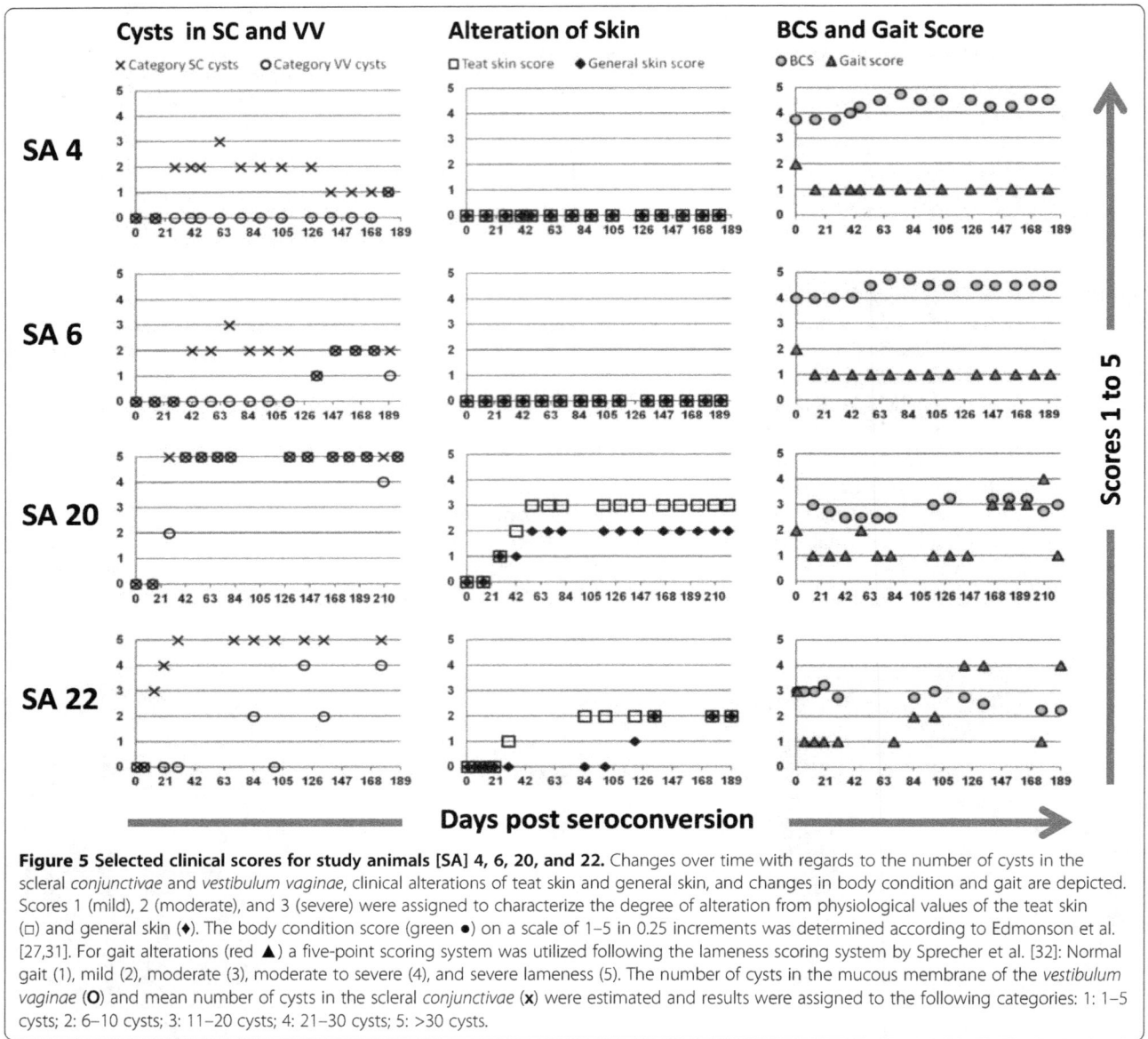

Figure 5 Selected clinical scores for study animals [SA] 4, 6, 20, and 22. Changes over time with regards to the number of cysts in the scleral *conjunctivae* and *vestibulum vaginae*, clinical alterations of teat skin and general skin, and changes in body condition and gait are depicted. Scores 1 (mild), 2 (moderate), and 3 (severe) were assigned to characterize the degree of alteration from physiological values of the teat skin (□) and general skin (♦). The body condition score (green ●) on a scale of 1–5 in 0.25 increments was determined according to Edmonson et al. [27,31]. For gait alterations (red ▲) a five-point scoring system was utilized following the lameness scoring system by Sprecher et al. [32]: Normal gait (1), mild (2), moderate (3), moderate to severe (4), and severe lameness (5). The number of cysts in the mucous membrane of the *vestibulum vaginae* (O) and mean number of cysts in the scleral *conjunctivae* (x) were estimated and results were assigned to the following categories: 1: 1–5 cysts; 2: 6–10 cysts; 3: 11–20 cysts; 4: 21–30 cysts; 5: >30 cysts.

Claw disease associated with B. besnoiti infections

For SA 4 and 6, lameness was not recorded any time after the acute stage of disease (Figure 5).

SA 20 presented moderate changes in gait and stance 166 *dps*. The animal walked with an arched back, keeping its head low during movement. All limbs were clearly abducted during the protraction phase. At rest, the animal presented a wide stance in both front and hind limbs. The head was kept low and the cow appeared depressed. Functional claw trimming of all feet revealed signs of chronic laminitis on all four lateral claws (Figure 6L) and sole ulcers on both lateral front claws. Keeping the animal on deep straw bedding did

not lead to improvement of its overall condition. Shortly after, SA 20 delivered a healthy calf 212 *dps*, a second claw treatment was performed, and the animal was transferred to pasture where lameness receded (Figure 5).

Eighty-four *dps*, SA 22 presented mild supporting leg lameness on the left hind leg. Further, it walked carefully and stiffly on hard concrete surface. A lameness score of 4 was recorded 120 *dps* (Figure 5). The protraction phase of both hind limbs was shortened. While standing, the animal shifted its weight from one hind leg to the other a few times per minute. During movement, front feet were placed carefully, and the head of the animal was kept low. Functional claw trimming of the hind

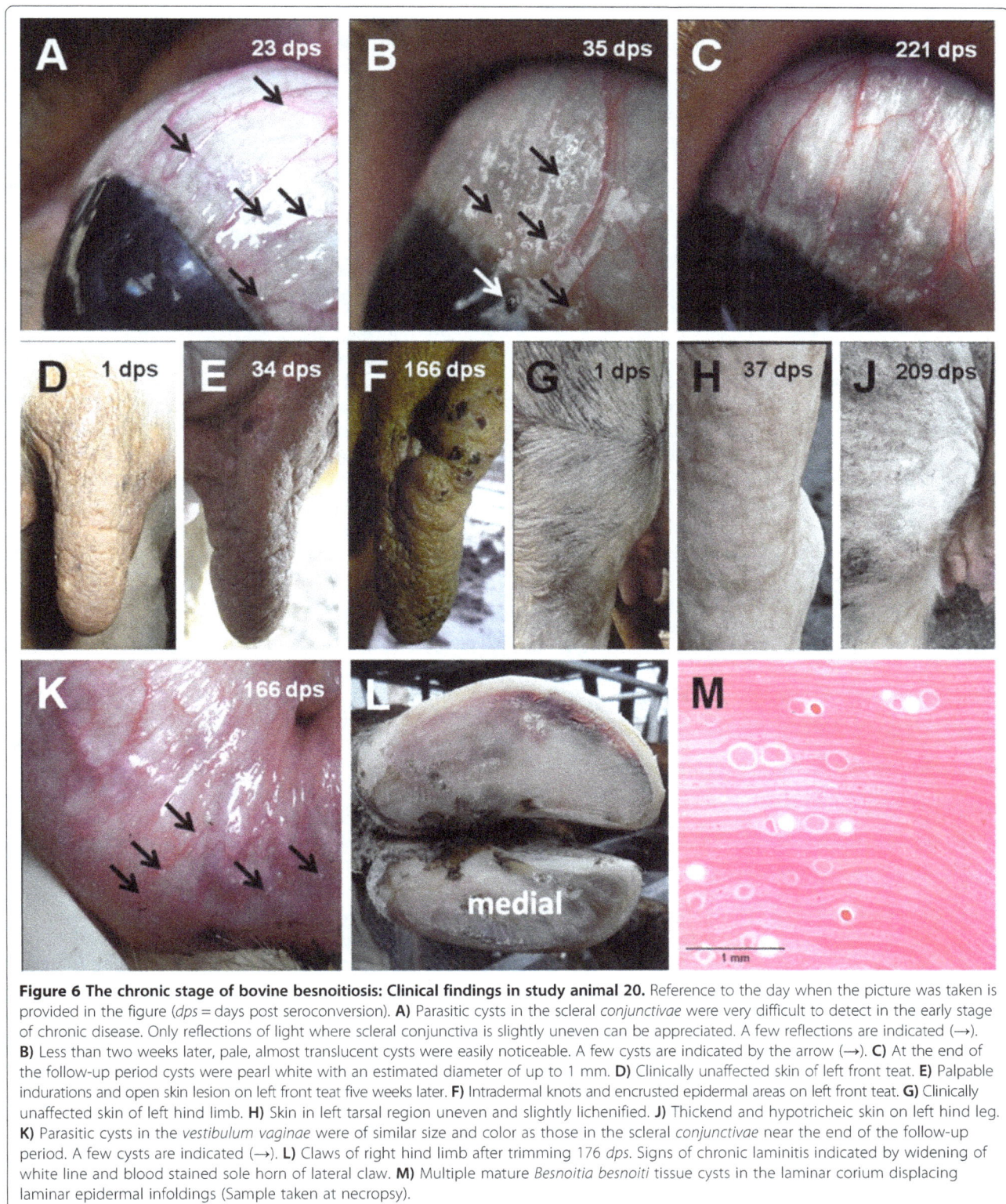

Figure 6 The chronic stage of bovine besnoitiosis: Clinical findings in study animal 20. Reference to the day when the picture was taken is provided in the figure (*dps* = days post seroconversion). **A)** Parasitic cysts in the scleral *conjunctivae* were very difficult to detect in the early stage of chronic disease. Only reflections of light where scleral conjunctiva is slightly uneven can be appreciated. A few reflections are indicated (→). **B)** Less than two weeks later, pale, almost translucent cysts were easily noticeable. A few cysts are indicated by the arrow (→). **C)** At the end of the follow-up period cysts were pearl white with an estimated diameter of up to 1 mm. **D)** Clinically unaffected skin of left front teat. **E)** Palpable indurations and open skin lesion on left front teat five weeks later. **F)** Intradermal knots and encrusted epidermal areas on left front teat. **G)** Clinically unaffected skin of left hind limb. **H)** Skin in left tarsal region uneven and slightly lichenified. **J)** Thickend and hypotricheic skin on left hind leg. **K)** Parasitic cysts in the *vestibulum vaginae* were of similar size and color as those in the scleral *conjunctivae* near the end of the follow-up period. A few cysts are indicated (→). **L)** Claws of right hind limb after trimming 176 *dps*. Signs of chronic laminitis indicated by widening of white line and blood stained sole horn of lateral claw. **M)** Multiple mature *Besnoitia besnoiti* tissue cysts in the laminar corium displacing laminar epidermal infoldings (Sample taken at necropsy).

claws revealed chronic laminitis and Rusterholz sole ulcers on the lateral claws. After claw treatment, the animal was housed on deep straw bedding and delivered a healthy calf 152 *dps*. On the last day of the follow-up period, SA 22 was examined on pasture and was found to be free of lameness (Figure 5).

After the follow-up period ended, SA 20 and 22 were rejoined with Herd-BbGer1. However, when signs of severe lameness reappeared, both cattle were submitted to necropsy. Examination of the claws of SA 20 and 22 revealed moderate to severe rotation of the distal phalanges. In several claws, maceration of claw horn was present, and in few claws, a purulent and necrotizing inflammation of the laminar corium and the distal phalanx. Histological examination of the laminar corium revealed multiple *B. besnoiti* tissue cysts leading to distension of the laminar papillae and lamellae and deviation or displacement of the laminar epidermal infoldings (Figure 6M) [33].

Cattle and insect behavior

Intense mating activity of SA 1 was noted whenever a heifer or cow in the pasture group, irrespective of disease status, was in spontaneous or hormone-induced estrus. With the exception of SA 6 and 9 on td 38, Simmental heifers were not served by the bull on the same day as cows in the chronic stage of bovine besnoitiosis (see Figure 2 for details). Physiological grooming and reproductive behavior of cattle were observed throughout the study. It is noteworthy that animals licked each other's skin biopsy wounds until potential residual bleeding subsided. Insects were frequently observed feeding on ocular and nasal secretions and on skin wounds after sampling. Healthy cattle reacted to biting insect activity by stamping, kicking, head shaking, frequent tail flicking and contractions of the *musculus cutaneus trunci*. In animals with acute bovine besnoitiosis, reactions to ward off insects were less distinct and numbers of insects on these cattle were noticeably greater than on healthy animals.

Insect species collected

The following species of the family *Muscidae* (Diptera) were caught on td 24 and 32: Two secretophagous insect species *Musca domestica* Linnaeus 1758 (td 24: n = 40; td 32: n = 2), and *Musca autumnalis* De Geer 1776 (td 24: n = 23; td 32: n = 2); and two hematophagous insect species *Haematobia irritans* Linnaeus 1758 (td 24: n = 10; td 32: n = 34), and *Stomoxys calcitrans* Linnaeus 1758 (td 24: n = 0; td 32: n = 48). One *S. calcitrans*, caught directly on SA 6 during acute besnoitiosis tested positive for *B. besnoiti* DNA in two repetitive examinations (ct-value: 29.99).

Discussion

In this paper, we present results of the first longitudinal clinical study of cattle monitored in acute, subacute and chronic stages of naturally acquired bovine besnoitiosis in which clinical findings could be correlated with results of current state-of-the-art laboratory tests. The reported 12-week cohabitation experiment of six healthy

Simmentals kept with five clinically affected Limousins (three chronic cases, two recently infected animals) resulted in one subclinical case and two mild cases with clinical signs observed in the acute and chronic stage of disease. Major differences between the study described here and a previous cohabitation study [2], are the duration of the experiment (12 weeks compared to 2 years), the frequency of animal sampling, a clinically apparent acute stage, the opportunity to confirm infection after only a few days with serological and molecular techniques, and disease progression monitored in detail.

Clinical findings

Authors studying the clinical signs of experimentally and naturally acquired acute bovine besnoitiosis report that pyrexia is one of the first signs to appear in the acute stage. Shortly after that anorexia, polypnoe, hyperemia of unpigmented skin and mucous membranes, conjunctivitis, and photophobia develop [1,8,21]. In this study, pyrexia developed one day before (SA 4) or together (SA 6) with the appearance of other clinical signs/diagnoses typical for bovine besnoitiosis, like anorexia, depression, conjunctivitis, and ocular discharge (Figure 3). The duration of pyrexia was comparable with the data obtained by Bigalke (1968) [2], where cattle were 'naturally' infected via insects harboring parasites or nasal administration of skin suspensions containing cysts. Interestingly, the hallmark feature of acute bovine besnoitiosis, subcutaneous edema, was only observed in SA 20. As SA 4 and 6 both displayed edema in histological skin sections as well [33], edema in these cases were most likely too subtle to be noticed clinically. *Petechiae*, which are described in experimental bovine besnoitiosis [8] were only observed on a few days in SA 4 (Figure 3). As SA 20 and 22 both displayed multifocal hemorrhages in histological skin sections [33], *petechiae* in these cases were most likely obscured by skin pigmentation. Only SA 20, severely affected by *B. besnoiti*, displayed a palpable increase in synovial joint fluid (Figure 3), which is indicative of arthritis, a lesion which is described in experimental bovine besnoitiosis as well [8].

In the chronic stage of bovine besnoitiosis, all animals developed typical minute parasitic cysts in the nonintestinal mucous membranes. Interestingly, in all four cases, cysts in the scleral *conjunctivae* appeared before cysts in the *vestibula vaginae* became visible (Figure 5). Typical skin lesions associated with bovine besnoitiosis like thickening, folding and reduced elasticity [1,6] developed only in SA 20 and 22.

Cysts in the scleral *conjunctivae* developed 28 and 38 days after first fever in SA 4 and 6, respectively, which is twelve respectively two days shorter compared with the mean reported in Bigalke's 'natural' infections [2]. Interestingly, measurement of cyst diameter in histology revealed smaller cysts around the time point of first detection of cysts in the scleral *conjunctivae* than reported by Bigalke (1968) [2,33]. The course of besnoitiosis in this study reflected those of South African 'natural' cases, as SA 4 and 6 developed mild and SA 20 and 22 fairly severe besnoitiosis.

Clinical signs of chronic laminitis during chronic bovine besnoitiosis were only noted in SA 20 and 22. Although lameness or reluctance to move are common clinical signs during acute bovine besnoitiosis [1,21], an association between chronic bovine besnoitiosis and chronic laminitis has only recently been made [33]. Steric interference of tissue cysts with epidermal lamellae and dermal vessels most likely propagates development of chronic laminitis. Inappropriate weight distribution and secondary changes like rotation of the third phalanx and reduction in horn quality then facilitate the formation of lesions like (Rusterholz) sole ulcers. Persistence of parasitic cysts in the dermis followed by chronic inflammation may explain why sole ulcers did not heal in SA 20 and 22 even after appropriate treatment.

Disease stages of bovine besnoitiosis are often not clearly defined in the literature. In accordance with many other authors, we use the onset of pyrexia and other common clinical findings such as depression, conjunctivitis, subcutaneous edema, lymphadenitis, and lameness to define the acute stage [1,12,21]. As scleroderma is a striking feature in chronic besnoitiosis, but not very common in mildly affected animals [2], we used the typical cysts in the scleral *conjunctivae* as determinant of the chronic stage, which is widely accepted and a common tool to detect infected animals and assess disease severity [1,2,22].

Correlation of clinical findings and laboratory test results
Results of serological and PCR examinations correlated with the course of bovine besnoitiosis in SA 6, 8, 20, and 22 (Table 2). Not surprisingly, IFAT and real-time PCR results reflected the massive parasitism in SA 20 and 22 which is in accordance with previous findings [22,36]. From a 25 mg skin sample 100 µl DNA was extracted. Hereafter, 1 µl was used for PCR. Based on previously published titrations and the assumption that a single parasite contains about 0.01 pg DNA, the number of parasites/25 mg biopsy were estimated [36]. It is possible to estimate that during the acute stage of infection SA 20 and 22 contained the DNA of between ~10^3 (equals ct-value 32.0) and ~10^4 (equals ct-value 29.0) parasites/ 25 mg of biopsy [36]. By contrast, in SA 4, less than the DNA of 10^3 parasites/25 mg skin sample (equivalent to ct-values > 32.0) was detectable during the acute stage. In SA 8 (ct-value 39.1) even less than 10^1 parasites/ 25 mg sample were found. As shown by Langenmayer et al. [33], tachyzoites disappear until the end of the acute stage and the number of cystozoites increases due

to intracystic multiplication of *B. besnoiti*. During that stage, parasite DNA per 25 mg sample in SA 20 and 22 remained almost constant (ct-values between 29.5 and 31.5, ~10^3 - 10^4 parasites per 25 mg). However, in the remaining animals with low parasite DNA skin levels in the acute stage, there was a clear decrease in the specific DNA levels during the subacute stage. Finally during the chronic stage of disease in SA 20 and 22, the mean estimate increased up to about 10^7 – 10^{10} parasites per 25 mg sample (ct-values between 11.6 and 19.5).

Although PCR suggests only a mild infection (ct-values between 23.2 and 37.6; ~ 10^1-10^6 parasites/25 mg sample) in the chronic stage, SA 6 showed a similar pattern in IFAT as SA 20 and 22. The reciprocal IFAT titer increased over time. Further, in this animal, the estimated number of parasites per 25 µg sample increased from below 10^3 in the acute stage up to 10^6 in the chronic stage (minimum ct-value: 23.2). By contrast, SA 4, which showed similar clinical signs as SA 6 during the acute stage, appeared to have successfully eliminated the parasites from the skin over time (no PCR positive skin samples in the chronic stage). This is most probably because of a pronounced immune reaction indicated by high specific antibody titers and early recognition and destruction of dermal cysts [33], leaving only few cysts behind for bradyzoites to proliferate. This pattern is further reflected by the decrease in the number of cysts found in the scleral *conjunctivae* (Figure 5), and supports findings of other studies where clinically infected animals reduce parasite load over time and remain parasite carriers [22]. Interestingly, in subclinically infected SA 8, real-time PCR of skin samples revealed that despite PCR negative results during the subacute stage, and mostly PCR negative results during the chronic stage, up to an estimate of ~10^4-10^5 parasites per 25 mg sample (minimum ct-value: 27.4) could be found in 3 of 9 samples. This supports the hypothesis that even subclinically infected cattle may contribute to the propagation of the parasite [22].

It is not clear which factor influenced the high parasite load in two animals (SA 20 and 22) during the chronic stage compared with the remaining animals. Since SA 20 and 22 were the animals with slightly higher parasite loads in the acute stage, it is tempting to speculate that higher loads in the acute stage of infection are determinant for extreme parasite loads in the chronic stage. To confirm this hypothesis and to identify the triggers, further studies analyzing cattle in both the acute and the chronic stage of infection are needed.

A potential effect of meloxicam treatment on disease progression/zoite proliferation is open to debate. However, at present, there are no such studies suggesting such an effect. In this study, Meloxicam treatment of animals was required due to animal welfare regulations (see Ethical statement). Its use most likely affected clinical signs and the sickness behavior response of affected cattle; an effect on parasite propagation, however, is most likely minor.

Disease transmission

It was beyond the scope of this study to determine routes of parasite transmission and to identify the source of *B. besnoiti* in acutely infected Simmentals. It has previously been demonstrated that *B. besnoiti* can be transmitted mechanically by hematophagous insects and also directly between cattle via the naso-pharyngeal route [2]. In this context a few possible interpretations of the circumstantial data are worth mentioning: Considering the results of PCR and histological examinations [33,34], study animals in the subacute and chronic stage exposed numerous parasitic cysts in biopsy wounds when skin samples were taken at least every other day. Thus, uptake of parasites by naïve cattle licking such wounds and by hematophagous and secretophagous insects feeding on blood and ichor may be presumed. Caught on SA 6 on the day after seroconversion, one out of 48 *S. calcitrans* specimen tested positive for *B. besnoiti* DNA. This further supports the hypothesis that this insect species may contribute to mechanical *B. besnoiti* transmission in the field.

Interestingly, SA 4 and 6 became clinically infected, when only SA 20 (in subacute stage) was frequently biopsied (Figure 2). SA 8, however, became only subclinically infected, even though four cattle in the subacute and chronic stage were frequently sampled during the assumed period of infection (> td 45). The chance for oral uptake of parasites had to be considerably higher for SA 8 compared with SA 4 and 6 (Figure 2). However, insect activity had substantially declined after td 45 when SA 8 became infected (data not shown), which fosters the hypothesis that mechanical transmission by insects may play a role in *B. besnoiti* transmission [2,37,38].

It has been suggested that close contact of cattle is pivotal for insect transmission [2,20,39]. This is supported by the finding that none of six similarly managed and sampled heifers kept at a minimal distance of 20 m to infected cattle seroconverted (Figure 1).

It is widely accepted, despite the lack of well controlled studies, that reproductive activity of cattle may represent a risk factor for parasite transmission. Some authors report that especially bulls become infected with the parasite in *B. besnoiti* affected herds [20,40], and that males may suffer from a more severe course of disease [15,26,41,42]. However, Bigalke (1968) could not confirm an effect of sex with regards to disease incidence [2]. In this particular study, reproductive activity of cattle could not be identified as a factor of parasite propagation. Chronically infected Limousins and SA 4, 6, and 8 had not been simultaneously in estrus during the respective

assumed time of infection; the bull SA 1 remained healthy (Figures 1 and 2).

In beef cattle herds, a single mature bull may serve up to 60 cows, often facilitating sexual encounters with multiple females on the same day [43]. This may not only increase the risk of indirect transmission of *B. besnoiti* but also represent an increased hazard for trauma to the mucous membranes of the bull's penis and prepuce. In this study, only eight females were served by bull SA 1. Even though the reproductive cycles of females were shortened by inducing estrus, there were periods of 24 hours and more when no heifer or cow was in heat (see Figure 2), thus the overall mechanical stress to the bull's penis and prepuce was low. Additionally, it has to be considered that encounters with chronically affected cows presenting parasitic cysts in the mucous membranes of their *vestibulum vaginae* were only observed on 17 of 84 days (Figure 2).

Conclusions

This longitudinal study provides detailed results of clinical examinations, serological and PCR tests performed on cattle in all stages of naturally acquired severe, mild and subclinical bovine besnoitiosis. It was demonstrated that recently infected animals can easily be identified by testing blood serum for antibodies twice within a 28 day interval by IFAT and/or western immunoblot. It was further shown that spatial separation of *B. besnoiti* infected and naïve cattle by at least 20 meters may minimize the risk for agent transmission. Reciprocal IFAT titers and parasite DNA loads in skin samples corresponded well with the clinical course of bovine besnoitiosis, representing an important means for herd screening tests and assessment of severity of disease. It was shown that bovine besnoitiosis-associated laminitis represents an important complication in severe chronic disease, which severely impairs animal welfare.

Additional file

> **Additional file 1: Disease history of chronically *Besnoitia besnoiti* infected study animals [SA] 13, 15, and 16: Supplementary table providing results of clinical, serological, PCR, and histological examinations of three chronically *Besnoitia besnoiti* infected, non-pregnant Limousin cows used in the cohabitation trial.**

Abbreviations
SA: Study animals; td: Trial day; *dps*: Days post seroconversion; Herd-BbGer1: First cattle herd diagnosed with cases of bovine besnoitiosis in Germany.

Competing interests
All authors declare that they or their institutions have no financial and personal relationship with other people or organizations that could inappropriately influence their work. Prionics AG, Schlieren, Switzerland, which partially funded the cohabitation study, had no influence on study design, data evaluation or writing of the manuscript.

Authors' contributions

NSG conceived of the study, designed and coordinated the clinical aspects of the investigation, performed the data analysis and wrote the manuscript. MCL and JCS carried out clinical examinations and sampling, were responsible for animal care and data management. MCL performed pathological examinations and helped to draft the manuscript. GS designed and coordinated the laboratory investigations (serology and PCR), helped to draft the manuscript and performed the respective data analysis. All authors read and approved the final manuscript.

Acknowledgements

The authors like to express their gratitude for scientific support to Dr. Burkhard Bauer and Dr. Carola Sauter-Louis, PhD. Further, we like to acknowledge the excellent technical support provided by the owner of Herd-BbGer1, Georg Muehrer, Ingrid Hartmann, Sonja Heinze, Lieselotte Minke, Andrea Bärwald, Susann Schares, Dr. Pavlo Maksimov, Aline Maksimov, Doris Merl, Michaela Nuetzel, and Heike Sperling. The authors also like to thank the owner of the Herd-BbGer1 and Prionics AG, Schlieren, Switzerland for financial support. NSG was supported by the BGF research stipend provided by the federal state of Bavaria.

Author details

[1]Clinic for Ruminants with Ambulatory and Herd Health Services at the Centre for Clinical Veterinary Medicine, Veterinary Faculty, Ludwig-Maximilians-Universitaet Muenchen, Sonnenstrasse 16, 85764 Oberschleissheim, Germany. [2]89129 Rammingen, Germany. [3]Friedrich-Loeffler-Institut, Federal Research Institute for Animal Health, Institute of Epidemiology, Suedufer 10, 17493 Greifswald-Insel Riems, Germany. [4]Institute of Veterinary Pathology at the Centre for Clinical Veterinary Medicine, Veterinary Faculty, Ludwig-Maximilians-Universitaet Muenchen, Veterinaerstr. 13, 80539 Munich, Germany.

References

1. Bigalke RD, Prozesky L. Besnoitiosis. In: Coetzer JAW, Tuskin RC, editors. Infectious diseases of livestock. Volume 1, 2nd edn. Cape Town: Oxford University Press Southern Africa; 2004. p. 351–9.
2. Bigalke RD. New concepts on the epidemiological features of bovine besnoitiosis as determined by laboratory and field investigations. Onderstepoort J Vet Res. 1968;35(1):3–137.
3. Cuillé J, Chelle PL, Berlureau F. Transmission expèrimentale de la maladie dènommèe "Sarcosporidiose cutanée" du boeuf (Besnoit et Robin) et déterminée par "Globidium Besnoiti". Bull Acad Med. 1936;115:161–3.
4. Pols JW. The artificical transmission of Globidium besnoiti (Marotel) 1912, to cattle and rabbits. J S Afr Vet Assoc. 1954;25(2):37.
5. Alvarez-Garcia G, Garcia-Lunar P, Gutierrez-Exposito D, Shkap V, Ortega-Mora LM. Dynamics of Besnoitia besnoiti infection in cattle. Parasitology. 2014;141(11):1419–35.
6. Cortes H, Leitao A, Gottstein B, Hemphill A. A review on bovine besnoitiosis: a disease with economic impact in herd health management, caused by Besnoitia besnoiti (Franco and Borges). Parasitology. 2014;141(11):1406–17.
7. Majzoub M, Breuer W, Gollnick NS, Rostaher A, Schares G, Hermanns W. Ein Ausbruch von boviner Besnoitiose bei Rindern in Deutschland; pathomorphologische, ultrastrukturelle und molekularbiologische Untersuchungen. Wien Tierärztl Mschr Vet Med Austria. 2010;97(1–2):9–15.
8. Basson PA, McCully RM, Bigalke RD. Observations on the pathogenesis of bovine and antelope strains of Besnoitia besnoiti (Marotel, 1912) infection in cattle and rabbits. Onderstepoort J Vet Res. 1970;37(2):105–26.
9. Bigalke RD, Naudé TW. The diagnostic value of cysts in the scleral conjunctiva in bovine besnoitiosis. Jl S Afr Vet Med Ass. 1962;33:21–7.
10. Rostaher A, Mueller RS, Majzoub M, Schares G, Gollnick NS. Bovine besnoitiosis in Germany. Vet Dermatol. 2010;21(4):329–34.
11. Gentile A, Militerno G, Schares G, Nanni A, Testoni S, Bassi P, et al. Evidence for bovine besnoitiosis being endemic in Italy - first in vitro isolation of Besnoitia besnoiti from cattle born in Italy. Vet Parasitol. 2012;184(2–4):108–15.
12. Alvarez-Garcia G, Frey CF, Mora LM, Schares G. A century of bovine besnoitiosis: an unknown disease re-emerging in Europe. Trends Parasitol. 2013;29(8):407–15.
13. Diesing L, Heydorn AO, Matuschka FR, Bauer C, Pipano E, de Waal DT, et al. Besnoitia besnoiti: studies on the definitive host and experimental infections in cattle. Parasitol Res. 1988;75(2):114–7.
14. Basso W, Schares G, Gollnick NS, Rutten M, Deplazes P. Exploring the life cycle of Besnoitia besnoiti - experimental infection of putative definitive and intermediate host species. Vet Parasitol. 2011;178(3–4):223–34.
15. Cortes H, Leitao A, Vidal R, Vila-Vicosa MJ, Ferreira ML, Caeiro V, et al. Besnoitiosis in bulls in Portugal. Vet Rec. 2005;157(9):262–4.
16. Besnoit C, Robin V. Sarcosporidiose cutanée chez une vache. Rev Vét. 1912;37(11):649–63.
17. McCully RM, Basson PA, Van Niekerk JW, Bigalke RD. Observations on Besnoitia cysts in the cardio-vascular system of some wild antelopes and cattle. Onderstepoort J Vet Res. 1966;33:245–76.
18. Pols JW. Studies on bovine besnoitiosis with special reference to the aetiology. Onderstepoort J Vet Res. 1960;28:265–356.
19. Hofmeyr CFB. Globidiosis in cattle. JS Afr Vet Med Assoc. 1945;16:102–9.
20. Schulz KCA. A report on naturally acquired besnoitiosis in bovines with special reference to its pathology. JS Afr Vet Med Assoc. 1960;31:21–35.
21. Jacquiet P, Lienard E, Franc M. Bovine besnoitiosis: epidemiological and clinical aspects. Vet Parasitol. 2010;174(1–2):30–6.
22. Frey CF, Gutierrez-Exposito D, Ortega-Mora LM, Benavides J, Marcen JM, Castillo JA, et al. Chronic bovine besnoitiosis: Intra-organ parasite distribution, parasite loads and parasite-associated lesions in subclinical cases. Vet Parasitol. 2013;197:95–103.
23. Hornok S, Fedak A, Baska F, Hofmann-Lehmann R, Basso W. Bovine besnoitiosis emerging in Central-Eastern Europe, Hungary. Parasites Vectors. 2014;7(1):20.
24. Basso W, Lesser M, Grimm F, Hilbe M, Sydler T, Trosch L, et al. Bovine besnoitiosis in Switzerland: imported cases and local transmission. Vet Parasitol. 2013;198(3–4):265–73.
25. Fernandez-Garcia A, Alvarez-Garcia G, Risco-Castillo V, Aguado-Martinez A, Marcen JM, Rojo-Montejo S, et al. Development and use of an indirect ELISA in an outbreak of bovine besnoitiosis in Spain. Vet Rec. 2010;166(26):818–22.
26. Gollnick NS, Gentile A, Schares G. Diagnosis of bovine besnoitiosis in a bull born in Italy. Vet Rec. 2010;166(19):599.
27. EFSA. Bovine besnoitiosis: an emerging disease in Europe. Scientific statement on bovine besnoitiosis of the European Food Safety Authority. EFSA J. 2010;8(2):1499.
28. Schares G, Basso W, Majzoub M, Cortes HC, Rostaher A, Selmair J, et al. First in vitro isolation of Besnoitia besnoiti from chronically infected cattle in Germany. Vet Parasitol. 2009;163(4):315–22.
29. Schares G, Basso W, Majzoub M, Rostaher A, Scharr JC, Langenmayer MC, et al. Comparative evaluation of immunofluorescent antibody and new immunoblot tests for the specific detection of antibodies against Besnoitia besnoiti tachyzoites and bradyzoites in bovine sera. Vet Parasitol. 2010;171(1–2):32–40.
30. Schares G, Peters M, Wurm R, Barwald A, Conraths FJ. The efficiency of vertical transmission of Neospora caninum in dairy cattle analysed by serological techniques. Vet Parasitol. 1998;80(1):87–98.
31. Edmonson AJ, Lean IJ, Weaver LD, Farver T, Webster G. A body condition scoring chart for Holstein dairy cows. J Dairy Sci. 1989;72:68–78.
32. Sprecher DJ, Hostetler DE, Kaneene JB. A lameness scoring system that uses posture and gait to predict dairy cattle reproductive performance. Theriogenology. 1997;47(6):1179–87.
33. Langenmayer MC, Gollnick NS, Majzoub-Altweck M, Scharr JC, Schares G, Hermanns W. Naturally acquired bovine besnoitiosis: histological and immunohistochemical findings in acute, subacute, and chronic disease. Vet Pathol. 2014. [Epub ahead of print].
34. Schares G, Langenmayer MC, Scharr JC, Minke L, Maksimov P, Maksimov A, et al. Novel tools for the diagnosis and differentiation of acute and chronic bovine besnoitiosis. Int J Parasitol. 2013;43:143–54.
35. Hermanns W, Liebig K, Schulz LC. Postembedding immunohistochemical demonstration of antigen in experimental polyarthritis using plastic embedded whole joints. Histochemistry. 1981;73(3):439–46.
36. Schares G, Maksimov A, Basso W, More G, Dubey JP, Rosenthal B, et al. Quantitative real time polymerase chain reaction assays for the sensitive detection of Besnoitia besnoiti infection in cattle. Vet Parasitol. 2011;178(3–4):208–16.
37. Lienard E, Salem A, Grisez C, Prevot F, Bergeaud JP, Franc M, et al. A longitudinal study of Besnoitia besnoiti infections and seasonal abundance of Stomoxys calcitrans in a dairy cattle farm of southwest France. Vet Parasitol. 2011;177(1–2):20–7.

38. Olias P, Schade B, Mehlhorn H. Molecular pathology, taxonomy and epidemiology of *Besnoitia* species (Protozoa: Sarcocystidae). Infect Genet Evol. 2011;11(7):1564–76.

39. Alzieu JP, Jaquiet P, Lienard E, Franc M. New data on kinetics of infection by besnoitiosis in cattle herds from endemic and non-endemic french areas. In: Proceedings of the European Buiatrics Forum: November 16–18 2011; Marceille, France. 2011. p. 25.

40. Neuman M. Serological survey of *Besnoitia besnoiti* (Marotel 1912) infection in Israel by immunofluorescence. Zentralbl Veterinarmed B. 1972;19:391–6.

41. Ferrié JJ. La besnoitiose bovine. Revue bibliographique. Observations personelles. France: Thesis, Ecole Nationale Vétérinaire de Toulouse; 1984. p. 288.

42. Legrand P. La besnoitiose bovine en Ariège. France: Thesis. Ecole Nationale Vétérinaire de Toulouse; 2003. p. 87.

43. Chenoweth PJ. Bull libido/serving capacity. Vet Clin North Am Food Anim Pract. 1997;13(2):331–44.

11

Feasibility and safety of intrathecal transplantation of autologous bone marrow mesenchymal stem cells in horses

Leandro Maia[1], Fernanda da Cruz Landim- Alvarenga[1], Marilda Onghero Taffarel[2], Carolina Nogueira de Moraes[1], Gisele Fabrino Machado[3], Guilherme Dias Melo[3] and Rogério Martins Amorim[4*]

Abstract

Background: Recent studies have demonstrated numerous biological properties of mesenchymal stem cells and their potential application in treating complex diseases or injuries to tissues that have difficulty regenerating, such as those affecting the central and peripheral nervous system. Thus, therapies that use mesenchymal stem cells are promising because of their high capacity for self-regeneration, their low immunogenicity, and their paracrine, anti-inflammatory, immunomodulatory, anti-apoptotic and neuroprotective effects. In this context, the purpose of this study was to evaluate the feasibility and safety of intrathecal transplantation of bone marrow-derived mesenchymal stem cells in horses, for future application in the treatment of neurological diseases.

Results: During the neurological evaluations, no clinical signs were observed that were related to brain and/or spinal cord injury of the animals from the control group or the treated group. The hematological and cerebrospinal fluid results from day 1 and day 6 showed no significant differences ($P > 0.05$) between the treated group and the control group. Additionally, analysis of the expression of matrix metalloproteinase (MMP) -2 and −9 in the cerebrospinal fluid revealed only the presence of pro-MMP-2 (latent), with no significant difference ($P > 0.05$) between the studied groups.

Conclusions: The results of the present study support the hypothesis of the feasibility and safety of intrathecal transplantation of autologous bone marrow-derived mesenchymal stem cells, indicating that it is a promising pathway for cell delivery for the treatment of neurological disorders in horses.

Keywords: Mesenchymal stem cells, Transplantation, Horse, Matrix metalloproteinases, Neurology

Background

Recent studies have demonstrated numerous biological properties of mesenchymal stem cells (MSCs), as well their potential application to treat complex diseases or injuries to tissues that have difficulty regenerating, such as those that affect the central and peripheral nervous system. Thus, stem cell therapy is a promising alternative for the treatment of these diseases because of the high capacity for self-regeneration, the low immunogenicity, and the paracrine, anti-inflammatory, immunomodulatory, anti-apoptotic and neuroprotective effects of MSCs.

During ischemic damage or severe tissue damage, MSCs can be attracted to the site of injury, where they secrete bioactive factors that influence the process of tissue repair and regeneration [1]. According to Baraniak and McDevitt [2], stem and progenitor cells are able to produce and secrete a large number of factors, including growth, angiogenic, antifibrotic, anti-inflammatory and immunosuppressive factors and compounds responsible for the homeostasis of the extracellular matrix (collagen, TIMPs and matrix metalloproteinases (MMPs), as well as antioxidants and anti-apoptotic molecules that play important roles in the regenerative process. In addition to producing cytokines, chemokines, growth factors and extracellular matrix molecules, it is noteworthy that stem/progenitor cells play an important role in the consume of

* Correspondence: rmamorim@fmvz.unesp.br
[4]Department of Veterinary Clinics, São Paulo State University, District of Rubião Júnior, n/n, CEP: 18618970, Botucatu, São Paulo, Brazil
Full list of author information is available at the end of the article

pro-apoptotic factors and inflammatory molecules [2]. All these properties are great attractions for the use of cell therapy in many diseases that affect animals and humans. However, preclinical and clinical trial data are fundamental to provide the scientific basis in support of stem cell therapy. The therapeutic window, the strategy of cell delivery, the cell doses and the possible secondary effects should be evaluated in clinical studies [1]. Because horses are commonly affected by musculoskeletal, neurological and reproductive disorders, the equine species can be used as a model for experimental MSCs therapy.

MSCs derived from the bone marrow (BM) and adipose tissue are the two most common types of stem cells used in therapeutic approaches to repair and/or regenerate tissues in horses [3]. The studies involving MSCs therapy of horses have focused mainly on osteoarticular and tendon injuries [4-9], with few reports of its use in other tissues, such as the nervous system. Thus, the application pathways most used until now for the clinical treatment of horses are intralesional and intra-articular. Preclinical studies that evaluated the safety of MSCs transplantation by other pathways, such as intrathecal, are lacking in equine medicine. An intrathecal injection is less invasive than an intralesional injection, can extensively deliver cells through the cerebrospinal fluid (CSF) [10] and is a more feasible routine for treatment of equine CNS injuries.

In this context, the purpose of this study was to evaluate the feasibility and safety of intrathecal transplantation of autologous bone marrow mesenchymal stem cells (BM-MSCs) in horses.

Results
Cultivation, characterization and differentiation capacities of the BM-MSCs
The cells from the mononuclear fraction of the BM exhibited adherence to the culture dish between 24 and 48 hours and fibroblastoid morphology starting at four days of cultivation. Confluence ($\geq$80%) and homogeneity of the culture were obtained after approximately three week of cell culture.

The immunophenotyping analysis revealed a high level of expression of the CD90 marker ($\bar{x} = 97 \pm 1.3\%$), a lower level of expression of the CD44 marker ($\bar{x} = 71 \pm 10.7\%$) and the lack of expression of the CD34 marker ($\bar{x} = 0.8 \pm 0.2\%$).

The differentiation potential of the MSCs was demonstrated *in vitro* by a positive response to the osteogenic, adipogenic and chondrogenic differentiation media by the tenth, eighth and twenty-first day of exposure, respectively.

The MSCs that initially had a fibroblastoid morphology acquired a predominantly polygonal morphology after exposure to the osteogenic medium and deposited large amounts of calcium-rich extracellular matrix, as shown by positive staining with Alizarin red (Figure 1a).

Adipogenic differentiation was confirmed by the deposition of lipid droplets in the cytoplasm, as demonstrated by positive staining with oil red O (Figure 1b). Chondrogenic differentiation was confirmed by the deposition of a hyaline matrix rich in proteoglycans, as demonstrated by positive staining with toluidine blue and Alcian blue (Figures 1c and d).

BM-MSCs transplantation
The anesthetic protocol used for the BM-MSC transplantation, including the CSF tap, proved to be appropriate and safe for both groups. No animal showed clinical alterations or allergic reactions that could be attributed to the BM-MSC transplantation, compared with the control group (CG).

Clinical and neurological evaluations
Neither clinical nor neurological alterations were observed in the treated group (TG) or CG animals during the exams conducted pre- and post-transplantation. All the animals exhibited a normal locomotion pattern (grade 0), and neurological deficits were not detected, according to the classification of Mayhew *et al.* [11]. In addition, no significant alterations in the integrity of the brain (mental state, behavior, head position and cranial nerve functions) were observed during the neurological examinations performed for both groups.

Hematological analysis
The median values obtained for the hematological variables (hematocrit, total protein, platelets, fibrinogen, total leukocytes, neutrophils, lymphocytes, basophils and monocytes) before (Day 1) and after transplantation (Day 6) are presented in Table 1. There were no significant differences ($P > 0.05$) between the values for the TG and CG groups or between the values at the chosen time points. However, the only variable that increased ($p < 0.05$) in both groups pre and post-transplantation was basophil, but there was no difference between groups. It is noteworthy that this increase was not accompanied by eosinophilia.

CSF analysis
The CSF samples collected from the animals in both groups were clear, colorless and not coagulated, both pre- and post-transplantation.

No significant differences ($p > 0.05$) between the CG and the TG pre- (day 1) and post-transplantation (day 6) were observed in the CSF density or pH, or the contents of red blood cells, nucleated cells, globulins, proteins, glucose, and pro-MMP-2, as shown in Table 2. Moreover, no significant changes ($p > 0.05$) in the CSF data obtained pre- and post-BM-MSC transplantation were observed in the TG or the CG.

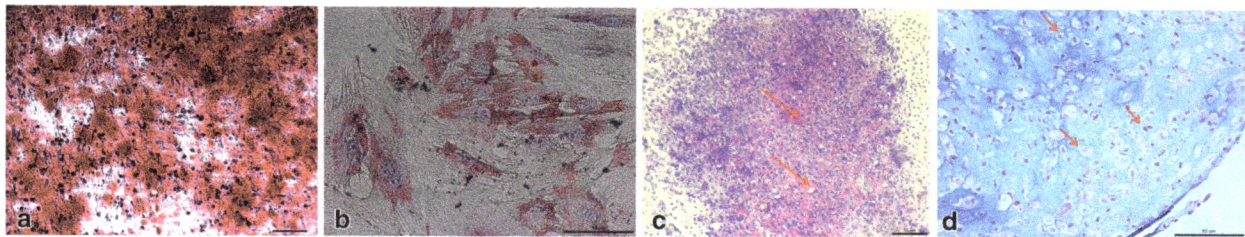

Figure 1 Differentiation assay of mesenchymal stem cells for osteogenic, adipogenic and chondrogenic lineages. (a) Osteogenic differentiation. Note calcium deposits stained with Alizarin red. **(b)** Adipogenic differentiation. Note the intracellular presence of lipid droplets stained with Oil red. **(c, d)** Chondrogenic differentiation. **(c)** Toluidin blue staining. Note the presence of metachromatic areas in pink (red arrow) indicating the presence of extracellular matrix containing proteoglycans. **(d)** Alcian blue staining. Note the presence of areas in blue indicating the presence of extracellular matrix containing proteoglycans beyond the presence of gaps (red arrow) possibly containing chondrocytes. Bar = 50 μm.

Expression of MMP-2 and -9 in CSF

Only the presence of pro-MMP-2 (inactive/latent) was detected in the CSF from the animals in the two groups; the differences between the values for the groups and the values for the same group at the different time points were not significant (P > 0.05) (Table 2). Latent or activated forms of MMP-9 were not detected in any of the CSF samples.

Discussion

In the present study, the safety of MSCs transplantation through the CSF was demonstrated by the results obtained from laboratory analysis and by the absence of alterations in the studied groups. The most interesting finding of our study was the absence of the expression of MMP-2 and MMP-9 in the CSF, particularly in their activated forms, after BM-MSC transplantation.

Characterization and differentiation assays of the MSCs

In the present study, the BM-MSCs isolated from the horses were characterized according to the criteria established by the International Society of Cellular Therapy for human MSCs [12]; i.e., they demonstrated the characteristics of adherence to plastic, fibroblastoid morphology, high expression of the CD90 marker (>95% positive), no expression of the hematopoietic cell marker CD34, and they responded positively to osteogenic, adipogenic and chondrogenic differentiation media. Furthermore, the expression of CD44 (hyaluronic acid-receptor), a surface glycoprotein important for the interactions and cell adhesion of MSCs, was also observed.

Some of these characteristics of the MSCs observed by our group have also been reported in studies that characterized the MSCs from equine adipose tissue [8,13],

Table 1 Median of hematological variables before and after the treatments of treated groups (TG) and control (CG)

Variables	Before transplantation			After transplantation	
	Groups			Groups	
	CG	TG		CG	TG
Hematocrit (%)	36	33		29	32
Protein (mg/dL)	7.2	7.6		7.0	7.6
Platelets (plt/μL^{-1})	182000	151000		193000	176000
Fibrinogen (mg/dL)	200	200		400	400
Leukocytes (cells μL^{-1})	7300	11000		7300	8700
Neutrophils (cells μL^{-1})	3790	4290		4200	5307
Lymphocytes (cells μL^{-1})	2714	4712		2709	3132
Eosinophils (cells μL^{-1})	448	284		248	174
Basophils (cells μL^{-1})	0	0		126*	315*
Monocytes (cells μL^{-1})	192	426		248	312

*Asterisk represents difference (P < 0.05) between moments (before and after transplantation) by the Wilcoxon test.
All values were presented as median.

Table 2 Median of CFS variables before and after the treatments of treated groups (TG) and control (CG)

Variables	Before transplantation		After transplantation	
	Groups		Groups	
	CG	TG	CG	TG
Density	1006	1006	1006	1006
pH	8.5	8.5	8.5	8.5
Red blood cells (cells μL^{-1})	0	1	3	1
Nucleated cells (cells μL^{-1})	0	0	4	0
Globulins	0	0	0	0
Proteins ($mg\ dL^{-1}$)	34	46.1	42.5	58.2
Glucose ($mg\ dL^{-1}$)	54	57	57	55
pro-MMP2 (AU)	34.43	31.86	42.8	28.69

Differences (P < 0.05) between moments and treatments were not observed for none of the variables.
AU: arbitrary units.
All values were presented as median.

bone marrow [14-16], peripheral blood [17], the matrix of the umbilical cord [18], amniotic fluid [19], gingival tissue and periodontal ligaments [20].

BM-MSC transplantation

Concern with the safety of BM-MSCs intrathecal transplantation through the atlanto-occipital space of the horses in the TG guided the selection of the vehicle to be for the cells and the method of preparing the cells. Thus, the BM-MSCs were washed three times to remove residual fetal bovine serum (FBS) that could induce an immune response in the animals. This measure appeared to be adequate because the animals displayed no changes after the transplantation. There is strong concern regarding the use of FBS in the culture medium, particularly for humans, considering that in addition to the possibility of immune reactions, prions, viruses and zoonotic agents could be transferred [21,22]. According to Dimarakis and Levicar [21], serum contains a variety of proteins that can bind to the cultured cells, thereby serving as antigens for immunological reactions after transplantation. Due to the controversy regarding the use of FBS, Toupadaskis et al. [23] used equine MSCs to study the possibility of substituting FBS with autologous serum (AS), and showed that the rate of cell proliferation with FBS was higher (P <0.05) than with AS. Therefore, the authors suggested that substituting only AS may not be a viable alternative for cell expansion under the current experimental conditions and that further studies must be directed at determining methods whereby immunogenicity can be reduced without affecting the growth rate of the MSCs. Additionally, these methods could include the initial culture and cell expansion with FBS and subsequent cell expansion with AS to reduce the immunogenic potential [23].

The phosphate-buffered solution (PBS) vehicle used for transplantation/in both groups was shown to be adequate

and safe, as demonstrated by the absence of complications, particularly in the CG. This vehicle has been used in experimentally induced tendinopathy in horses [7].

The concentration of the BM-MSCs transplanted in this pre-clinical study was similar to that used by Lim et al. [24] for lumbar administration to a rat model of stroke induced by occlusion of the middle cerebral artery. In their study, doses of 10^5 and 10^6 MSCs derived from the blood of human umbilical cords that were administered intrathecally had significant effects on recovery from ischemic damage. These findings support the hypothesis that BM-MSC transplantation via an intrathecal pathway is feasible and safe, and suggest great prospects for the use of cell therapy in treating neurological diseases in other species.

Clinical evaluation

The absence of clinical alterations, including neurological signs, observed in the TG under the conditions of this study demonstrated that the procedures performed did not dramatically change the neural environment, indicating that a CSF pathway can be used for BM-MSCs transplantation in horses. In laboratory studies of animals and humans, the CSF pathway has been used for the transplantation of mononuclear cells and allogeneic MSCs, without evidence of serious adverse effects [24,25].

In a study conducted with 114 humans affected by degenerative conditions (paraplegia, ataxia and multiple sclerosis), Yang et al. [25] performed a total of 592 intrathecal and intravenous administrations of allogeneic mononuclear cells from umbilical cord blood without observing serious adverse effects. The most common collateral effect (19/592, 3.2%) was headache, which was attributed to postural hypotension, a known complication of lumbar puncture that resolves spontaneously without the need for drastic interventions.

Hematological and CSF analyses

The CSF performs four major functions in the central nervous system (CNS), including the physical support of the neural structure, excretion, intracerebral transport and control of the chemical environment of the CNS [26]. Among these functions, the one that motivated us to conduct this study was the possibility of the CSF transporting MSCs, which have the potential to migrate, to sites of injury.

The transplantations performed in our study did not cause significant differences in the CSF values (p > 0.05) of the TG and CG. The density of the CSF [27] and its contents of erythrocytes, nucleated cells, protein and glucose [28] pre- and post-transplantation were within the normal ranges for the equine species. The pre- and post-transplantation pH values obtained using reagent strips were also considered normal in the laboratory where the analysis was conducted.

The median pre- and post-transplantation values for the pro-MMP-2 contents of the CSF from the CG and TG were similar to the average value (43.12 ± 13.90) determined by Melo *et al.* [29] in healthy dogs that were used as controls in a study conducted recently to evaluate the expression of MMP-2 and MMP-9 in the CSF and serum of dogs with neurological signs and visceral leishmaniasis. Our results cannot be compared with those of other studies conducted with equine species due to the difficulty of finding information in the literature about the MMP contents in the CSF of this species. Thus, the values obtained, particularly the pre-transplantation values for pro-MMP-2, will serve as a reference for further studies.

Similarly, the values for the hematological variables also did not differ (P > 0.05) between the groups or between the time points studied, demonstrating that the treatments did not affect those variables.

Expression of MMP-2 and -9 in CSF

MMPs are a family of zinc- and calcium-dependent endopeptidases that are responsible for degrading and remodeling the extracellular matrix, including its collagen, elastin, gelatin, proteoglycan and glycoprotein components [30]. An important characteristic of MMPs is their latency. These proteases are secreted in a pro-form (inactive/latent), requiring activation by a variety of mechanisms before becoming functional [31]. In the present study, the activity of only pro-MMP-2 (gelatinase A) was identified in the CSF, with no difference (P > 0,05) between the values of the groups or of each group at the two time points studied. According to Rosenberg [31], gelatinase A is a constitutively expressed molecule that is normally found in brain tissue and CSF. MMP-2 has been demonstrated in the astrocytic processes of normal brain, particularly those adjacent to vessels, the ependymal cells and the pia mater. The presence of MMP-2 in the astrocytic processes near the surface of the brain suggests that this metalloenzyme may play a role in the homeostasis of the brain fluid or in regulating the blood–brain barrier. Bergman *et al.* [32], who studied 23 clinically healthy dogs, also obtained results similar to ours, observing only the presence of pro-MMP-2 and the absence of MMP-9 in the CSF.

The lack of evidence for latent or active MMP-9 (gelatinase B), particularly in the group treated with MSCs, supports the hypothesis that the transplantation pathway tested by our group is safe, considering that according to Rosenberg [31], MMP-9 is markedly dysregulated under the inflammatory conditions of many diseases. High levels of MMP-9 have been observed in the CSF of human patients and animals affected by neurological diseases that involve intense neuroinflammation, such as visceral leishmaniasis [29], traumatic cerebral injury [33], meningitis [34,35] and multiple sclerosis [36].

Conclusion

Intrathecal transplantation of autologous BM-MSCs in horses does not cause clinical alterations, particularly in the variables evaluated in the neurological examinations and the hematological and CSF analyses, including the expression of MMPs. Therefore, this pathway for the delivery BM-MSCs was shown to be feasible and safe, raising the possibility of performing future clinical trials to treat neurological diseases in horses.

Methods

Animals

Ten healthy crossbred horses of both sexes (5 males and 5 females), aged between 4 and 12 years 300 to 500 Kg were used. The animals were selected based on prior clinical, hematological and neurological evaluations.

The experimental protocol (number 76/2009 - CEUA) was approved by the ethics committee of São Paulo State University, Botucatu, Brazil. All the procedures were performed according to the international guidelines for the care and use of experimental animals.

Experimental delineation

The selected animals were randomly divided into two groups; one group was transplanted with BM-MSC (TG, n = 5) and the other, which was the control group, received PBS (CG, n = 5). First, the bone marrow (BM) obtained using needle aspiration was used for to isolate, expand and characterize the BM-MSCs. After the characterization, the cells were transplanted intrathecally into the TG through the cisterna magna. In this same period, the animals from the CG received the same volume of PBS by the same pathway.

The safety of intrathecal BM-MSC transplantation was monitored by daily clinical and neurological examinations during the period of thirty days (day 1 until day 31), as well as by hematological and CSF analysis, including examining the expression of the latent and activated forms MMP-2 and −9 in the CSF (Figure 2).

Bone marrow collection

BM aspiration was performed according to the methodology described by Barreira *et al.* [37], with modifications. For this, the animals were maintained on quadrupedal position, physically restrained and sedated with 0.5 mg kg^{-1} xylazine (Sedomin®, Koning, ARG). Then it was performed shaving of an area of 5 × 20 cm related to the sternum of each horse. After identification of the fifth sternebrae it was performed antisepsis and local anesthetic block (Xylestesin® 2% Cristália, BRA). Once fixed, the bone marrow needle, Komiyashiki model, within the sternum, the mandrel was removed and proceeded to the aspiration of BM with the aid of two 20 mL syringes containing 2 mL of heparin (Hemofol, Cristália, BRA) and 2 mL of PBS, pH 7.2 (PBS 1×, LCG Biotechnology, BRA). After collection, the samples were identified and forwarded to the laboratory for processing.

Isolation and cultivation of BM- MSC

The isolation and cultivation of BM-MSCs were performed according to the methodology described by Maia *et al.* [38]. The mononuclear fraction from the samples of BM was cultured in low-glucose DMEM /F12 (1:1), 20% fetal bovine serum, penicillin/streptomycin (1%) and amphotericin B (1.2%) (Gibco Invitrogen, USA) at 37.5°C in a humid atmosphere containing 95% air and 5% CO2. The maintenance medium was changed every 2 or 3 days until a minimum of 80% cellular confluence was reached, and then the cells were recovered by trypsinization for characterization and use in treatment.

Flow cytometric analysis of cell surface markers

The immunophenotypic analysis of the BM-MSCs was performed on the primary cultured cells, using a FACS-Calibur cytometer (Becton Dickinson and Company, USA) using monoclonal mouse anti-rat CD90 (clone OX7, 1:100, Caltag Laboratories, USA) and mouse anti-human CD34 (clone 581/CD34, 1:50, Becton Dickinson and Company, USA) antibodies labeled with fluorescein isothiocyanate (FITC) and a mouse anti-horse CD44 (clone CVS18, 1:100, AbD Serotec, USA) antibody that was detected using an FITC-conjugated goat anti-mouse secondary antibody (1:200, Molecular Probes, USA). During the analysis, 10,000 events were recorded.

Assays of osteogenic, adipogenic and chondrogenic differentiation

After reaching confluence in the primary culture, BM-MSCs were trypsinized and seeded at a density of 2 × 10^5 MSCs/well, in six-well plates (Sarstedt, USA). After 48 hours, the maintenance medium was removed and media for osteogenic or adipogenic differentiation StemPro (Gibco Invitrogen, USA) were added to the subcultures, in triplicate, according to the manufacturer's recommendation with modifications. The adipogenic medium was supplemented with 5% rabbit serum. The media were changed every 2 to 3 days and confirmation of osteogenic and adipogenic differentiation was obtained, respectively, by demonstrating the deposition of a calcium-containing matrix using the histological method of staining with 2% Alizarin red, pH 4.2 and the presence of intracytoplasmic lipid droplets by staining with 0.5% oil red O (Sigma-Aldrich Corp., USA).

For chondrogenic differentiation, the BM-MSCs were cultivated at a density of 10^6 MSCs/mL in a 3D pellet in a Falcon tube (15 mL) for 21 days in StemPro chondrogenic differentiation medium that was changed every three days. To confirm that chondrogenic differentiation

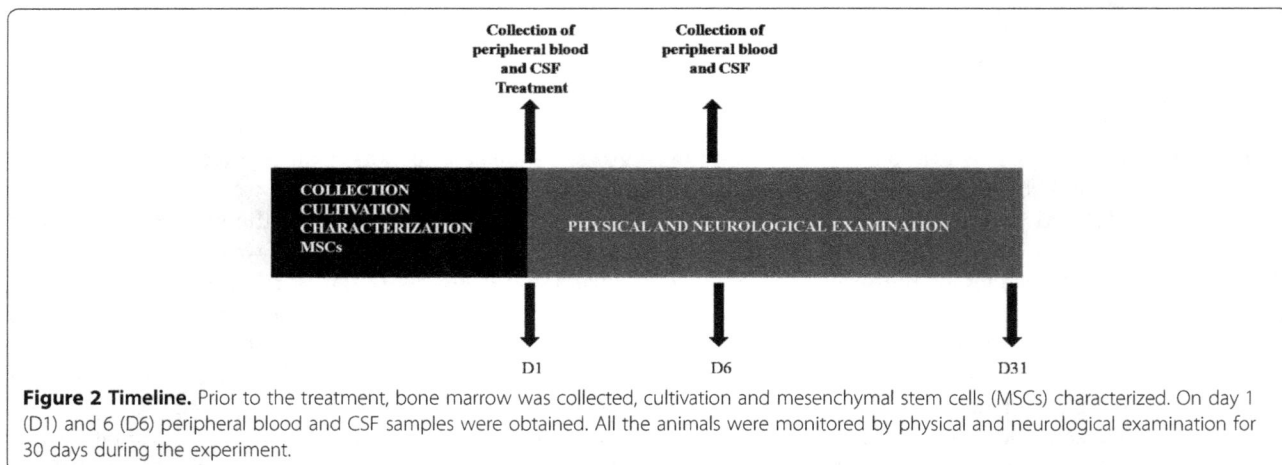

Figure 2 Timeline. Prior to the treatment, bone marrow was collected, cultivation and mesenchymal stem cells (MSCs) characterized. On day 1 (D1) and 6 (D6) peripheral blood and CSF samples were obtained. All the animals were monitored by physical and neurological examination for 30 days during the experiment.

had occurred, the pellets were stained with Alcian Blue, pH 2.5, and toluidine blue, pH 1, which detect proteoglycans [39].

Collection of blood and hematological analysis

The blood samples for the hematological analyses were collected from the TG and CG animals immediately before (day 1) and on six days (day 6) after the intrathecal transplantation.

Aliquots of 4 mL of blood were collected by puncture of the external jugular vein into tubes containing anticoagulant (Vacutainer BD, USA). The blood in the EDTA-containing tubes were used to determine the hematocrit, total plasma protein, number of platelets, fibrinogen content, total leukocyte count and the differential cell count. The total leukocytes and platelet counts were performed using a cell counter (HemaScreen 18, Ebram, BRA).

Collection and analysis of CSF

CSF was collected from the animals in both groups through the atlanto-occipital space, according to the technique described by Mayhew [40], immediately before BM-MSC transplantation (TG) or PBS inoculation (CG) (day 1) and subsequently in day 6. All horses were sedated with 0.5 mg/kg xylazine (Sedomin®, Koning, ARG), followed by induction of anaesthesia with ketamine (3 mg/kg) (Cetamin, Rhobifarma, BRA) associate with diazepan (0,1 mg/kg) (Compaz, Cristália, BRA). After orotracheal intubation, anaesthesia was maintained with isoflurane (Isoforine, Cristália, BRA) in oxygen. Ventilation was controlled with a tidal volume of 10 ml/kg and 10 breaths per minute.

The physical variables of the CSF that were evaluated were the appearance, color and coagulation; the density was determined using refractometry and the pH determined using a reagent strip. For the cytological analysis, the total number of cells in the undiluted CSF samples was counted using a Neubauer chamber, and the differential counts were performed after cytocentrifugation (Revan centrifuge 2000 D).

In the biochemical analysis, the concentrations of protein and glucose in the CSF samples were determined using commercial kits (Micropote kit, Doles, BRA and Glucose kit, Katal, BRA, respectively), according to the manufacturers' recommendations.

The possible presence of globulins in the CSF was determined by the Pandy test, in which 1 mL of Pandy reagent is mixed and homogenized with a few drops of CSF. In the case of a positive test, the results for the intensity of the turbidity observed macroscopically were represented using one to four crosses.

Immediately after the collection, CSF samples from each of the animals in the TG and the CG were cryopreserved for subsequent evaluation of their contents of MMP-2 and MMP-9 using zymography.

BM-MSC transplantation

Prior to transplantation, the BM-MSCs were trypsinized and washed three times with filtered DMEM medium by centrifugation at 250 g to remove residual fetal bovine serum which could induce allergic and/or immune responses in the animals in the treated group (TG, n = 5). After this procedure, the pelleted BM-MSCs were suspended in 2 mL of PBS for immediate transplantation. The TG received on average approximately 1×10^6 BM-MSCs suspended in 2 mL of PBS intrathecally through the atlanto-occipital space using the technique and anesthesia described previously. The control group (CG, N = 5) received 2 mL of PBS (placebo) by the same pathway.

Clinical and neurological evaluations

After treating of the CG and TG animals, physical examinations were performed daily for thirty days, to evaluate behavior, posture, degree of hydration, staining of the mucosa, capillary refill time, heart rate, respiratory rate, body temperature and bowel movements and to determine the body condition score.

The evaluation of the integrity of the brain (mental state, behavior, head position and cranial nerve functions) and spinal cord was performed as described by Malikides et al. [41] and Mayhew [42].

During the neurological examinations of the TG and CG animals, locomotion was evaluated using the classification system of ataxia and paresis described by Mayhew et al. [11], as follows:

Degree 0 (normal) – deficit not detected.
Degree 1 – deficit barely detected at a normal gait or posture.
Degree 2 – deficit easily detected, and exaggerated by backing, turning, swaying, loin pressure and neck extension.
Degree 3 – deficit very prominent at a normal gait with a tendency to buckle or fall with backing, turning, swaying, loin pressure and neck extension.
Degree 4 – stumbling, tripping and falling spontaneously at a normal gait, and more severe deficits.

Analysis of MMPs using the technique of gelatin zymography

The latent (pro-) and activated forms of MMP-2 and –9 were analyzed using zymography and densitometry, according to the methods described by Melo et al. [29] and Marangoni et al. [43]. Briefly, a volume containing an equal amount of total protein was incubated in the sample buffer (125 mM Tris–HCl, pH 6.8; 20% v/v glycerol, 4% w/v SDS, 0.2% w/v bromophenol blue) without boiling and submitted to electrophoresis with polyacrylamide gels (10%) copolymerized with gelatin (G8150-100G, Sigma–Aldrich). The gels were rinsed in 2.5% Triton X-100 for 30 min and incubated in the enzymatic activation buffer (50 mM Tris, 200 mM NaCl, 5 mM CaCl$_2$, 0.2% w/v Brij-35, pH 7.5), for 20 h at 37°C with gentle shaking, which allows gelatin digestion by both latent and active forms of MMPs. The gels were stained (0.5% w/v Coomassie brilliant blue R-250, 45% v/v methanol, 10% v/v glacial acetic acid) for 30 min, and destained in the same solution without the dye for 45 min. MMP levels were assessed using gelatinolytic activity, indicated as clear bands against the dark blue background. MMP identity and normalization between gels was achieved with human recombinant MMP-2 (PF037, Calbiochem) and MMP-9 (PF038, Calbiochem). The gels were digitalized and the integrated density of the bands, expressed as arbitrary units, was calculated using the open-access software ImageJ 1.41o (Wayne Rasband, National Institutes of Health; http://rsb.info.nih.gov/ij).

Data analysis

The data regarding the immunophenotypic analysis were expressed descriptively as the mean values ($\bar{x}$) and standard error of the means. The Wilcoxon rank-sum test was used to compare the values of the CG and TG for the hematological and CSF variables at the two time points (pre- and post-transplantation). To compare the values for the CSF and hematological variables at the two time points, the Wilcoxon signed rank test for paired samples was used. All analyses were conducted using SAS statistical software version 9.3 [44], with probability set at 5%.

Abbreviations
MSCs: Mesenchymal stem cells; MMP: Matrix metalloproteinases; BM: Bone marrow; CSF: Cerebrospinal fluid; BM-MSCs: Bone marrow mesenchymal stem cells; CG: Control group; TG: Treated group; FBS: Fetal bovine serum; AS: Autologous serum; CNS: Central nervous system; PBS: Phosphate-buffered solution.

Competing interests
The authors declare that they have no competing interests.

Authors' contributions
LM participated in the research design, in the writing of the paper, in the performance of the research and participated in data analysis. FCLA participated in the research design and participated in the writing of the paper. MOT participated in the performance of the research. CNM participated in the writing of the paper. GFM participated in the performance of the research. GDM participated in the performance of the research. RMA participated in the research design and participated in the writing of the paper. All authors read and approved the final manuscript.

Acknowledgements
To FAPESP for the PhD scholarship (Proc.2009/51431-6) and to Fundunesp (Proc.00571/09), and CNPQ (Proc. 481350/2009-8) for the financial support.

Author details
[1]Department of Animal Reproduction, São Paulo State University, District of Rubião Júnior, n/n, CEP: 18618970, Botucatu, São Paulo, Brazil. [2]Department of Veterinary Medicine, Maringá State University, Av. Colombo, 5.790, CEP: 87020-900, Maringá, Paraná, Brazil. [3]Department of Clinic, Surgery and Animal Reproduction, São Paulo State University, Clóvis Pestano, 793, CEP: 16050-680, Araçatuba, São Paulo, Brazil. [4]Department of Veterinary Clinics, São Paulo State University, District of Rubião Júnior, n/n, CEP: 18618970, Botucatu, São Paulo, Brazil.

References
1. Wright KT, Masri WE, Osman A, Chowdhury J, Johnson WEB. Concise review: bone marrow for the treatment of spinal cord injury: mechanisms and clinical applications. Stem Cell. 2011;29:169–78.
2. Baraniak PR, McDevitt TC. Stem cell paracrine actions and tissue regeneration. Regen Med. 2010;5:121–43.
3. Vidal MA, Robinson SO, Lopez MJ, Paulsen DB, Borkhsenious Johnson JR, Moore RM, et al. Comparison of chondrogenic potential in equine mesenchymal stromal cells derived from adipose tissue and bone marrow. Vet Surg. 2008;37:713–24.
4. Crovace A, Lacitignola L, De Siena R, Rossi G, Francioso E. Cell therapy for tendon repairin horses: an experimental study. Vet Res Commun. 2007;31:281–3.
5. Pacini S, Spinabella S, Trombi L, Galimberti S, Dini F, Carulicci F, et al. Suspension of bone marrow-derived undifferentiae mesenchymal stromal cells for repair of superficial digital flexor tendon in race horses. Tissue Eng. 2007;13:2949–55.
6. Wilke MM, Nydam DV, Nixon AJ. Enhanced early chondrogenesis in articular defects following arthroscopic mesenchymal stem cell implantation in an equine model. J Orthop Res. 2007;25:913–25.
7. Nixon AJ, Dahlgren LA, Haupt JL, Yeager AE, Ward DL. Effect of adipose-derived nucleated cell fractions on tendon repair in horseswith collagenase-induced tendinitis. Am J Vet Res. 2008;69:928–37.
8. Carvalho AM, Alves ALG, Oliveira PGG, Alvarez LEC, Laufer-Amorim R, Hussni CA, et al. Use of adipose tissue-derived mesenchymal stem cells for experimental tendinitis therapy in equines. J Equine Vet Sci. 2011;31:26–34.
9. McIlwraith CW, Frisbie DD, Rodkey WG, Kisiday JD, Werpy NM, Kawcak CE, et al. Evaluation of intra-articular mesenchymal stem cells to augment healing of microfractured chondral defects. Arthroscopic. 2011;27:1552–61.
10. Zhang J, Li Y, Chen J, Lu M, Elias SB, Mitchell JB, et al. Human bone marrow stromal cell treatment improves neurological functional recovery in EAE mice. Exp Neurol. 2005;195:16–26.
11. Mayhew IG, De Lahunta A, Whitlock RH. Spinal cord disease in the horse. The Cornell Vet. 1978;68:1–207.
12. Dominici M, Le Blanc K, Mueller I, Slaper-Cortenbach I, Marini FC, Krauses D, et al. Minimal criteria for defining multipotent mesenchymal stromal cells. The international society for cellular therapy position statement. Cytotherapy. 2006;8:315–7.
13. Carvalho AM, Alves ALG, Golim MA, Moroz A, Hussni CA, Oliveira PGG, et al. Isolation and immunophenotypic characterization of mesenchymal stem cells derived from equine species adipose tissue. Vet Immunol Immunop. 2009;132:303–6.
14. Arnhold SJ, Goletz I, Klein H, Stumpf G, Beluche LA, Rohde C, et al. Isolation and characterization of bone marrow–derived equine mesenchymal stem cells. Am J Vet Res. 2007;68:1095–105.
15. Guest DJ, Ousey JC, Smith MRW. Defining the expression of marker genes in equine mesenchymal stromal cells. Stem Cells and Cloning: Adv Appl. 2008;2008:1–9.
16. Radcliffe CH, Flaminio JBF, Fortier L. Temporal analysis of equine bone marrow aspirate during establishment of putative mesenchymal progenitor cell populations. Stem Cells Dev. 2010;19:269–82.
17. Martinello T, Bronzini I, Maccatrozzo L, Iacopetti I, Sampaolesi M, Mascarello F, et al. Cryopreservation does not affect the stem characteristics of multipotent cells isolated from equine peripheral blood. Tissue Eng Part C. 2010;16:771–81.
18. Hoynowski SM, Fry MM, Gardner BM, Leming MT, Tucker JR, Black L, et al. Characterization and differentiation of equine umbilical cord-derived matrix cells. Biochem Biophys Res Commun. 2007;362:347–53.

19. Iacono E, Brunori L, Pirrone A, Pagliaro PP, Ricci F, Tazzari PL, et al. Isolation, characterization and differentiation of mesenchymal stem cells from amniotic fluid, umbilical cord blood and Wharton's jelly in the horse. Reproduction. 2012;143:455–68.

20. Mensing N, Gasse H, Hambruch N, Haeger JD, Pfarrer C, Staszyk C. Isolation and characterization of multipotent mesenchymal stromal cells from the gingiva and the periodontal ligament of the horse. BMC Vet Res. 2011;7:1–42.

21. Dimarakis I, Levicar N. Cell culture medium composítion and translational adult bone marrow-derived stem cell research. Stem Cells. 2006;24:1407–8.

22. Sotiropoulou PA, Perez SA, Salagianni M, Baxevanis CN, Papamichail M. Cell culture medium composítion and translational adult bone marrow-derived stem cell research. Stem Cells. 2006;24:1409–10.

23. Toupadakis CA, Woung A, Genetos DC, Cheung WK, Borjesson DL, Leach JK, et al. Comparison of the osteogenic potential of equine mesenchymal stem cells from bone marrow, adipose tissue, umbilical cord blood, and umbilical cord tissue. Am J Vet Res. 2010;71:1237–45.

24. Lim JY, Jeong CH, Jun JA, Kim SM, Ryu CH, Hou Y, et al. Therapeutic effects of human umbilical cord blood-derived mesenchymal stem cells after intrathecal administration by lumbar puncture in a rat model of cerebral ischemia. Stem Cell Res Ther. 2011;2:1–13.

25. Yang WZ, Zhang Y, Wu F, Min WP, Minev B, Zhang M, et al. Safety evaluation of allogeneic umbilical cord blood mononuclear cell therapy form degenerative conditions. J Transl Med. 2010;8:1–6.

26. Kaneko JJ, Harvey JW, Bruss ML. Clinical biochemistry of domestic animals. Burlington: Elsevier; 2008.

27. Green E, Constantinescu G, Kroll R. Equine cerebrospinal fluid: Analysis. Compend Contin Educ Pract Vet. 1993;15:288–301.

28. Mayhew IG, Whitlock RH, Tasker JB. Equine cerebrospinal fluid: reference values of normal horses. Am J Vet Res. 1977;38:1271–4.

29. Melo GD, Marcondes M, Machado GF. Canine cerebral leishmaniasis: potential role of matrix metalloproteinase-2 in the development of neurological disease. Vet Immunol Immunopathol. 2012;148:260–6.

30. Verma PR, Hansch C. Matrix metalloproteinases (MMPs): chemical–biological functions and (Q) SARs. Bioorg Med Chem. 2007;15:2223–68.

31. Rosenberg GA. Matrix metalloproteinases in neuroinflammation. Glia. 2002;39:279–91.

32. Bergman RL, Inzana KD, Inzana TJ. Characterization of matrix metalloproteinase-2 and –9 in cerebrospinal fluid of clinically normal dogs. Am J Vet Res. 2002;63:1359–62.

33. Grossete M, Phelps J, Arko L, Yonas H, Rosemberg GA. Elevation of MMP-3 and MMP-9 in CSF and blood in patients with severe traumatic brain injury. Neurosurgery. 2009;65:702–4.

34. Leppert D, Leib SL, Grygar C, Miller KM, Schaad UB, Holländer GA. Matrix metalloproteinase (MMP)-8 and MMP-9 in cerebrospinal fluid during bacterial meningitis: association with blood–brain barrier damage and neurological sequelae. Clin Infect Dis. 2000;31:80–4.

35. Williams PL, Leib SL, Kamberi P, Leppert D, Sobel RA, Bifrare Y, et al. Levels of matrix metalloproteinase–9 within cerebrospinal fluid in a rabbit model of coccidioidal meningitis and vasculitis. J Infect Dis. 2002;186:1692–5.

36. Leppert D, Ford J, Stabler G, Grygar C, Lienert C, Huber S, et al. Matrix metalloproteinase-9 (gelatinase B) is selectively elevated in CSF during relapses and stable phases of multiple sclerosis. Brain. 1998;121:2327–34.

37. Barreira APB, Bacellar DTL, Kiffer RG, Alves ALG. Punção aspirativa de medula óssea em equinos adultos para obtenção de células-tronco. Rev Bras Ciênc. 2008;15:56–9.

38. Maia L, Landim-Alvarenga FC, Golim MA, Sudano MJ, Taffarel MO, De Vita B, et al. Potential of neural transdifferentiation of mesenchymal stem cells from equine bone marrow. Pesq Vet Bras. 2012;32:444–52.

39. Maia L, Landim-Alvarenga FC, Da Mota LS, De Assis Golim M, Laufer-Amorim R, De Vita B, et al. Immunophenotypic, immunocytochemistry, ultrastructural, and cytogenetic characterization of mesenchymal stem cells from equine bone marrow. Microsc Res Tech. 2013;5:618–24.

40. Mayhew IG. Collection of cerebrospinal fluid from the horse. Cornell Vet. 1975;65:500–11.

41. Malikides N, Hodgson DR, Rose RJ. Neurology. In: Rose RJ, Hodgson DR, editors. Manual Equine Practice. 2nd ed. Philadelphia: Saunders; 2000. p. 503–75.

42. Mayhew IGJ. Neurologic Evaluation. In: Mayhew IGJ, editor. Large Animal Neurology. 2nd ed. West Sussex: Wiley-Blackwell Publishing; 2009. p. 11–46.

43. Marangoni NR, Melo GD, Moraes OC, Souza MS, Perri SHV, Machado GF. Levels of matrix metalloproteinase-2 and –9 in the cerebrospinal fluid of dogs with visceral leishmaniasis. Parasite Immunol. 2011;33:330–4.

44. SAS Institute Inc. SAS/IML 9.3 User's Guide. Cary, NC: SAS Institute Inc; 2011.

12

First report of junctional epidermolysis bullosa (JEB) in the Italian draft horse

Katia Cappelli[1*], Chiara Brachelente[1], Fabrizio Passamonti[1], Alessandro Flati[2], Maurizio Silvestrelli[1] and Stefano Capomaccio[3]

Abstract

Background: Epitheliogenesis imperfecta in horses was first recognized at the beginning of the 20th century when it was proposed that the disease could have a genetic cause and an autosomal recessive inheritance pattern. Electron microscopy studies confirmed that the lesions were characterized by a defect in the lamina propria and the disease was therefore reclassified as epidermolysis bullosa. Molecular studies targeted two mutations affecting genes involved in dermal–epidermal junction: an insertion in *LAMC2* in Belgians and other draft breeds and one large deletion in *LAMA3* in American Saddlebred.

Case presentation: A mechanobullous disease was suspected in a newborn, Italian draft horse foal, which presented with multifocal to coalescing erosions and ulceration on the distal extremities. Histological examination of skin biopsies revealed a subepidermal cleft formation and transmission electron microscopy demonstrated that the lamina densa of the basement membrane remained attached to the dermis. According to clinical, histological and ultrastructural findings, a diagnosis of junctional epidermolysis bullosa (JEB) was made. Genetic tests confirmed the presence of 1368insC in *LAMC2* in the foal and its relatives.

Conclusion: This is the first report of JEB in Italy. The disease was characterized by typical macroscopic, histologic and ultrastructural findings. Genetic tests confirmed the presence of the 1368insC in *LAMC2* in this case: further investigations are required to assess if the mutation could be present at a low frequency in the Italian draft horse population. Atypical breeding practices are responsible in this case and played a role as odds enhancer for unfavourable alleles. Identification of carriers is fundamental in order to prevent economic loss for the horse industry.

Keywords: Junctional epidermolysis bullosa, Horse, Mechanobullous disease, Electron microscopy, Lamina densa, *LAMC2*, Italian draft horse, Inbreeding

Background

Junctional epidermolysis bullosa (JEB) belongs to the group of vesiculo-bullous diseases of the epidermis. With this term, several diseases are encompassed that are all characterized by the formation of a split (vesicle or bulla) in any layer of the epidermis or beneath it, at the dermoepidermal junction. This split occurs in two ways: as a consequence of an immune-mediated attack to components of the intercellular and cell-basement membrane adhesion system or as a result of an inherited condition resulting in a lack of any of these components.

In this second case, epidermolysis bullosa (EB) is a recessive inherited disease characterized by a genetic defect leading to an inadequate synthesis of structural components of intercellular adhesions such as keratin filaments, desmosomes and hemi-desmosome proteins and anchoring fibrils such as collagen VII [1]. In humans, three subtypes of EB are described that are classified according to the distribution of the lesions and the location of the split in the epidermis and dermis: in simplex EB, the split forms in the basal keratinocyte layer; in junctional EB the split forms in the lamina lucida, leaving the lamina densa anchored to the underlying dermis; in dystrophic EB the split forms within or below the lamina densa which therefore remains attached to the overlying epidermis [2].

* Correspondence: katia.cappelli@unipg.it
[1]Department of Veterinary Medicine, University of Perugia, Via San Costanzo 4, 06126 Perugia, Italy
Full list of author information is available at the end of the article

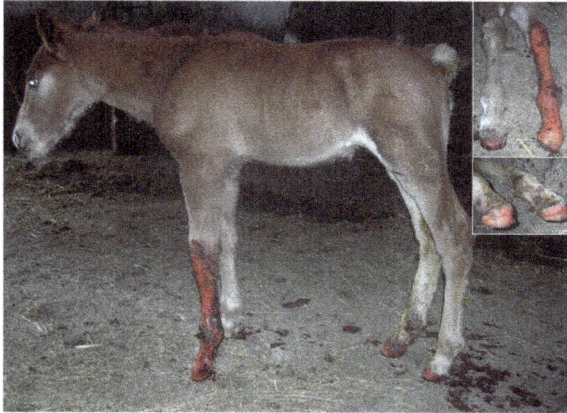

Figure 1 Italian draft horse foal, male, 4-day-old: Focal extensive, erosive to ulcerative lesions were present in all four legs and particularly severe in the left front leg. Lesions were covered by crusts and were associated with sloughing of the hoof and bleeding.

Epidermolysis bullosa is recognized in dogs, sheep, horses, cattle, goats and cats [3-7]. Lesions can be present at birth or develop in a short period of time and are characterized by the development of vesicles and bullae that rapidly progress to erosions and ulceration at sites of minor trauma such as the lips, the oral mucosa, the distal extremities and the coronary band, with resulting sloughing of the hoof or claws. Lesions can be secondarily infected and become pustules. Affected animals may die soon after birth due to inability to suckle. Histologically, the lesions show a split that can be intraepidermal, at the dermoepidermal junction or subepidermal. The anatomical location of the

split is an important diagnostic criterion because it reflects a different pathogenesis of lesion formation [3].

In horses, two mutations have been associated with the disease, involving two different genes coding for the Laminin 332 protein complex [4,8]. Laminin is a heterotrimeric basement membrane protein integral to the structure and function of the dermal–epidermal junction consisting of three glycoprotein subunits: the α3, β3 and γ2 chains, which are encoded by the *LAMA3*, *LAMB3* and *LAMC2* respectively [9]. A mutation in any of these genes results in the condition known as hereditary junctional epidermolysis bullosa (JEB). An insertion of a cytosine (1368insC) in the *LAMC2* was found in 2002 in draft horses (Belgian Horse, Trait Breton and Trait Comtois) [4,10]. This mutation is responsible for a frameshift, with consequent premature stop codon formation, leading to a truncated form of the Laminin 332 chain. In 2009, a 6589-bp deletion spanning exons 24 and 27 was found in the *LAMA3* in American Saddlebred foals born with the skin-blistering condition formerly known as epitheliogenesis imperfecta. The deletion confirms that the disease can be classified as JEB and corresponds to Herlitz JEB in humans [8]. In both cases, the inheritance of the disease is a classic Mendelian autosomal recessive.

Case presentation

A male foal coming from a horse farm with 25 animals was born at term with eutocic delivery. The foal, at birth, showed the presence of lesions affecting the distal extremities of all four legs. From the carpus of the left foreleg and from the coronet of the other three legs, the

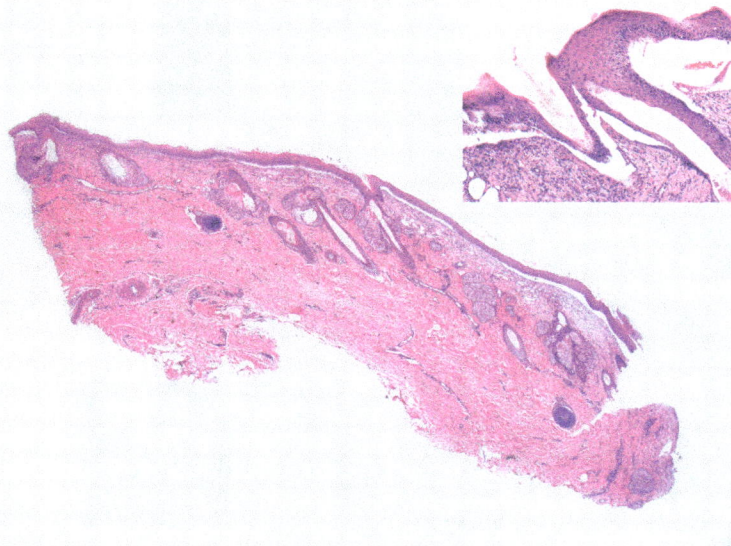

Figure 2 Italian draft horse foal, male, 6-day-old, biopsy from the coronet: Histological examination showed the presence of a subepidermal cleft with little or no underlying dermal inflammation. The dermoepidermal separation involved the hair follicle infundibulum as well (insert). HE. 1,25x (insert 10x).

skin was missing and the denuded dermis was covered by debris (Figure 1). No lesions were observed at the mucocutaneous junctions or in oral mucosa. The foal was treated with IV antibiotics (cefquinome 1 mg/kg twice a day and amikacin 15 mg/kg once a day) and a hoof boot was applied to the foot that had lost the hoof. Two days later, four skin biopsies were taken with the owner's consent from the dorsal and palmar surface of the carpus, from the coronary band and from the coronet at the transition between affected and unaffected areas. Despite treatment, the foal died after 6 days and the owner declined the necropsy. Histologic examination of skin biopsies revealed the presence of vesiculobullous lesions characterized by a complete separation of the epidermis from the dermis at the level of the dermoepidermal junction. The blister formation also involved the infundibular portion of hair follicles and ulcerated areas were covered by thick serocellular crusts. Periodic acid-Schiff (PAS) staining revealed a PAS positive lamina densa at the pavement of the blister, attached to the underlying dermis. The macroscopic and histologic lesions were compatible with a hereditary epidermolysis bullosa. According to the PAS staining results, our case

was compatible with a junctional epidermolysis bullosa (Figure 2). Transmission electron microscopy from formalin fixed skin biopsies confirmed the presence of a splitting between the epidermis and dermis. Basal keratinocytes were intact and demonstrated normal desmosomes but no hemidesmosomes were identifiable. The lamina densa was present on the pavement, at the dermal side of the blister, consistent with a splitting at the level of the lamina lucida (Figure 3).

Based on the macroscopic and histologic findings as well as the ultrastructural features, a diagnosis of hereditary junctional epidermolysis bullosa was made. Molecular tests aimed at the detection of known mutations associated with the disease, involving the Laminin 5 protein complex, were performed in order to confirm the diagnosis. Nucleic acids were extracted from 200 µl of total blood using the QIAamp DNA Mini Kit (Qiagen) following the manufacturer's instructions. Since the disease has a Mendelian autosomal recessive inheritance, foal's DNA together with the DNA of the mother (admixed horse), of the father (heavy horse who was also the grandfather) and of the maternal grandmother (light horse) was tested at the cited loci. PCR was performed as previously described [4,8] using 30 ng of DNA as template for the amplification of *LAMC2* and *LAMA3* regions where the known mutations rely, and amplicons directly sequenced. PCR results were negative for *LAMA3* deletion in all samples. The affected foal was homozygous for 1368insC in *LAMC2* whereas the sire and the dam were heterozygous for the insertion (Figure 4).

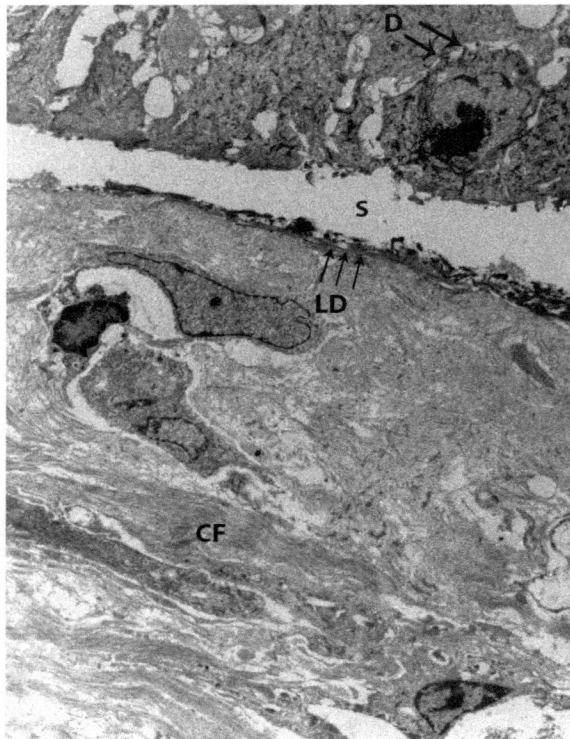

Figure 3 Transmission electron micrograph of the skin biopsy. Normal keratinocytes form the roof of the split (S) and the dermis is at its base. Desmosomes (D) are still visible whereas hemidesmosomes are not present. The lamina densa (LD) is located at the base of the split. Normal collagen fibers (CF) are visible in the superficial dermis. TEM. 2,800x.

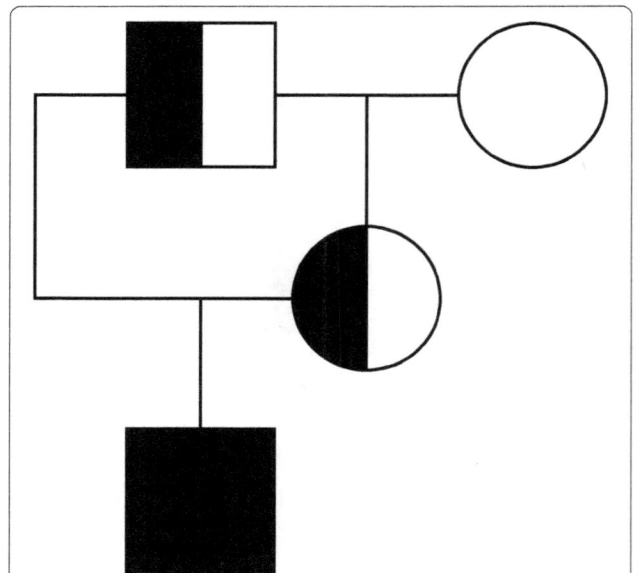

Figure 4 Pedigree tree of the affected foal, homozygous for the mutation in *LAMC2* gene (full black square). Half black figures indicate carrier subjects while open figure equates to the wild type. Squares indicate males while circle female subjects.

These results confirmed that the mutation causing junctional epidermolysis bullosa in the foal was localized in the *LAMC2*, as already described in northern Europe's coldblood breeds (Belgian Horse, Trait Breton and Trait Comtois) [4,10], which participated, with some lines, to the creation of Italian draft horses [11]; since the disease has a classical autosomal recessive Mendelian inheritance, both parents must be heterozygous (carriers).

Inbreeding, enhanced by erroneous breeding practices, should always be avoided as it can increase the frequency of potentially deleterious recessive alleles in the population and their phenotypic manifestation at individual level [12].

Conclusion

This is the first report of JEB in Italy. The disease was histologically described as having the typical pathognomonic features and assessed via molecular tests.

Future studies should include genotyping the 1368insC mutation in *LAMC2* in a larger population of Italian Draft horses to determine the allele frequency within this population, and avoid other episodes of JEB.

Identification of carriers is crucial as much as breeder awareness about the avoidance of certain mates in order to prevent economic loss for the horse industry.

Competing interests
The authors declare that they have no competing interests.

Authors' contributions
Conceived and designed the study: SC, MS. FP, AF retrieved the case and made the clinic diagnosis. KC and SC wrote the manuscript and perform molecular tests and diagnosis. CB wrote the manuscript, read the histopathology and the transmission electron microscopy, made the histological and ultrastructural diagnosis. All authors read and approved the final manuscript.

Acknowledgements
The authors would like to acknowledge Gianluca Alunni for his technical help and Paola Coliolo for her excellent work in the preparation of the ultrastructural samples.

Author details
[1]Department of Veterinary Medicine, University of Perugia, Via San Costanzo 4, 06126 Perugia, Italy. [2]Private Practitioner, via Roma 193, Scoppito, L'Aquila, Italy. [3]Institute of Zootechnics, UCSC, via Emilia Parmense 84, 29122 Piacenza, Italy.

References
1. Intong LRA, Murrell DF. Inherited epidermolysis bullosa: New diagnostic criteria and classification. Clin Dermatol. 2012;30:70–7 [Bullous Skin Diseases: Part II].
2. Sawamura D, Nakano H, Matsuzaki Y. Overview of epidermolysis bullosa. J Dermatol. 2010;37:214–9.
3. Scott D, Miller W. Congenital and Hereditary Skin Diseases. 2nd Edition. Saunders; 2011.
4. Spirito F, Charlesworth A, Linder K, Ortonne J-P, Baird J, Meneguzzi G. Animal models for skin blistering conditions: absence of laminin 5 causes hereditary junctional mechanobullous disease in the Belgian horse. J Investig Dermatol. 2002;119:684–91.
5. Kerkmann A, Ganter M, Frase R, Ostmeier M, Hewicker-Trautwein M, Distl O. Epidermolysis bullosa in German black headed mutton sheep. Berl Munch Tierarztl Wochenschr. 2010;123:413–21.
6. Medeiros GX, Riet-Correa F, Armién AG, Dantas AF, de Galiza GJ, Simões SV. Junctional epidermolysis bullosa in a calf. J Vet Diagn Invest. 2012;24:231–4.
7. Medeiros GX, Riet-Correa F, Barros SS, Soares MP, Dantas AF, Galiza GJ, et al. Dystrophic epidermolysis bullosa in goats. J Comp Pathol. 2013;148:354–60.
8. Graves KT, Henney PJ, Ennis RB. Partial deletion of the LAMA3 gene is responsible for hereditary junctional epidermolysis bullosa in the American Saddlebred Horse. Anim Genet. 2009;40:35–41.
9. Finno CJ, Spier SJ, Valberg SJ. Equine diseases caused by known genetic mutations. Vet J. 2009;179:336–47.
10. Milenkovic D, Chaffaux S, Taourit S, Guérin G. A mutation in the LAMC2 gene causes the Herlitz junctional epidermolysis bullosa (H-JEB) in two French draft horse breeds. Genet Sel Evol. 2003;35:249–56.
11. Hendricks B. International Encyclopedia of Horse Breeds. University of Oklahoma Press; 2007.
12. Hartl DL, Clark AG. Principles of population genetics. 4th ed. Sunderland, Massachusetts: Sinauer Associates, Inc. Publishers; 2007.

13

Effects of sodium citrate and acid citrate dextrose solutions on cell counts and growth factor release from equine pure-platelet rich plasma and pure-platelet rich gel

Carlos E Giraldo[*], María E Álvarez and Jorge U Carmona

Abstract

Background: There is a lack information on the effects of the most commonly used anticoagulants for equine platelet rich plasmas (PRPs) elaboration on cell counts and growth factor release from platelet rich gels (PRGs). The aims of this study were 1) to compare the effects of the anticoagulants sodium citrate (SC), acid citrate dextrose solution A (ACD-A) and ACD-B on platelet (PLT), leukocyte (WBC) and on some parameters associated to platelet activation including mean platelet volume (MPV) and platelet distribution width (PDW) between whole blood, pure PRP (P-PRP) and platelet-poor plasma (PPP); 2) to compare transforming growth factor beta 1 (TGF-β_1) and platelet-derived growth factor isoform BB (PDGF-BB) concentrations in supernatants from pure PRG (P-PRG), platelet-poor gel (PPG), P-PRP lysate (positive control) and plasma (negative control); 3) to establish the possible correlations between all the studied cellular and molecular parameters.

Results: In all cases the three anticoagulants produced P-PRPs with significantly higher PLT counts compared with whole blood and PPP. The concentrations of WBCs were similar between P-PRP and whole blood, but significantly lower in PPP. The type of anticoagulant did not significantly affect the cell counts for each blood component. The anticoagulants also did not affect the MPV and PDW parameters. Independently of the anticoagulant used, all blood components presented significantly different concentrations of PDGF-BB and TGF-β_1. The highest growth factor (GF) concentrations were observed from P-PRP lysates, followed by PRG supernatants, PPP lysates, PPG supernatants and plasma. Significant correlations were observed between PLT and WBC counts ($\rho = 0.80$), PLT count and TGF-β_1 concentration ($\rho = 0.85$), PLT count and PDGF-BB concentration ($\rho = 0.80$) and PDGF-BB and TGF-β_1 concentrations ($\rho = 0.75$). The type of anticoagulant was not correlated with any of the variables evaluated.

Conclusions: The anticoagulants did not significantly influence cell counts or GF concentrations in equine PRP. However, ACD-B was apparently the worst anticoagulant evaluated. It is necessary to perform additional research to determine the effect of anticoagulants on the kinetics of GF elution from P-PRG.

Keywords: Anticoagulant, Horse, Platelet concentrate, Transforming growth factor beta 1, Platelet derived growth factor isoform BB, Regenerative therapy

* Correspondence: cgiraldo@ucaldas.edu.co
Grupo de Investigación Terapia Regenerativa, Departamento de Salud Animal, Universidad de Caldas, Manizales, Colombia

Background

There is an increased use of platelet-rich plasma (PRP) as a treatment for musculoskeletal diseases and severe wounds in horses [1-4]. It was recognized that among the regenerative therapies, platelet-rich plasma (PRP) is an autologous platelet concentrate suspended in plasma that, administrated in the wound site, releases growth factors and promotes the wound healing cascade [2,5]. Platelets contain a pool of growth factors, including transforming growth factor-b (TGF-β), platelet derived growth factor (PDGF) and vascular endothelial growth factor (VEGF), mainly contained in platelet alpha granules [6] that are released after platelet degranulation in the damage site and enhance tissue regeneration by stimulating cell proliferation, increasing extracellular matrix synthesis, promoting vascular ingrowth and reducing catabolic matrix-degrading cytokines such as interleukins and matrix metalloproteinases [5,7].

PRP intended for regenerative proposes may be classified as: pure-platelet rich plasma (P-PRP) or leukoreduced PRP, leukocyte- and platelet-rich plasma (L-PRP) and platelet rich fibrin (PRF). P-PRP and L-PRP are obtained in a liquid form by using anticoagulants [8]. PRF is a second generation platelet concentrate, which does not require anticoagulant for its elaboration. In horses, P-PRP displays slightly higher platelet counts (1.3 - 4.0 fold) and leukocyte (WBC) counts (0.5 - 2.0 fold) than whole blood, whereas L-PRP has increased platelet (5 fold) and leukocyte (3 - fold or more) counts when compared with whole blood. There is not a complete consensus regarding the role of leukocyte concentrations in PRP [2]. However, *in vitro* evidence suggests that leukoreduced PRP could be more suitable for the treatment of tendon and soft tissue injuries in horses, as this substance induces tendon anabolism and decreases the expression of catabolic cytokines when compared with L-PRP [9].

Although PRP (either L-PRP or P-PRP) is employed as a promising treatment in equine practice [5], there are some controversial issues that should solved to improve the clinical use of this substance in horses and other animals. There are a plethora of PRP products and PRP-associated technologies that are used in human and equine practices [2,8,10]. However, little is known regarding the cellular and molecular quality of these substances, as they are influenced by intrinsic factors that are dependent on the patient, such as gender, age, breed [6] and pathological conditions [11], amongst others and by extrinsic factors, such as the type of anticoagulant used [12], the relative centrifugation forces (rcf or g) used for cell concentration [2,13,14], the type and form of the kit used for PRP preparation and the activating substance used for PRP activation and growth factor release [2,15].

Recent equine PRP studies have showed that the cell and growth factor release profiles are influenced by the intrinsic factors of the patients [6]. Furthermore, it has also been observed that activating substances, including calcium salts and thrombin, affect the growth factor release profile from equine PRP [15]. However, there is a lack of information of the effect on the most commonly used anticoagulants for PRP elaboration on cell counts and growth factor release. Although, a human study indicated that acid citrate dextrose solution A (ACD-A) was better than sodium citrate (SC) for PRP preparation [12], there is no information regarding the effect of the type of anticoagulant used for PRP preparation in horses on cell counts from PRP or growth factor release from PRG.

The aims of this study were: 1) to compare the effects of the anticoagulants SC, ACD-A and ACD-B on platelet and leukocyte counts and platelet activation associated parameters, such as mean platelet volume (MPV) and platelet distribution width (PDW) between whole blood, P-PRP and platelet-poor plasma (PPP); 2) to compare the PDGF-BB and TGF-β_1 concentrations in the supernatants from pure platelet-rich gel (P-PRG), platelet-poor gel (PPG), P-PRP lysate (positive control) and plasma (negative control); 3) to establish the possible correlations between all the studied cellular and molecular parameters.

The hypothesis of this study was that anticoagulants do not influence cell counts and PDGF-BB and TGF-β_1 release from equine P-PRP/P-PRG.

Methods

This study was approved by the Ethical Committee of the Universidad de Caldas.

Horses

Eighteen clinically normal Argentinean Creole horses (geldings) were used. The horses had a mean age of 12.5 (± standard deviation (s.d) 6.3) years old. All the horses were from the same farm, and the owner did know the nature of the study and authorized the blood extraction accordingly.

Blood collection and preparation of platelet concentrates

From each animal blood samples were collected in triplicate by jugular venipuncture and deposited randomly in tubes with either sodium citrate (SC) (12.35 mg sodium citrate and 2.21 mg citric acid [BD Vacutainer®, Becton Drive, Franklin Lakes, NJ, USA]) or acid citrate dextrose (ACD) solution A (ACD-A) (22.0 g/L trisodium citrate, 8.0 g/L citric acid and 24.5 g/L dextrose [BD Vacutainer®, Becton Drive, Franklin Lakes, NJ, USA]) or ACD solution B (ACD-B) (13.2 g/L trisodium citrate 4.8 g/L citric acid and 14.7 g/L dextrose [BD Vacutainer®, Becton Drive, Franklin Lakes, NJ, USA]).

Tubes with each anticoagulant were randomly processed for P-PRP production. The total whole blood used for P-PRP preparation using each anticoagulant varied between 110 and 140 mL. Briefly, after centrifugation at 120 g for 5 min, the first 50% of the top supernatant plasma fraction, adjacent to the buffy coat, was collected. This fraction was then centrifuged at 240 g for 5 min and the bottom quarter fraction was collected [16]. This fraction was considered to be P-PRP. The upper plasma fraction P-PRP was considered to be PPP (Figure 1). Plasma was obtained by centrifugation from each anticoagulated blood at 3500 g for 8 min. The time between blood collection and processing was approximately 1 h. All the samples were deposited and transported from the farm to the laboratory in an icebox.

Haematological analysis

Complete, automated haemograms (Celltac-α MEK 6450, Nihon Kodhen, Japan) were performed in duplicate for whole blood, P-PRPs and PPPs obtained from each anticoagulant. Platelet (PLT) counts, mean platelet volume (MPV fL), platelet distribution width (PDW %) and total leukocyte (WBC) counts were determined.

Activation of platelet concentrates

Four hundred μL of a 10% calcium gluconate (CG) solution (9.3 mg/mL) (Ropsohn Therapeutics Ltda®, Bogotá, Colombia) was added to 4 mL of P-PRP or PPP obtained with each anticoagulant to produce the P-PRGs and PPGs, respectively. P-PRGs and PPGs were incubated at 37°C for 3 h to stimulate GF release. Clots were mechanically released from the walls of the tubes and centrifuged at 3500 g for 8 min. The resulting supernatant was aliquoted, and frozen at −82°C for later determination of TGF-β_1 and PDGF-BB concentrations.

Lysis of platelet concentrates

Samples of 4 mL of P-PRPs and PPPs obtained using each anticoagulant were incubated at 37°C for 15 min with 400 μL of a solution containing 0.5% of a non-ionic detergent (NID) (Triton® X100, Panreac Química, Barcelona, Spain). Platelet concentrates treated with NID were used as a positive control for GF release [11]. Lysates were processed in a similar fashion to supernatants from P-PRGs and PPGs.

Total protein determination

Total protein (TP) concentration from all the samples were determined using the biuret method (Proteína total (Biuret), BioSystems, Barcelona, Spain) [17], followed by spectrophotometric quantifications.

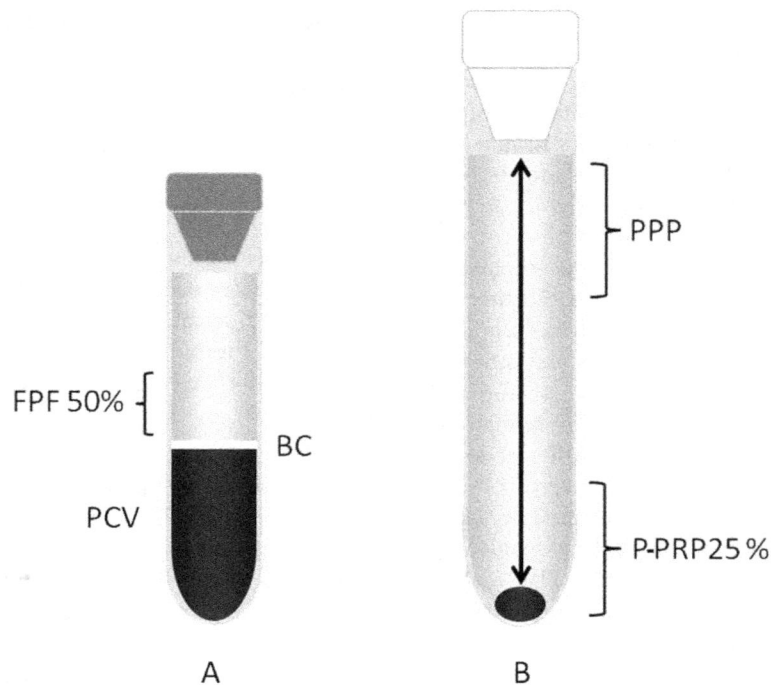

Figure 1 Schematic representation of the plasma fractions obtained with the tube method protocol. Left tube **(A)** containing the first fraction of plasma (50%) (PFP) obtained by the single centrifugation tube method. Right tube **(B)** containing platelet-rich plasma (PRP) obtained by the double centrifugation tube method. BC: buffy coat. PCV: packed cell volume.

Determination of TGF-β_1 and PDGF-BB concentrations by ELISA

The TGF-β_1 and PDGF-BB concentrations from the supernatants and lysates of each blood component were determined in duplicate by a sandwich ELISA using commercially available antibodies against human TGF-β_1 (Human TGF-β1, DY240E, R&D Systems, Inc., Minneapolis, MN USA) and PDGF-BB (Human PDGF-BB, DY220, R&D Systems, Inc.). Both ELISAs were performed according to the manufacturer's instructions. Readings were performed at 450 nm. Both ELISAs were determined with human antibodies because there is a high homology of these growth factors between equines and humans [18,19]. Further, several equine PRP studies have validated these ELISA kits [6,14-16].

Statistical analysis

Data were analysed using commercial software (SPSS 18.0, IBM, Chicago, IL, USA). Data were initially assessed for normality (goodness of fit) by a Shapiro-Wilk test and a direct plot analysis of each evaluated variable. When the variables had a normal distribution (Shapiro-Wilk test, P > 0.05), they were presented as means (± s.d.) and evaluated by parametric tests (e.g., Student's t-test for paired samples, and one way analysis of variance (ANOVA) and Tukey's test (for $post-hoc$ paired comparisons). Non-parametric variables (Shapiro-Wilk test, P <0.05) were presented as medians (interquartile range -IR-) and evaluated using a Kruskal-Wallis test followed, when necessary, by a Mann–Whitney U-test. A Wilcoxon test was used for non-related paired comparisons. All the variables were analysed for general and specific correlations using a Spearman (r_s) test. A P value ≤0.05 was considered to be significant for all tests.

Results

Haematological findings

In all cases, the three anticoagulants produced P-PRPs with significantly (P < 0.001) higher PLT counts compared with whole blood and PPP. The concentrations of WBCs were similar between P-PRP and whole blood, but significantly (P < 0.001) lower in PPP. The type of anticoagulant did not significantly affect the cell counts for each blood component. The anticoagulants also did not affect the MPV and PDW parameters. However, in general, these platelet activation parameters were significantly higher in P-PRP than in PPP. A summary of the haematological results is shown in Table 1.

Growth factor release from blood components

Independently of the anticoagulant used, all blood components presented significantly different concentrations of PDGF-BB and TGF-β_1. The highest GF concentrations were observed from P-PRP lysates, followed by PRG supernatants, PPP lysates, PPG supernatants and plasma (Table 2). However, when data were plotted, a statistical trend (P = 0.20) was observed for PDGF-BB concentrations in P-PRG from SC in comparison with ACD-B (Figure 2). In contrast, this trend was not observed for TGF-β_1 released from P-PRG (Figure 3).

Correlations

Significant correlations were observed between PLT and WBC counts ($\rho = 0.80$, P <0.01), PLT counts and TGF-β_1 concentrations ($\rho = 0.85$, P <0.01), PLT counts and PDGF-BB concentrations ($\rho = 0.80$, P <0.01) and PDGF-BB and TGF-β_1 concentrations ($\rho = 0.75$, P <0.01). The type of anticoagulant was not correlated with any of the variables evaluated.

Discussion

To our knowledge, this is the first study to evaluate the effects of several anticoagulants used for producing equine PRP as a regenerative therapy. The cellular results from this study were similar to those previously reported by other equine PRP studies, in which the double centrifugation tube method was used [6,13].

The parameters associated with platelet activation, such as MPV and PDW were not affected by the type of anticoagulant evaluated in this study. However, MPV and PDW values were significantly lower in PPP when compared with whole blood and P-PRP, although they

Table 1 Means (± s.d) of the haematological variables for each blood component obtained with every anticoagulant

Variable	Anticoagulant								
	Sodium citrate (SC)			ACD-A			ACD-B		
	Whole blood	P-PRP	PPP	Whole blood	P-PRP	PPP	Whole blood	P-PRP	PPP
PLT (10^3/μL)	143.8 (19.4)[a,b]	390.6 (57.6)[c]	111.0 (22.6)	137.0 (21.3)[a]	399.1 (62.8)[c]	112.6 (23.7)	137.1 (25.4)[a]	398.5 (48.0)[c]	111.2 (18.5)
MPV (fL)	3.8 (0.4)	4.1 (0.6)[b]	3.6 (0.3)	3.8 (0.4)	4.2 (0.6)[b]	3.7 (0.4)	3.8 (0.4)[d]	4.2 (0.5)[b]	3.7 (0.4)
PDW (%)	16.5 (0.5)[c]	16.8 (0.5)[c]	17.8 (0.5)	16.3 (0.5)[c]	16.5 (0.6)[c]	17.6 (0.7)	16.1 (0.6)[c]	16.7 (0.6)[c]	17.8 (0.7)
WBC (10^3/μL)*	8.4 (1.7)[c,d]	9.5 (3.0)[c]	0.1 (0.0)	7.9 (2.0)[c,d]	9.8 (5.0)[c]	0.1 (0.0)	8.3 (2.3)[e]	10.6 (4.0)[c]	0.1 (0.0)

ACD: acid citrate dextrose (solution-A,-B); P-PRP: pure platelet-rich plasma; PPP: platelet-poor plasma; PLT, platelets; MPV: mean platelet volume; PDW: platelet distribution width; WBC: white blood cells. Lower-case letters represent significant differences between blood components for every independent anticoagulant. Blood components significantly different with a: P-PRP (P <0.001); b: PPP (P <0.05); c: PPP (P <0.001); d: P-PRP (P <0.05); and e: P-PRP PPP (P <0.001); *Data are presented as medians (interquartile range (IR).

Table 2 Means (± s.d) of the TGF-$\beta_1$and PDGF-BB concentrations (pg/mg of total protein (TP)) in every blood component obtained with every anticoagulant

Variable	Blood component				
	Plasma	P-PRP lysate	P-PRG	PPP lysate	PPG
SC					
PDGF-BB (pg/mg of TP)	0.9 (0.6)[a,b]	25.2 (14.4)[c]	19.0 (29.4)[d]	8.3 (5.4)[d]	4.5 (5.5)
TGF-β1(pg/mg of TP)*	26.8 (10.4)[a,e]	90.7 (30.7)[c,e]	54.5 (33.1)	45.2 (10.3)[d]	29.2 (17.1)
ACD-A					
PDGF-BB (pg/mg of PT)	1.0 (0.6)[a,b]	28.2 (20.1)[c]	11.3 (30.6)	8.2 (5.0)	5.8 (8.0)
TGF-β1(pg/mg of TP)*	30.0 (8.7)[a]	101.5 (31.2)[c,e]	56.4 (39.1)	47.8 (12.2)	33.3 (17.9)
ACD-B					
PDGF-BB (pg/mg of TP)	1.1 (0.9)[a]	18.4 (13.4)[b]	6.6 (17.3)	7.2 (4.1)	4.8 (6.5)
TGF-β1(pg/mg of TP)*	27.5 (10.0)[c]	87.8 (23.0)[d]	50.8 (31.2)	44.6 (12.9)	31.3 (12.7)

*Data are presented as medians (IR). P-PRG: pure platelet-rich gel; PPG: platelet-poor gel. Lowercase letters represent independent significant differences for every blood component obtained with a specific anticoagulant. SC: blood component different with a: P-PRP and PPP lysates (P <0.001); b: P-PRG and PPG (P <0.05); c: PPP lysate and PPG (P <0.001); d: PPG (P <0.05); and e: P-PRG (P <0.05). ACD-A: blood component different with a: P-PRP and PPP lysates (P <0.001); b: P-PRG and PPG (P <0.05); c: PPP lysate and PPG (P <0.001); d: PPG; and e: P-PRG (P <0.05). ACD-B: blood component different a: all blood components (P <0.05); b: PPP lysate and PPP (P <0.05); c: P-PRP lysate (P <0.05); d: PPP lysate and PPG (P <0.05).

remained within the normal physiological values for this species [6]. It is known, that ACD is a very good anticoagulant, compared to SC for preserving the structural and physiological properties of platelets after two or more hours of blood collection [20]. From a regenerative medicine perspective, ACD should be used to conserve PLT integrity in situations in which the processing (and transporting) of the blood samples could take two or more hours before the PRP can be used.

Although the type of anticoagulant did not significantly influence the PDGF-BB and TGF-β_1 concentrations in the different blood components in the present study, there was a better apparent concentration of PDGF-BB in the blood components processed with SC, followed by ACD-A and ACD-B. In contrast, when TGF-β_1 concentrations were evaluated, there were better apparent concentrations of this GF in the blood components processed with ACD-A, followed by SC and ACD-

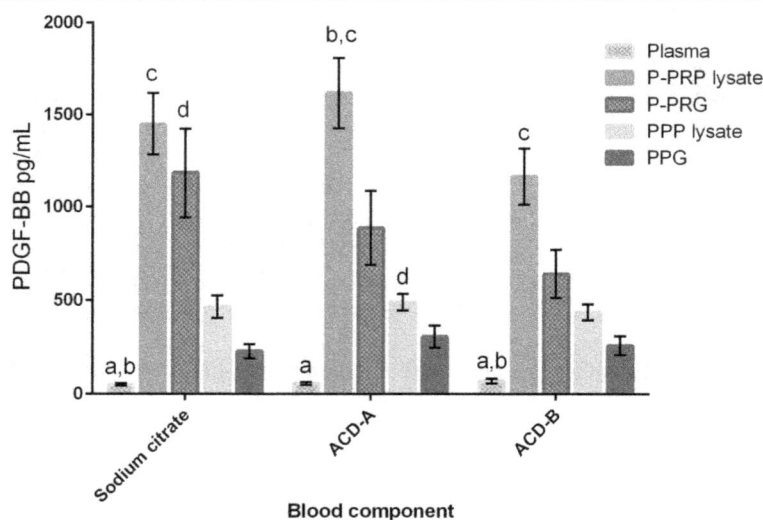

Figure 2 Means (standard error of the mean (s.e.m)) of PDGF-BB concentration (pg/mL) in the different blood components. Lower-case letters denote significant differences between blood components for every independent anticoagulant. Sodium citrate (SC): blood component significantly different with a: pure platelet-rich plasma (P-PRP) lysate and platelet poor plasma (PPP) lysate (P <0.001); b: pure platelet-rich gel (P-PRG) and platelet poor gel (PPG) (P <0.05); c: PPG and PPP lysate (P <0.001); and d: PPG (P <0.05). Acid citrate dextrose solution A (ACD-A): blood component significantly different with a: P-PRP lysate, PPP lysate, P-PRG and PPG (P <0.001); b: PPG and PPP lysates (P <0.001); and c: P-PRG (P <0.05). ACD-B: blood component significantly different with a: P-PRP and PPP lysates (P <0.001); b: P-PRG and PPG (P <0.05); and c: PPG and PPP lysates (P <0.001).

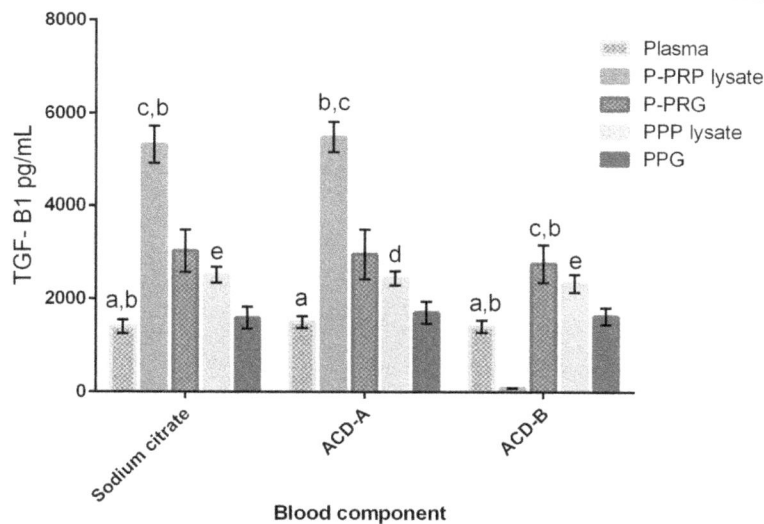

Figure 3 Means (s.e.m) of TGF-β₁concentration (pg/mL) in the different blood components. Lower-case letters denote significant differences between blood components for every independent anticoagulant. SC: blood component significantly different with a: P-PRP lysate (P <0.001); b: P-PRG and PPP lysates (P <0.05); c: PPG and PPP lysates (P <0.001); d: P-PRG (P <0.05); and e: PPG (P <0.05). ACD-A: blood component significantly different with a: P-PRP and PPP lysates (P <0.001); b: PPG and PPP lysates (P <0.001); c: P-PRG (P <0.05); and d: PPG (P <0.05). ACD-B: blood component significantly different with a: PRP and PPP lysates (P <0.001); b: P-PRG (P <0.05); c: PPG and PPP lysates (P <0.001); d: P-PRG (P <0.001); and e: PPG (P <0.05).

B. The same finding was reported for human PRP obtained with ACD-A and SC [12].

Notably, ACD-B had a very negative influence on GF concentrations when compared with the other anticoagulants. It is possible that the type of anticoagulant influenced (albeit not significantly) the release patterns of both GFs from all P-PRGs, as PDGF-BB release was substantially larger from platelet clots processed with SC in comparison with ACD-A and ACD-B. In contrast, TGF-β₁ release was more uniform (50% of the concentration with respect to P-PRP lysates) from the P-PRGs obtained with any of the three anticoagulants.

Despite the intriguing results observed regarding GF release from P-PRGs, the present study may have had some methodological limitations. For instance, perhaps measuring GF release at a single time point is not appropriate for determining the exact influence of the anticoagulants on GF release from P-PRGs [15]. In this situation, it is imperative to perform a study that evaluates the elution kinetics of both GFs at several time points. This study is necessary to determine whether the type of anticoagulant could produce GF loss (degradation) or GF absorption in the P-PRGs.

Many P-PRPs produced by manual tube protocols in different species (including equines) are performed with commercial vacuum tubes for *in vitro* diagnoses, not for therapeutic purposes [6,13,21,22]. This is a well-manifested concern by researches defending the use of commercial kits for producing platelet concentrates [23]. However, in the experience of the authors, the only problem with using commercial tubes with anticoagulants for

equine PRP processing is that the PLT collection efficiency is very low [6,16]. The use of many tubes during PRP preparation could be associated with a risk of bacterial contamination [24] and with a major time expenditure for PRP processing [2]. However, it is well recognized that the main source for bacterial contamination during PRP processing is the skin of the venipuncture site, not the tubes [24]. In view of these limitations, it is possible that the use of ACD-A tubes could be more suitable for manual PRP processing, as the volume capacity of the tubes is almost 44% greater than that of sodium citrate tubes.

The correlations obtained in this study were similar to those obtained in previous equine PRP studies, which evaluated manual protocols [6,16]. In general, there were moderate to strong correlations between cell (PLT and WBC) counts and GF concentrations. These findings are in agreement with several procedures for obtaining PRP in humans [25], dogs [26] and cattle [27]. The role of WBCs in PRP is controversial because there are data supporting the catabolic effect of these cells in equine tendon explants [9]. However, this situation could be more clinically relevant when L-PRP preparations are used [28]. The authors believe that the number of WBCs concentrated in the P-PRPs from this study could be beneficial for treating tissues because these cells are correlated with GF concentrations, especially TGF-β₁ [6].

Conclusions

This study presents new information regarding the effect of the anticoagulants: SC, ACD-A and ACD-B, for the elaboration of equine P-PRP. The results obtained in the study confirm the working hypothesis that the anticoagulants evaluated did not significantly influence cell counts or GF concentrations in equine P-PRP. However, ACD-B was apparently the worst anticoagulant evaluated, because it produced the lower cell counts and GF concentrations when compared with the other two anticoagulants. It is necessary to perform additional research to determine the GF elution kinetics from P-PRGs obtained with the anticoagulants evaluated in this study.

Abbreviations

ACD-A(B): Acid citrate dextrose solution A(B); BC: Buffy coat; CG: Calcium gluconate; COL1: Collagen type I; EOS: Eosinophils; FPF: First plasma fraction; GF: Growth factors; WBC: Leukocytes (white blood cells); L-PRP: Leukocyte-platelet rich plasma; LY: Lymphocytes; MPV: Mean platelet volume; NID: Non-ionic detergent; PLT: Platelet; PC: Platelet concentrates; PDGF-BB: Platelet derived growth factor isoform BB; PDW: Platelet distribution width; PG: Platelet gels; PPG: Platelet poor plasma gel; PPP: Platelet poor plasma; PRF: Platelet rich fibrin; P-PRP: Pure platelet-rich plasma; P-PRG: Pure platelet-rich gel; SC: Sodium citrate; TP: Total protein; TGF-β_1: Transforming growth factor beta 1.

Competing interests

The authors declare that they have no competing interests.

Authors' contributions

This manuscript represents a part of the PhD Thesis submitted by CEG to the Agrarian Sciences Doctoral Program of the Universidad de Caldas, Manizales, Colombia. JUC and CEG conceived of the study. JUC and CEG collected samples. CEG, MEA performed the laboratory tests. CEG and JUC performed the statistical analysis. All the authors participated in the drafting of the manuscript. JUC coordinated the study. All authors read and approved the final manuscript.

Acknowledgements

The Authors thank Catalina López, MVZ, PhD for her technical assistance. This research was supported by a grant of the Vicerrectoría de Investigaciones y Postgrados of the Universidad de Caldas. The authors also thank Policia Nacional de Colombia.

References

1. Castelijns G, Crawford A, Schaffer J, Ortolano GA, Beauregard T, Smith RKW. Evaluation of a filter-prepared platelet concentrate for the treatment of suspensory branch injuries in horses. Vet Comp OrthopTraumatol. 2011;24(5):363–9.
2. Carmona JU, López C, Sandoval JA. Review of the currently available systems to obtain platelet related products to treat equine musculoskeletal injuries. Rec Pat Reg Med. 2013;3(2):148–59.
3. López C, Carmona JU. Platelet-rich plasma as an adjunctive therapy for the management of a severe chronic distal limb wound in a foal. J Equine Vet Sci. 2014;34(9):1128–33.
4. Iacopetti I, Perazzi A, Ferrari V, Busetto R. Application of platelet-rich gel to enhance wound healing in the horse: a case report. J Equine Vet Sci. 2012;32(3):123–8.
5. Bazzano M, Piccione G, Giannetto C, Tosto F, Di Pietro S, E. G. Platelet rich plasma intralesional injection as bedside therapy for tendinitis in athletic horse. Acta Sci Vet. 2013;41:1145.
6. Giraldo CE, López C, Álvarez ME, Samudio IJ, Prades M, Carmona JU. Effects of the breed, sex and age on cellular content and growth factor release from equine pure-platelet rich plasma and pure-platelet rich gel. BMC Vet Res. 2013;9:29.
7. Carmona J, López C, Giraldo C. Uso de concentrados autólogos de plaquetas como terapia regenerativa de enfermedades crónicas del aparato musculoesquelético equino. Arch Med Vet. 2011;43(1):1–10.
8. Dohan Ehrenfest DM, Bielecki T, Mishra A, Borzini P, Inchingolo F, Sammartino G, et al. In search of a consensus terminology in the field of platelet concentrates for surgical use: platelet-rich plasma (PRP), platelet-rich

fibrin (PRF), fibrin gel polymerization and leukocytes. Currt Pharm Biotechnol. 2012;13(7):1131–7.
9. McCarrel TM, Minas T, Fortier LA. Optimization of leukocyte concentration in platelet-rich plasma for the treatment of tendinopathy. J Bone Joint Surg Am. 2012;94(19):e143.141–8.
10. Mazzucco L, Balbo V, Cattana E, Guaschino R, Borzini P. Not every PRP-gel is born equal Evaluation of growth factor availability for tissues through four PRP-gel preparations: Fibrinet®; RegenPRP-Kit®; Plateltex®; and one manual procedure. Vox Sang. 2009;97(2):110–8.
11. O'Shaughnessey K, Matuska A, Hoeppner J, Farr J, Klaassen M, Kaeding C, et al. Autologous protein solution prepared from the blood of osteoarthritic patients contains an enhanced profile of anti-inflammatory cytokines and anabolic growth factors. J Orthop Res. 2014;32(10):1349–55.
12. Lei H, Gui L, Xiao R. The effect of anticoagulants on the quality and biological efficacy of platelet-rich plasma. Clin Biochem. 2009;42(13–14):1452–60.
13. Vendruscolo CP, Carvalho AM, Moraes LF, Maia L, Queiroz DL, Watanabe MJ, et al. Evaluating the effectiveness of different protocols for preparation of platelet rich plasma for use in equine medicine. Pesq Vet Bras. 2012;32(2):106–10.
14. Textor JA, Norris JW, Tablin F. Effects of preparation method, shear force, and exposure to collagen on release of growth factors from equine platelet-rich plasma. Am J Vet Res. 2011;72(2):271–8.
15. Textor JA, Tablin F. Activation of equine platelet-rich plasma: Comparison of methods and characterization of equine autologous thrombin. Vet Surg. 2012;41(7):784–94.
16. Argüelles D, Carmona JU, Pastor J, Iborra A, Viñals L, Martínez P, et al. Evaluation of single and double centrifugation tube methods for concentrating equine platelets. Res Vet Sci. 2006;81(2):237–45.
17. Gornall AG, Bardawill CJ, David MM. Determination of serum proteins by means of the biuret reaction. J BiolChem. 1949;177(2):751–66.
18. Penha-goncalves MN, Onions DE, Nicolson L. Cloning and sequencing of equine transforming growth factor-beta 1 (TGF beta-1) cDNA. DNA Seq. 1997;7(6):375–8.
19. Donnelly BP, Nixon AJ, Haupt JL. Nucleotide structure of equine platelet-derived growth factor-A and –B and expression in horses with induced acute tendinitis. Am J Vet Res. 2006;67(7):1218–25.
20. Macey M, Azam U, McCarthy D, Webb L, Chapman ES, Okrongly D, et al. Evaluation of the Anticoagulants EDTA and Citrate, Theophylline, Adenosine, and Dipyridamole (CTAD) for Assessing Platelet Activation on the ADVIA 120 Hematology System. Clin Chem. 2002;48(6):891–9.
21. Fontenot RL, Sink CA, Werre SR, Weinstein NM, Dahlgren LA. Simple tube centrifugation for processing platelet-rich plasma in the horse. Can Vet J. 2012;53(12):1266–72.
22. Silva RF, Carmona JU, Rezende CMF. Intra-articular injections of autologous platelet concentrates in dogs with surgical reparation of cranial cruciate ligament rupture. Vet Comp Orthop Traumatol. 2013;26(4):285–90.
23. O'Connell SM. Safety Issues Associated With Platelet-Rich Fibrin Method. Oral Surg, Oral Med, Oral Pathol, Oral Radiol Endodontol. 2007;103(5):587.
24. Álvarez ME, Giraldo CE, Carmona JU. Monitoring bacterial contamination in equine platelet concentrates obtained by the tube method in a clean laboratory environment under three different technical conditions. Equine Vet J. 2010;42(1):63–7.
25. Zimmermann R, Arnold D, Strasser E, Ringwald J, Schlegel A, Wiltfang J, et al. Sample preparation technique and white cell content influence the detectable levels of growth factors in platelet concentrates. Vox Sang. 2003;85(4):283–9.
26. Silva RF, Carmona JU, Rezende CMF. Comparison of the effect of calcium gluconate and batroxobin on the release of transforming growth factor beta 1 in canine platelet concentrates. BMC Vet Res. 2012;8:121.
27. López C, Giraldo CE, Carmona JU. Evaluation of a double centrifugation tube method for concentrating bovine platelets: Cellular study. Arch Med Vet. 2012;44(2):109–15.
28. Dragoo JL, Braun HJ, Durham JL, Ridley BA, Odegaard JI, Luong R, et al. Comparison of the acute inflammatory response of two commercial platelet-rich plasma systems in healthy rabbit tendons. Am J Sports Med. 2012;40(6):1274–81.

Use of a novel silk mesh for ventral midline hernioplasty in a mare

Jennifer Haupt, José M García-López[*] and Kate Chope

Abstract

Background: Ventral midline hernia formation following abdominal surgery in horses is an uncommon complication; however, it can have serious consequences leading to increased morbidity and mortality. Currently, mesh hernioplasty is the treatment of choice for large ventral midline hernias in horses to allow potential return to normal function. Complications following mesh hernioplasty using polypropylene or polyester mesh in horses can be serious and similar to complications seen in human patients, including persistent incisional drainage, mesh infection, hernia recurrence, intra-abdominal adhesions, mesh or body wall failure, recurrent abdominal pain (colic), and peritonitis. This report describes the use of a novel bioresorbable silk mesh for repair of a large ventral midline incisional hernia in a mature, 600-kg horse. To our knowledge, this is the first report of its kind in the literature.

Case presentation: A 9-year-old, 600-kg Warmblood mare presented with a ventral midline hernia following emergency exploratory celiotomy 20 months prior. The mare was anesthetized and a hernioplasty was performed using a novel bioresorbable silk mesh (SERI® Surgical Scaffold; Allergan Medical, Boston, MA). No complications were encountered either intra- or postoperatively. The mare was discharged from the hospital at 3 days postoperatively in an abdominal support bandage. At 8 and 20 weeks postoperatively, ultrasonographic assessment showed evidence of tissue ingrowth within and around the mesh. The mare was able to be bred 2 years in a row, carrying both foals to full gestation with no complications. Following both foalings, the abdomen has maintained a normal contour with no evidence of hernia recurrence.

Conclusions: Ventral abdominal hernias can be repaired in horses using a bioresorbable silk mesh, which provides adequate biomechanical strength while allowing for fibrous tissue ingrowth. The use of a bioresorbable silk mesh for the repair of ventral hernias can be considered as a realistic option as it potentially provides significant benefits over traditional non-resorbable mesh.

Keywords: Abdominal, Hernia, Hernioplasty, Horse, Mesh, Silk

Background

Ventral midline celiotomy is a common procedure for evaluation and treatment of abdominal pain in horses. Early incisional complications following colic surgery include incisional drainage in 29% of horses and subsequent incisional infection in 4% of horses [1]. Long-term complications following celiotomy for surgical treatment of colic in horses include ventral midline hernia formation in 8% to 16% of cases [2,3]. Factors that increase the likelihood for hernia formation include incisional drainage or infection and repeat laparotomy [2-4].

Although not all ventral midline hernias in horses require surgical repair, mesh hernioplasty is the treatment of choice for large defects, which can inhibit athletic activity, gestation and parturition, and can lead to bowel incarceration. Currently, the available mesh implants for use in equine hernioplasty are non-absorbable knitted polypropylene or polyester mesh. Open repair of large ventral midline hernias with subperitoneal mesh placement and hernia ring apposition is the most common surgical technique [5,6]. Major complications can occur in mesh hernioplasty in horses ranging from persistent incisional drainage, mesh infection, hernia recurrence, intra-abdominal adhesions, mesh or body wall failure, recurrent abdominal pain (colic), and peritonitis [5]. Based on the current literature, complication rates following mesh hernioplasty using synthetic,

---

[*] Correspondence: jose.garcia-lopez@tufts.edu
Department of Clinical Sciences, Cummings School of Veterinary Medicine, Tufts University, 200 Westboro Road, North Grafton, MA 01536, USA

non-absorbable mesh range from 20% to 60%, with mortality rates up to 50% following repair in large horses (>450 kg) [5,7]. The most significant complications leading to increased morbidity and mortality following mesh hernioplasty in horses include persistent mesh infection, rupture of the internal abdominal oblique muscle, and persistent colic [5]. Potential causes of recurrent colic and rupture of the internal abdominal oblique muscle include the rigidity of the synthetic mesh implant and tearing at the mesh-host tissue interface.

Bioresorbable surgical meshes are the ideal implant for mesh hernioplasty as they enhance the mechanical integrity of the body wall while supporting ingrowth of host tissue. In addition, the bioresorbable mesh should reduce postoperative complications including infection and recurrent pain associated with the rigidity of synthetic mesh implants. Recently, a novel bioresorbable silk mesh (SERI˚ Surgical Scaffold; Allergan Medical, Boston, MA) was evaluated in a rodent abdominal body wall defect model. In this animal model, the silk mesh demonstrated significantly greater ingrowth of fibrous tissue compared with polyester mesh [8]. The silk mesh also provided an ideal bioresorption rate, which allowed the ultimate load to be shared between the body wall, mesh implant, and repair tissue [8]. Based on the promising results of the rodent abdominal body wall defect study, we aimed to evaluate silk mesh for use in a large ventral body wall defect in a large horse with the hypothesis that silk mesh would minimize postoperative complications and provide adequate biomechanical properties during healing. This report describes the use of a novel silk mesh for ventral midline hernioplasty in a large horse.

Case presentation

A 9-year-old, 600-kg Warmblood mare was admitted for evaluation of a ventral midline hernia. The mare initially presented to the hospital 20 months previously for treatment of abdominal pain (colic) which was diagnosed as a left dorsal displacement of the large colon and was corrected by exploratory celiotomy and reduction of the displacement. Following the exploratory celiotomy, the mare developed an incisional infection and subsequent ventral midline hernia. A previous repair was attempted in the field by a referring veterinarian with no success. In addition, the owner reported no success with abdominal support bandaging.

On initial evaluation, a ventral midline hernia was palpable at the cranial aspect of the previous celiotomy incision. The hernia sac was soft with a palpable hernia ring and there was no obvious bowel present within the hernia sac (Figure 1). Ultrasonography was used to further evaluate the size of the defect as well as the quality of the hernia ring and surrounding tissues in preparation for mesh hernioplasty. It revealed that the hernia sac contained primarily peritoneal fluid, with the hernia ring being well-demarcated with thick, fibrous edges; the hernia measured 4.2 cm (width) by 7.4 cm (length) (Figure 1). No obvious intra-abdominal adhesions were present either associated with the hernia or surrounding ventral midline. Due to the large size of the hernia defect, the desire to retain the mare for breeding, and the concern about potential herniation of bowel within the hernia sac during gestation or foaling, mesh hernioplasty was elected by the owner.

Surgery was planned for the following day, and food but not water was withheld for 6 hours before anesthesia. Ceftiofur sodium (2.2 mg/kg, IV q12h), gentamicin (6.6 mg/kg, IV q24h), and flunixin meglumine (1.1 mg/kg IV q12h) were administered before surgery and continued for 3 days postoperatively.

Surgical procedure

The mare was sedated with xylazine hydrochloride (1 mg/kg, IV) and then induced with a combination of ketamine (2.2 mg/kg, IV) and midazolam (0.1 mg/kg, IV). Anesthesia was maintained with isoflurane delivered in 100% oxygen in a semi-closed system. The mare was placed under general anesthesia in dorsal recumbency

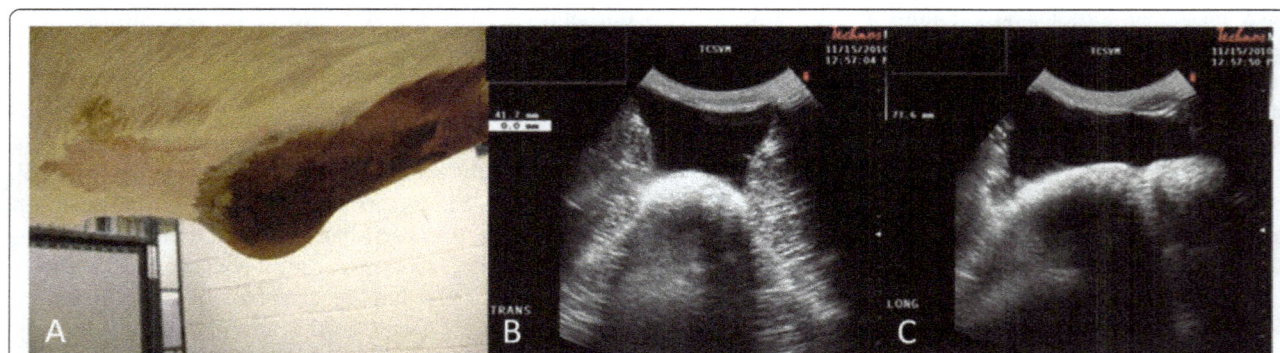

Figure 1 Preoperative gross (A) and ultrasonographic appearance of the ventral midline hernia using a 5 MHz convex abdominal ultrasound probe in transverse (B) and longitudinal (C) planes revealing peritoneal fluid filling the hernia sac. Measurement markings on right side of the ultrasound images indicate 0.5-cm intervals. E indicates the cranial and lateral margins of the defect.

with routine surgical preparation and draping of the ventral abdomen.

A 7-cm semielliptical incision through skin and subcutaneous tissues was made slightly to the right of midline at the edge of the hernia (Figure 2). The fibrous tissue of the hernia was visualized directly deep to the subcutaneous tissue with an approximate thickness of 2 cm. The fascial planes between skin and hernia fibrous tissue were bluntly dissected. A 6-cm semielliptical incision paralleling the skin incision was made through the fibrous tissue of the hernia sac. The peritoneum was visible deep to the hernia but did not appear to be involved or adhered. The body wall was located at edges of fibrous hernia tissue. A 6-cm (width) by 9-cm (length) square of silk mesh (SERI® Surgical Scaffold) was placed in a retroperitoneal position within the hernia ring with pre-placement of 11 individual sutures of #2 nylon encircling the hernia followed by sequential tightening (Figure 2). The fibrous tissue of the hernia sac was closed with 2 polydioxanone (PDS II; Ethicon, Bridgewater, NJ) in a horizontal mattress pattern, interspersed with simple interrupted followed by simple interrupted tacking sutures using 0 poliglecaprone 25 (Monocryl Plus; Ethicon, Bridgewater, NJ), which were placed through the hernia sac and subcutaneous tissue to reduce dead space

(Figure 2). Subcutaneous tissue was closed in two layers with 0 poliglecaprone 25 using a simple continuous pattern. The skin was apposed using surgical staples, and the incision was protected in a commercial hernia belt (CM Equine Products, Norco, CA) for recovery. The mare recovered from anesthesia without complications.

Postoperative care
The mare was discharged from the hospital 3 days postoperatively on a course of parenteral antibiotics (ceftiofur) and anti-inflammatories (flunixin meglumine) with management in an abdominal support bandage. At 8 and 20 weeks postoperatively, ultrasonography was conducted to evaluate healing based on tissue ingrowth of the mesh and fibrous tissue formation around the mesh (Figure 3). No complications were reported at either time point. Furthermore, the ventral abdomen was observed to have a normal contour at both time points. Based on the formation of fibrous tissue surrounding the mesh, the mare was bred 2 years in a row, carrying both foals to full gestation with no complications. Following both foalings, the abdomen has maintained a normal contour with no evidence of hernia recurrence (Figure 4).

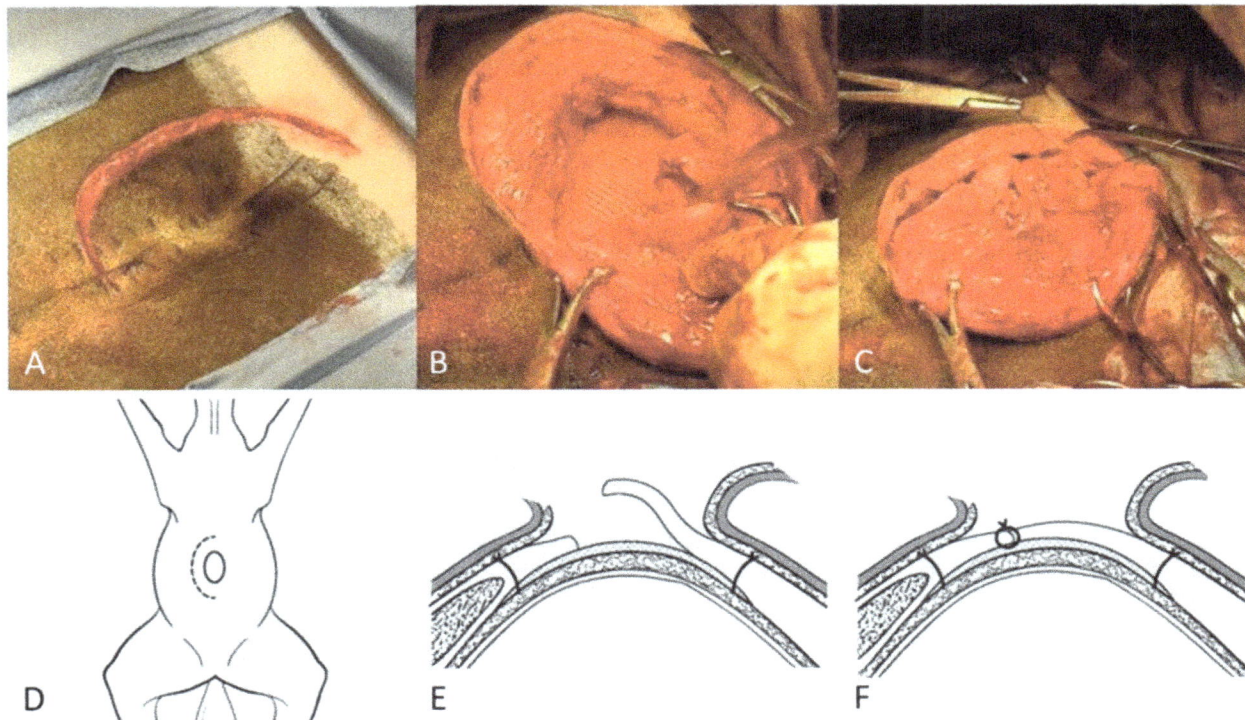

Figure 2 Intraoperative photographs and corresponding cross-sectional drawings revealing the various stages of intraoperative repair using silk mesh. Initial elliptical skin incision around the hernia revealing the ventral midline incision from the previous exploratory celiotomy and incision from the previous repair attempt **(A)**. Implantation and suturing of the silk mesh extraperitoneally under the hernia sac **(B)**. Closure of the hernia sac overlying the silk mesh **(C)**. Corresponding figures depict tissue layers **(D–F)**.

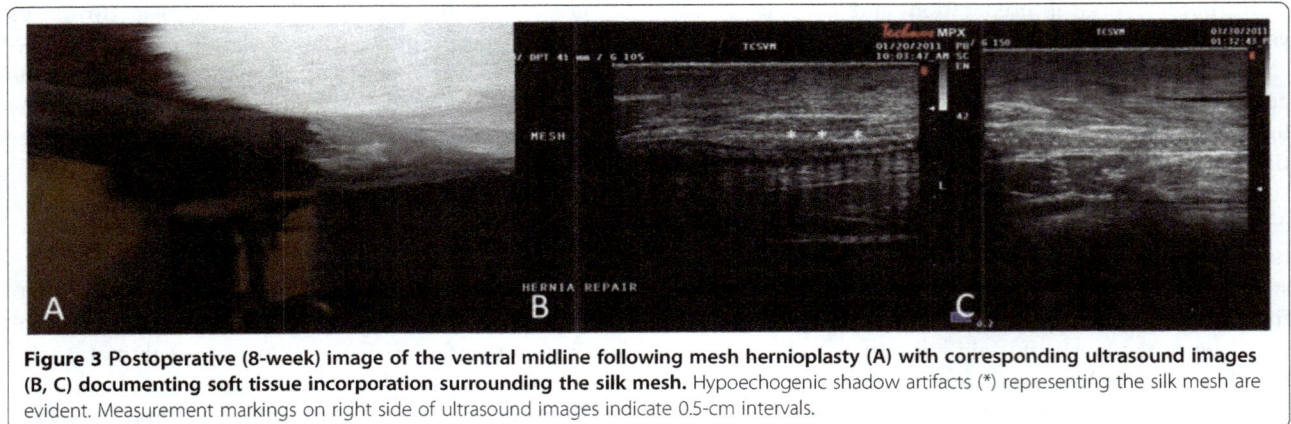

Figure 3 Postoperative (8-week) image of the ventral midline following mesh hernioplasty (A) with corresponding ultrasound images (B, C) documenting soft tissue incorporation surrounding the silk mesh. Hypoechogenic shadow artifacts (*) representing the silk mesh are evident. Measurement markings on right side of ultrasound images indicate 0.5-cm intervals.

Discussion

Ventral midline hernia formation is a complication following surgical management of abdominal pain in horses with incisional drainage and incisional infection being the largest risk factor for hernia formation [1,2]. In the case presented here, the development of a ventral midline hernia was subsequent to infection of the body wall associated with a previous exploratory celiotomy for treatment of colic. Conventional repair of large ventral midline hernia defects in horses involves subperitoneal implantation of non-absorbable knitted polypropylene or polyester mesh and hernia ring apposition. However, this repair technique has high complication rates (20%–60%), with mortality rates up to 50% due to persistent infection of the implant, rupture of the internal abdominal oblique muscle, and persistent colic, which are all potentially due to the rigidity of synthetic, non-resorbable mesh implants [5,7]. Further concerns regarding currently used non-absorbable mesh implants include tissue erosion, persistent inflammation, infection, and pain following mesh hernioplasty as well as difficulties with potential surgical revision.

Alternative surgical techniques for repair of ventral midline hernias include attempted primary closure of the defect without mesh implantation, subperitoneal mesh placement with fascial overlay, and subcutaneous mesh placement with hernia ring apposition [5-7]. In this case, primary closure of the defect without mesh was previously attempted and likely failed due to the large size of the defect, in addition to the large size of the patient. Subperitoneal placement with fascial overlay involves more aggressive dissection of the hernia sac, allowing more potential exposure of the peritoneal cavity to the mesh implant. Consequences of peritoneal contact with the surface of the mesh include intra-abdominal adhesion of the bowel to the mesh implant, which can lead to chronic colic. In addition, mesh infection would have dire consequences leading to potential septic peritonitis, for which mortality rates range from 40% to 60% in equine patients [9,10]. To help minimize these complications, implantation of subcutaneous mesh following primary closure of the defect has been described [6]. This procedure was not elected in this case, as the significant

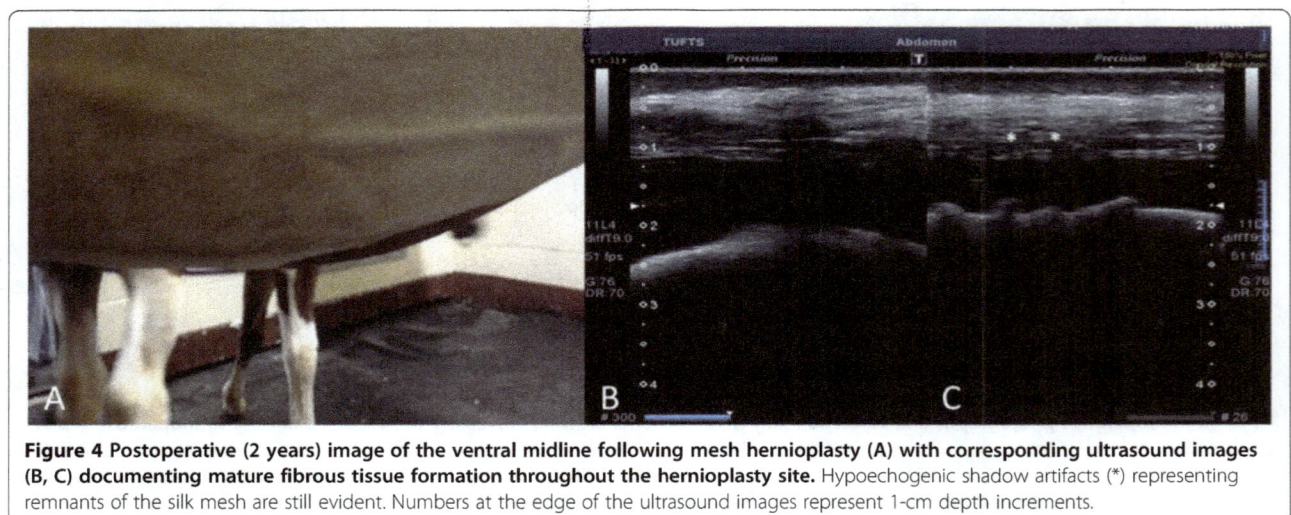

Figure 4 Postoperative (2 years) image of the ventral midline following mesh hernioplasty (A) with corresponding ultrasound images (B, C) documenting mature fibrous tissue formation throughout the hernioplasty site. Hypoechogenic shadow artifacts (*) representing remnants of the silk mesh are still evident. Numbers at the edge of the ultrasound images represent 1-cm depth increments.

size of the defect and large patient size would have created a large amount of tension on the ventral midline and body wall, likely causing dehiscence of the primary closure as well as potential failure of the mesh. In addition, as the mesh is placed subcutaneously, there is greater concern for mesh infection.

To our knowledge, this is the first published report describing the use of silk mesh for ventral midline hernioplasty in a large animal. The mesh used in this case is a novel silk-derived bioresorbable scaffold designed to support fibrous tissue ingrowth while allowing long-term bioresorption. Prior to the knitting of the mesh scaffold, the silk is processed to remove the outer sericin coat, which is the major cause of allergenic responses [11]. By removing the sericin, the silk has greater biocompatibility and thus enhanced bioresorption in vivo [8,11]. An earlier version of this silk mesh was evaluated for repair of body wall defects in rodents in comparison to the conventionally used polyester meshes [8]. In contrast to the polyester mesh, the silk mesh had higher reduction in the cross-sectional area over the course of the study, whereas the polyester mesh remained essentially unchanged [8]. Although the silk began to bioresorb, the mesh allowed for significantly greater fibrous tissue ingrowth with biomechanical properties comparable to the polyester mesh at the 3-month termination point of the study [8]. In addition, this study found the inflammatory reaction was similar with both silk mesh and polyester mesh [8]. Subjectively speaking, the silk mesh was extremely easy to work with, less rigid than standard polypropylene or polyester mesh, and less abrasive to the touch. We did not encounter any issues with how the silk mesh handled the suture bites and did not experience any pullout or ripping at the edges during application. Although we believe SERI silk mesh has a soft enough texture not to be abrasive to the bowel if placed intra-peritoneally, we cannot comment on its effect with regards to adhesion formation or bowel irritation.

Gross and colleagues recently published their results of the use of the silk mesh used in this case report for soft tissue support in two-stage breast reconstruction using an ovine model [12]. In their study they were able to demonstrate that the load-bearing responsibility which originally was provided by the mesh was gradually transferred to the new ingrown tissue consisting early on of collagen type 3 and later shifting to collagen type 1. The ingrowth of fibrous tissue resulted in a significant increase in the burst strength of the implant when compared to sham samples [12]. Such increase in strength of the implant has obvious benefits, especially when placed in dependent areas such as in this case report.

In this case report, we aimed to evaluate the potential use of silk mesh in a large horse for ventral midline hernioplasty. In this single case, no complications were encountered when implanting the silk mesh retroperitoneally with hernia ring apposition and closure of subcutaneous tissues and skin. The silk mesh allowed adequate sharing of load between the body wall and mesh, while allowing tissue remodeling and fibrous tissue formation around the defect, as documented by ultrasonography. In our study, remnants of the mesh were visible 2 years following hernioplasty with healthy and organized fibrous scar tissue. In their study, Gross and colleagues were able to document histologically the ingrowth of new collagen fibers, with silk fibrils still visible throughout their 12-month study without evidence of hypersensitivity or immune response [12]. Although we were unable to perform histologic and biomechanical analysis of the repair tissue, the outcome had adequate cosmesis of the ventral abdomen and provided enough biomechanical strength to support the ventral midline of a large horse throughout gestation and parturition of two foals.

Conclusions

In conclusion, we report the successful use of a novel bioresorbable silk mesh for repair of a large ventral midline hernia in a 600-kg mare. Although this is a single case report, the use of a bioresorbable mesh in a large animal has clinical significance not only for horses but also for humans, as the mesh was able to provide adequate biomechanical strength while allowing for fibrous tissue ingrowth with no complications.

Competing interests

JH and KC declare no conflict of interest. JGL makes known that he has a business relationship with Allergan Medical. Activity in connection to this company includes consulting and animal model design. JGL declares no conflict of interest that directly relates to this study. The silk mesh (SERI* Surgical Scaffold) was provided by Allergan for use in this case report. No additional financial support was provided for this case report.

Authors' contributions

JH and JGL were responsible for the surgical procedure. KC performed all sonographic examinations. JH, JGL, and KC were involved in the drafting and writing of the manuscript. All authors read and approved the final version of the manuscript.

Acknowledgements

The authors thank Mrs. Beth Mellor for her assistance with the illustrations. Editorial assistance was provided by Evidence Scientific Solutions and was funded by Allergan, Inc.

References

1. Mair TS, Smith LJ. Survival and complication rates in 300 horses undergoing surgical treatment of colic. Part 2: Short-term complications. Equine Vet J. 2005;37:303–9.
2. Mair TS, Smith LJ. Survival and complication rates in 300 horses undergoing surgical treatment of colic. Part 3: Long-term complications and survival. Equine Vet J. 2005;37:310–4.
3. Gibson KT, Curtis CR, Turner AS, McIlwraith CW, Aanes WA, Stashak TS. Incisional hernias in the horse. Incidence and predisposing factors. Vet Surg. 1989;18:360–6.

4.   French NP, Smith J, Edwards GB, Proudman CJ. Equine surgical colic: risk
      factors for postoperative complications. Equine Vet J. 2002;34:444–9.
5.   Elce YA, Kraus BM, Orsini JA. Mesh hernioplasty for repair of incisional hernias
      of the ventral body wall in large horses. Equine Vet Educ. 2005;17:252–6.
6.   Kelmer G, Schumacher J. Repair of abdominal wall hernias in horses using primary
      closure and subcutaneous implantation of mesh. Vet Rec. 2008;163:677–9.
7.   Tulleners EP, Fretz PB. Prosthetic repair of large abdominal wall defects in
      horses and food animals. J Am Vet Med Assoc. 1983;182:258–62.
8.   Horan RL, Bramono DS, Stanley JR, Simmons Q, Chen J, Boepple HE, et al.
      Biological and biomechanical assessment of a long-term bioresorbable
      silk-derived surgical mesh in an abdominal body wall defect model.
      Hernia. 2009;13:189–99.
9.   Hawkins JF, Bowman KF, Roberts MC, Cowen P. Peritonitis in horses:
      67 cases (1985-1990). J Am Vet Med Assoc. 1993;203:284–8.
10.   Mair TS, Hillyer MH, Taylor FG. Peritonitis in adult horses: a review of 21
      cases. Vet Rec. 1990;126:567–70.
11.   Altman GH, Diaz F, Jakuba C, Calabro T, Horan RL, Chen J, et al. Silk-based
      biomaterials. Biomaterials. 2003;24:401–16.
12.   Gross J, Horan R, Gaylord M, Olsen RE, McGill LD, García-López JM, et al. An
      evaluation of SERI Surgical Scaffold for soft-tissue support and repair in an
      ovine model of two-stage breast reconstruction. Plast Reconstr Surg.
      2014;134:700e–4.

15

Lipopolysaccharide derived from the rumen down-regulates stearoyl-CoA desaturase 1 expression and alters fatty acid composition in the liver of dairy cows fed a high-concentrate diet

Tianle Xu[†], Hui Tao[†], Guangjun Chang, Kai Zhang, Lei Xu and Xiangzhen Shen[*]

Abstract

Background: Dairy cows are often fed a high-concentrate diet to meet lactating demands, yet long-term concentrate feeding induces subacute ruminal acidosis (SARA) and leads to a decrease in milk fat. Stearoyl-CoA desaturase1 (SCD1) participates in fatty acid biosynthesis in the liver of lactating ruminants. Here, we conducted this study to investigate the impact of lipopolysaccharide derived from the rumen on SCD1 expression and on fatty acid composition in the liver of dairy cows fed a high-concentrate diet. Eight multiparous mid-lactating Holstein cows (455 ± 28 kg) were randomly assigned into two groups in the experiment and were fed a low-concentrate diet (LC) or high-concentrate diet (HC) for 18 weeks.

Results: The results showed that the total volatile fatty acids and lactic acid accumulated in the rumen, leading to a decreased rumen pH and elevated lipopolysaccharides (LPSs) in the HC group. The long chain fatty acid profile in the rumen and hepatic vein was remarkably altered in the animals fed the HC diet. The triglyceride (TG), non-esterified fatty acid (NEFA) and total cholesterol (TCH) content in the plasma was significantly decreased, whereas plasma glucose and insulin levels were increased. The expression of SCD1 in the liver was significantly down-regulated in the HC group. In regards to transcriptional regulators, the expression of sterol regulatory element binding transcription factors (SREBF1c, SREBF2) and SREBP cleavage activating protein (SCAP) was down-regulated, while peroxisome proliferator-activated receptor α (PPARα) was up-regulated.

Conclusions: These data indicate that lipopolysaccharide derived from the rumen down-regulates stearoyl-CoA desaturase 1 expression and alters fatty acid composition in the liver of dairy cows fed a high-concentrate diet.

Keywords: Lipopolysaccharide, Stearoyl-CoA desaturase 1, Long chain fatty acid, Liver, High concentrate diet, Dairy cows

Background

Dairy cows are often fed a high-concentrate diet to meet lactating requirements for high milk performance [1]. However, long-term feeding with a high-concentrate diet causes a decline in the rumen pH if organic acids, such as volatile fatty acids (VFAs) and lactic acid, accumulate in the rumen [2,3], and a chronic digestive disorder known as subacute ruminal acidosis (SARA) may occur. A rumen pH of less than 5.6 for over 3 h per day is used as a parameter to determine the occurrence of SARA [1]. Decreased rumen pH results in the release of lipopolysaccharides (LPSs), which originate from the cell-wall component of gram-negative bacteria [4].

Previous studies demonstrated that LPSs stimulate the gene expression of fatty acid synthetase (FAS) and acetyl-CoA carboxylase (ACC) in the liver of mice [5] but depressed stearoyl-CoA desaturase (SCD) expression in bovine hepatocytes [6]. SCD is a rate-limiting enzyme that catalyzes the synthesis of the monounsaturated fatty acids oleate (18:1) and palmitoleate (16:1) and forms triglycerides

* Correspondence: xzshen@njau.edu.cn
[†]Equal contributors
College of Veterinary Medicine, Nanjing Agricultural University, Nanjing 210095, China

and cholesterol esters [7]. Microarray assays have indicated that the gene expression profile was altered in the liver of SCD knockout mice, and the most obvious pattern was down-regulation of the genes involved in lipogenesis and up-regulation of the genes associated with fatty acid β-oxidation [8]. It was reported that LPS modulates lipid metabolism by inhibiting the clearance of triacylglycerol in the livers of bovine [9]. Furthermore, in a LPS-induced liver injury model, SCD1 expression was inhibited in the liver of mice, suggesting the potential action of LPS on SCD1 inhibition [10].

The liver is responsible for lipid metabolism in ruminant animals, and SARA is associated with liver abscesses, fatty liver and a whole-body inflammatory response when a high-grain diet is offered [11]. Therefore, the repartition of energy from production to anti-inflammation may exist in the liver and consequently lead to a negative energy balance during long-term high-concentrate supply. Many studies have been carried out on milk fat depression (MFD) in diet-induced SARA [12]. Some studies have focused on the *trans* fatty acid (i.e., *trans-10* C18:1n) pathway [13], while others have paid attention to LPS, which initiates the inflammatory response and influences the fatty acid profile in the rumen and milk [14]. Currently, several studies have been performed to evaluate hepatic lipid metabolism in dairy cows via exogenous LPS infusion [15].However, less information is available in regards to the alterations in hepatic lipid metabolism during long-term diet-induced SARA in dairy cows. Therefore, the present study was conducted to investigate the effects of a high-concentrate diet on the fatty acid composition and SCD1 expression in the liver of dairy cows.

Methods
Animals, diets and experimental design
Eight multiparous mid-lactating Holstein cows (455 ± 28 kg) were randomly assigned into two groups. One group was fed with a high-concentrate diet (HC) composed of 40% forage and 60% concentrate as a treatment, and the other group was offered a low-concentrate diet (LC) composed of 60% forage and 40% concentrate as a control for the 18-week experimental period. The ingredients and nutritional composition of the diets are presented in Table 1. The cows were fitted with a rumen fistula and hepatic catheters two weeks before the experiment and were ensured that they recovered from the surgery. The animals were maintained in individual tie stalls, fed at 0400, 1200, and 2000 h, and had free access to fresh water throughout the experimental time period.

The animal experiment was reviewed and approved by the Institutional Animal Care and Use Committee of Nanjing Agricultural University. The experiment was performed in accordance with the "Guidelines for Experimental Animals" of the Ministry of Science and Technology (Beijing, China).

Table 1 The ingredients in the diets and the nutritional composition

Ingredients, % of DM	LC[1]	HC[1]
Corn silage	30	20
Alfalfa	30	20
Maize	22.78	33.6
Wheat bran	5.15	15
Soybean meal	9.81	9
Calcium phosphate dibasic	0.92	0.53
Powder	0	0.52
Salt	0.35	0.35
Premix[2]	1	1
Total	100	100
Nutritional Composition[3]		
NE MJ/kg	6.32	6.74
CP %	16	16.2
EE %	3.96	4.15
NDF %	37.71	31.92
ADF %	22.75	17.55
NFC %	33.43	40.31
Ca %	0.9	0.8
P %	0.45	0.45

[1] LC, low concentrate; HC, high concentrate.
[2] The premix contained VA,1,900ku/kg; VD, 250ku/kg; VE, 3,000 mg/kg; Niacin, 4,000 mg/kg; Cu, 1,200 mg/kg; Fe, 525 mg/kg; Zn, 13,000 mg/kg; Mn, 5,500 mg/kg; I, 170 mg/kg; Co, 50 mg/kg; Se, 27 mg/kg.
[3] The calculated nutritional composition values.

Sample collection and analysis
The cows were milked at 0500, 1300, and 2100 h, and the milk yield was recorded daily. A 50-mL milk sample was taken to determine the milk fat and milk protein concentrations once a week (MilkoScan™ FT1, FOSS, Denmark). Samples of the ruminal fluid were taken via the rumen fistula for 3 consecutive days during the 18th week, at 2-h intervals starting at 0400 h (after the morning feeding) for 12 hours. The samples were filtered through 2 layers of cheesecloth and stored at −20°C for the LPS, VFA, lactic acid and long-chain fatty acid analyses. A blood sample was taken at the same time as the ruminal fluid collection via the hepatic vein catheter and from the jugular vein using 5-mL vacuum tubes containing sodium heparin as an anticoagulant. The plasma was isolated from the blood samples by centrifugation at 3000 × g at 4°C for 15 min and was stored at −20°C for the LPS, biochemical parameter, hormones and long chain fatty acid analyses. Liver tissue samples were taken using a punch biopsy with a local anesthesia, and the samples were frozen in liquid nitrogen and then stored at −70°C until the quantitative Real-Time PCR and western blotting analyses.

LPS and biochemical parameters in the plasma and ruminal fluid

The LPS concentration in the ruminal fluid and plasma were determined using a chromogenic endpoint assay (CE64406, Chinese Horseshoe Crab Reagent Manufactory Co., Ltd., Xiamen, China) with a minimum detection limit of 0.05 EU/mL. The procedures were performed according to the manufacturer's instructions.

The analyses for the triglyceride, NEFA, total cholesterol and glucose concentrations were performed using commercial kits (Glucose Assay Kit, Rongsheng, Shanghai, China; Nonesterified Free Fatty Acids Assay Kit, Jiancheng, Nanjing, China; Total Cholesterol Reagent Kit, Dongou, Zhejiang, China; Lactic Acid Assay Kit, Jiancheng, Nanjing, China; Triglyceride Reagent Kit, Jiancheng, Nanjing, China) that used an enzymatic colorimetric method read by a microplate reader (Epoch, BioTek, USA). Plasma insulin and glucagon concentration was determined using an Iodine (^{125}I) Insulin Radioimmunoassay (RIA) Kit and Iodine (^{125}I) Glucagon Radioimmunoassay (RIA) Kit (Beijing North Institute of Biological Technology, Beijing, China) with Gamma Radioimmunoassay Counter (SN-6105, Hesuo Rihuan Photoelectric Instrument Co., Ltd, Shanghai, China). All of the procedures were performed according to the manufacturer's instructions.

Fatty acid analysis via gas chromatography

The VFA concentration in the ruminal fluid was determined via gas chromatography (GC) using a FFAP 123–3233, 30-m × 0.32-mm × 0.5-µm, capillary column (Agilent J&W GC Columns, Netherlands) on an Agilent 7890A (Agilent Technologies, USA) as described before with some modifications [16]. Crotonate was used as the internal standard.

The total lipids were extracted from the ruminal fluid and plasma using a mixture of polar and non-polar solvents according to Folch *et al.* at room temperature [17]. The fatty acid methyl esters (FAMEs) were prepared via esterification using sodium methoxide, followed by 14% borontrifluoride in methanol [18]. Heptadecanoic acid methyl ester served as the internal standard and was added to the samples prior to extraction and methylation. The FAME extracts were used for the gas chromatographic analysis of the total fatty acids. The fatty acid composition was determined using GC with a CP 7489, 100-m × 0.25-mm × 0.25-µm, capillary column (Agilent J&W Advanced Capillary GC Columns, Netherlands) on an Agilent 7890A (Agilent Technologies, USA) with an autosampler, flame ionization detector and split injection. The temperature programming was optimal for the separation of the majority of the C18:1 *trans* isomers. The initial oven temperature was 150°C, held for 5 min, then increased to 200°C at a rate of 2°C/min, held for 10 min, then increased to 220°C at 5°C/min

and held for 35 min. Helium was used as carrier gas at a flow rate of 1 mL/min. The injector was set at 260°C and the detector at 280°C. The FAMEs were identified by comparing with the retention times of the standard.

RNA extraction, cDNA synthesis and quantitative real time PCR

The total RNA was extracted from 50 mg of liver tissue using the RNA iso Plus^{TM} reagent (Takara Co., Otsu, Japan) via homogenization on ice. The purity and concentration of the RNA were measured using an Eppendorf BioPhotometer Plus (Eppendorf AG, Hamburg, Germany). The first-strand cDNA was synthesized using 250 ng of the total RNA template using the PrimeScript RT Master Mix Perfect Real Time kit (Takara Co., Otsu, Japan). The primers were designed using Premier 6.0 (Premier Biosoft International, USA) and were based on known cattle sequences or those cited in the published literature [19-21] (Table 2), and the primer efficiencies were evaluated prior to use. The qPCR was performed using the SYBR Premix Ex Taq^{TM}kit (Takara Co., Otsu, Japan) on an ABI 7300 Real-Time PCR System (Applied Biosystems, Foster City, CA, USA) according to the recommendations in the instruction manual. The standard PCR protocol was described in the manual: denaturing at 95°C for 15 s, then 40 cycles at 95°C for 5 s, and 60°C for 31 s. Glyceraldehyde phosphate dehydrogenase (GAPDH) served as the housekeeping gene for normalization, and the $2^{-\Delta\Delta Ct}$ method was used for the relative quantification.

Western blotting analysis

The liver samples were homogenized in RIPA lysis buffer (Beyotime, Shanghai, China) using 0.1 M PMSF using a Dounce homogenizer, and the lysate was centrifuged at 15,000 × g at 4°C for 20 min. The protein concentration of the supernatant was determined using bicinchoninic acid (BCA) and bovine serum albumin as standards (Pierce, Rockford, IL, USA). Equal amounts of protein were separated using 10% SDS-polyacrylamide gel electrophoresis (PAGE) and transferred onto a nitrocellulose membrane (Millipore, Danvers, MA) at 4°C. After blocking with 10% nonfat dry milk in tris-buffered saline at 4°C overnight, the membrane was washed and incubated with a primary antibody directed against SCD (Polyclonal antibodies raised in goat;sc-23016,Santa Cruz Biotechnology, diluted to 1:200) and HRP affinipure rabbit anti-goat IgG as the secondary antibody (E030130-01, Earth Ox, CA, diluted to 1:10,000). Visualization of the SCD protein was performed using the ECL western blot detection system (ECL plus, Beyotime, Shanghai China). The same membrane was then stripped with striping buffer (AR0153, Boster, Wuhan, China)and was normalized against β-tubulin (Polyclonal antibodies raised in goat,sc-9935, Santa Cruz Biotechnology, diluted

Table 2 The gene name, GeneBank accession number, sequence and product size of the primers used for the qRT-PCR

Gene	Accession #[1]	Forward Primer (5'-3')	Reverse Primer (5'-3')	Product Size
GAPDH[§]	NM_001034034	GGGTCATCATCTCTGCACCT	GGTCATAAGTCCCTCCACGA	176
ACC-α[§]	NM_174224	AGCTGAATTTTCGCAGCAAT	GGTTTTCTCCCCAGGAAAAG	117
FASN[§]	AF285607	GCATCGCTGGCTACTCCTAC	GTGTAGGCCATCACGAAGGT	136
LPL[§]	NM_001075120	GGGTTTTGAGCAAGGGTACA	GCCACAATGACCTTTCCAGT	193
FABP1&	FJ415874.1	GTTCATCATCACCGCTGGCT	CCACTGCCTTGATCTTCTCCC	101
PLIN2&	NM_173980.2	TTTATGGCCTCATGCTTTTGC	CTCAGAGCAGACCCCAATTCA	100
ACOX1&	NM_001035289.3	ACCCAGACTTCCAGCATGAGA	TTCCTCATCTTCTGCACCATGA	100
CPT1α&	FJ415874.1	TCGCGATGGACTTGCTGTATA	CGGTCCAGTTTGCGTCTGTA	100
SCD[§]	NM_173959.4	TTATTCCGTTATGCCCTTGG	GGTAGTTGTGGAAGCCCTCA	151
DGAT1&	FJ415874.1	CCACTGGGACCTGAGGTGTC	GCATCACCACACACCAATTCA	101
DGAT2&	FJ415874.1	CATGTACACATTCTGCACCGATT	TGACCTCCTGCCACCTTTCT	100
SREBF1c	FJ415874.1	CACTCGTCTTCCTCTGTCTC	GAGTGACTGGTTCTCCATAG	243
SREBF2&	NM_001205600.1	AGAGCAAACTCCTGAAGGGC	GGAGGCGACATCAGAAGGAC	103
SCAP	NM_001101889.1	CATCAAGCTCTACTCCATCC	CAATGGCAGCGTTGTCCAGCA	206
LXRα&	NM_001014861.1	CCCCATGACCGACTGATGTT	TGTCCTTCATCTGGCTCCACC	241
PPARα&	FJ415874.1	CATAACGCGATTCGTTTTGGA	CGCGGTTTCGGAATCTTCT	102

[§]published in [19,20]. &published in [21].
[1]Entrez Gene, National Center for Biotechnology Information (NCBI).

to 1:200). The procedures for the secondary antibody and visualization were the same as that used for SCD. The ECL signals were recorded using an imaging system (LAS4000, USA) and analyzed using Quantity One (Bio-Rad, USA).

Statistical analysis

All of the data were expressed as the mean ± SEM. The statistical data analysis was conducted via unpaired or paired Student's t-tests using IBM SPSS 20.0 Statistics for mac (IBM Inc., New York, USA). A difference was considered to be significant when $p < 0.05$.

Results
Rumen pH, LPS content in the rumen and plasma, and the milk composition

The pH value in the ruminal fluid is shown in Figure 1. The dynamic pH curve in the HC group was lower than that in the LC group during the long-term experiment. It showed that a pH value under 5.6 lasted for 223 minutes in the HC group, which indicated that SARA was successfully induced. The pH value of the HC group was significantly lower than that of the LC group after the morning feeding for 8 h ($p < 0.05$).

The LPS concentration in the ruminal fluid of the HC group was significantly increased, from 47.17×10^3 EU/mL to 79.04×10^3 EU/mL, compared to the LC group ($p < 0.01$). In the peripheral plasma, the LPS level in the HC group was 0.86 EU/mL, while it was 0.47 EU/mL in the LC group ($p < 0.001$).

Milk samples were collected from the 1st week to the 18th week to determine the change in the milk composition. The results showed that the milk yield, the percentage of milk fat and the milk fat yield decreased significantly in the HC group compared to the LC group ($p < 0.01$). However, the percentage of milk protein increased remarkably in the HC group ($p < 0.05$; Table 3).

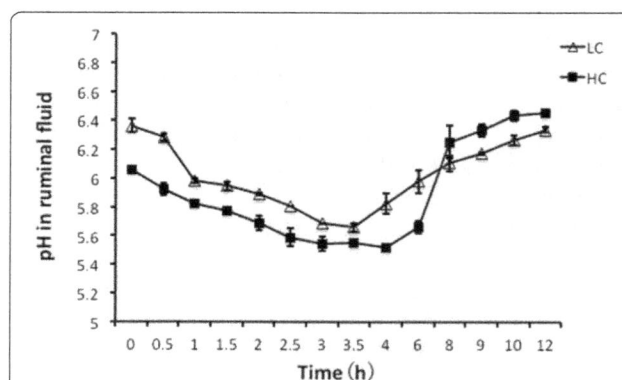

Figure 1 Comparison of the pH values in the ruminal fluid between the low-concentrate (LC) and high-concentrate (HC) groups. The data were measured using ruminal fluid samples collected at times ranging from 0 to 12 hours (shown on the x-axis) for three days during the 18th week. Significant differences were observed across all of the sampling times ($p < 0.05$), with the exception of 8 hours after the morning feeding. The error bars indicate the standard error of the mean. The data were compared using Student's t-test.

Table 3 The LPS, milk yield and milk composition in the dairy cows fed the low-concentrate (LC) and high-concentrate (HC) diets

Item	Treatment			
	LC	HC	SEM[1]	p-Value[2]
Rumen LPS, EU/mL[1] ($\times 10^3$)	47.17	79.04[b]	7.94	<0.01
Plasma LPS, EU/mL[2]	0.47	0.86[ab]	0.08	<0.001
Milk[3]				
Milk yield, kg	28.05	26.92[b]	0.30	<0.01
Fat, %	3.40	3.09[b]	0.03	<0.01
Fat yield, kg/d	0.95	0.84[b]	0.02	<0.01
Protein, %	3.04	3.16[a]	0.03	<0.05
Protein yield, kg/d	0.85	0.85	0.02	0.98

[1]SEM = Standard error of the mean between the two groups.
[2]The LPS data were compared using Student's t-test. The milk samples were compared using a paired t-test.
[3]The milk samples were obtained from the 1st week to the 18th week.
[ab]indicates $p < 0.001$; [a]indicates $p < 0.05$; [b]indicates $p < 0.01$.

The VFA profile in the ruminal fluid and the plasma biochemical parameters

The VFA profiles in the ruminal fluid and the biochemical parameters in the peripheral plasma between the LC and HC groups are presented in Table 4. When compared to the LC group, the total VFA and lactic acid concentration in the rumen was significantly elevated in the HC group (105.95 *vs.* 92.91, $p < 0.05$ and 1.55 *vs.* 0.96 mmol/L, $p < 0.01$, respectively). The molar proportion (mmol/mol) of propionate was increased in the dairy cows fed the high-concentrate diet (281.83 *vs.* 247.68, $p < 0.01$), but the other proportional concentrations of the individual VFAs were unchanged. The ratio of propionate to butyrate (1.18 *vs.* 1.44, $p < 0.05$) was significantly increased, while the ratio of acetate to propionate (1.84 *vs.* 1.57, $p < 0.05$) was significantly reduced.

When compared to the LC group, the triacylglycerol ($p < 0.05$), NEFA ($p < 0.01$) and total cholesterol ($p < 0.01$) concentrations were significantly decreased in the peripheral plasma of the HC group. However, the glucose and insulin concentration were significantly enhanced ($p < 0.01$, $p < 0.05$ respectively) in the plasma of the high-concentrate diet group.

The long-chain fatty acid profiles in the ruminal fluid and the hepatic vein plasma

The LCFA profiles in the ruminal fluid and the hepatic vein plasma are shown in Tables 5 and 6, respectively. The LCFA concentration in the ruminal fluid and the hepatic vein of the HC group was lower than that in the LC group, specifically for palmitate C16:0 ($p < 0.05$) and palmitoleate C18:0 ($p < 0.05$). The desaturation index that was determined by calculating the plasma C16:1n-9/C16:0 ratio was decreased in the HC group ($p = 0.087$).

Table 4 The ruminal fluid composition, blood metabolites and hormone level in the dairy cows fed the low-concentrate (LC) diet and high-concentrate (HC) diet

VFA profile[1]	Treatment			
	LC	HC	SEM[2]	p-value[3]
Total VFA(mmol/L)	92.91	107.64[a]	3.66	<0.05
Molar proportion, mmol/mol				
Acetate	454.51	440.55	3.10	0.47
Propionate	247.68	281.83[b]	2.41	<0.01
Isobutyrate	25.19	24.68	0.38	0.83
Butyrate	210.11	195.99	1.77	0.17
Isovalerate	36.31	34.52	0.67	0.67
Valerate	21.25	19.93	0.24	0.38
Caproate	4.95	2.49[b]	0.17	<0.01
Acetate:Propionate	1.84	1.57[a]	0.02	<0.05
Propionate:Butyrate	1.18	1.44[b]	0.05	<0.01
Lactic acid	0.96	1.55[b]	0.20	<0.01
Plasma biochemical parameter[4]				
TG (mmol/L)	0.28	0.21[a]	0.05	<0.05
NEFA (mmol/L)	1.16	0.48[ab]	0.07	<0.001
TCH (mmol/L)	2.21	1.69[b]	0.31	<0.01
GLU (mg/dL)	45.23	56.02[b]	4.54	<0.01
Hormone level[4]				
Insulin (μIU/mL)	16.95	21.57[a]	1.01	<0.05
Glucagon (pg/mL)	191.23	161.02	18.28	0.28
Insulin:Glucacon	0.10	0.16[c]	0.01	0.07

[1]The volatile fatty acid and lactic acid concentrations and the mean proportion across the sampling times during the 18th week.
[2]SEM = Standard error of the mean between the two treatments.
[3]The data were compared using a paired t-test.
[4]The mean metabolite concentration in the jugular plasma across the sampling times. TG, triglyceride; NEFA: non-esterified fatty acid; TCH, total cholesterol; GLU, glucose;
[a]indicates $p < 0.05$; [b]indicates $p < 0.01$; [ab]indicates <0.001.

Additionally, a decrease in the Δ^9 monounsaturated oleic acid (C18:1n-9) concentration was observed in the HC group. Compared with the LC group, the concentration of *cis9,trans 11* CLA was similar in the both rumen and plasma. The concentration of *trans11* C18:1 was increased in rumen of the HC group ($p = 0.067$), while in the plasma, the *trans11* C18:1 content was similar. In regards to α-linolenic acid (C18:3n-3), its content in the HC group was four-fold lower than that of the LC group. However, the content of both C22:0 and C22:1n-9 was significantly increased ($p < 0.05$) in the HC group. The desaturation index of C18:1n-9/C18:0 and *cis9, trans11* C18:2n/*trans11* C18:1n was decreased in the HC group, but no statistical significance was observed. Meanwhile, the presence of longer-chain saturated FAs (C20:0, $p < 0.01$; C21:0, $p < 0.01$), which are produced via ruminal microbial biohydrogenation, was decreased in the HC group.

Table 5 The fatty acid composition in the ruminal fluid of the dairy cows

µg/mL	Treatment		SEM[1]	p-Value[2]
	LC	HC		
C12:0	2.67	2.05	0.27	0.28
C13:0	3.31	2.92	0.30	0.56
C14:0	254.80	74.26	55.68	0.11
C15:0	6.25	3.47	1.05	0.21
C16:0	147.09	96.84[b]	10.48	<0.01
cis9C16:1	3.17	2.32	0.11	0.27
C18:0	473.48	281.65[ab]	38.02	<0.001
trans11C18:1n	4.53	11.40[c]	1.93	0.07
C18:1n-9	11.36	8.93	0.65	0.05
C18:2n-6	10.15	7.18[c]	0.89	0.09
C20:0	6.28	4.40[b]	0.40	<0.01
6C18:3n	0.55	0.75	0.09	0.27
C20:1	0.52	0.35[b]	0.04	<0.01
C18:3n-3	2.65	2.04	0.27	0.30
cis9, trans11C18:2n	6.61	5.27	0.45	0.15
C21:0	0.76	0.53[b]	0.05	<0.01
C22:0	3.53	3.10	0.17	0.23
C23:0	1.21	1.12	0.06	0.51
C24:0	4.26	3.83	0.19	0.29
C24:1	0.69	0.60	0.04	0.29
C22:6n-3	2.21	1.83	0.13	0.17

[1]SEM = Standard error of the mean between the two treatments.
[2]The data were compared using Student's t-test.
[a]indicates $p < 0.05$; [b]indicates $p < 0.01$; [ab]indicates $p < 0.001$;
[c]indicates $0.05 < p < 0.1$.

Table 6 The fatty acid composition in the hepatic vein plasma of the dairy cows

µg /mL	Treatment		SEM[1]	P-Value[2]
	LC	HC		
C12:0	3.57	4.04	0.20	0.26
C13:0	5.92	6.99	0.50	0.32
C14:0	66.06	74.32	13.66	0.79
C14:1	6.47	4.39[c]	0.57	0.06
C15:0	8.81	6.43	0.84	0.17
C15:1	1.39	1.25	0.09	0.49
C16:0	92.47	71.10[a]	5.14	<0.05
cis9C16:1	5.32	2.84[c]	0.64	0.05
C18:0	121.33	85.5[a]	8.81	<0.05
trans11C18:1n	2.92	2.93	0.09	0.96
C18:1n-9	62.24	40.28[a]	5.69	<0.05
C18:2n-6	277.99	71.13[a]	38.72	<0.05
C20:0	0.89	1.02[a]	0.03	<0.05
C20:1	0.45	0.61[c]	0.05	0.10
C18:3n-3	25.86	6.6[b]	3.74	<0.01
cis9, trans11C18:2n	4.56	4.57	0.07	0.98
C21:0	1.27	1.00	0.19	0.51
C22:0	0.97	1.31[a]	0.08	<0.05
C20:3n-6	27.01	10.80[c]	4.41	0.07
C22:1n-9	1.24	1.57[a]	0.08	<0.05
C20:4n-6	33.46	16.13[b]	3.84	<0.01
C22:6n-3	10.57	6.20[ab]	0.83	<0.001
Desaturation index				
cis9 C16:1/C16:0	0.05	0.04[c]	0.01	0.09
cis9 C18:1/C18:0	0.51	0.47	0.02	0.37
cis9,trans11 C18:2/tran11 C18:1	1.66	1.55	0.06	0.37

[1]SEM = Standard error of the mean between the two treatments.
[2]The data were compared using Student's t-test.
[a]indicates $p < 0.05$; [b]indicates $p < 0.01$; [ab]indicates $p < 0.001$;
[c]indicates $0.05 < p < 0.1$.

mRNA expression of the genes involved in lipid metabolism in the liver

The liver mRNA expression levels of the genes involved in lipid metabolism are presented in Figure 2. The expression levels of the genes associated with fatty acid uptake/transport, lipid formation, fatty acid oxidation and transcriptional regulators of lipogenic enzymes were remarkably altered between the HC and LC groups. There was a decrease in fatty acid binding protein 1 (FABP1) expression ($p = 0.09$) in the HC group compared to the LC group, and LPL was significantly down-regulated in the HC group. Compared with the LC group, the expression of perilipin 2 (PLIN2) ($p < 0.05$) was significantly decreased in the HC group, and there was 2-fold down regulation of SCD1 expression in the HC group. The expression of diacylglycerol acyltransferase (DGAT1 and DGAT2) was similar between the two groups, and the expression of ACCα and FAS, which are involved in *de novo* fatty acid synthesis, showed no significant difference between the HC and LC groups. However, the expression of carnitine palmitoyltransferase 1α (CPT1α)

was up-regulated in the HC group ($p < 0.05$), whereas the expression of acyl-CoA oxidase 1 (ACOX1) was increased in the HC group ($p = 0.10$).

With respect to transcriptional regulators, the mRNA level of SCAP was down-regulated in the HC group ($p < 0.05$). Meanwhile, both the SREBF1c ($p = 0.09$) and SREBF2 ($p = 0.08$) mRNA expression levels were decreased in the HC group. However, the mRNA expression of PPARα was significantly increased in the HC group ($p < 0.05$). The expression of liver X receptor α (LXRα) showed no significant difference.

The protein expression of SCD1 in the liver

The protein expression of SCD in the liver is shown in Figure 3. The results demonstrated that the expression

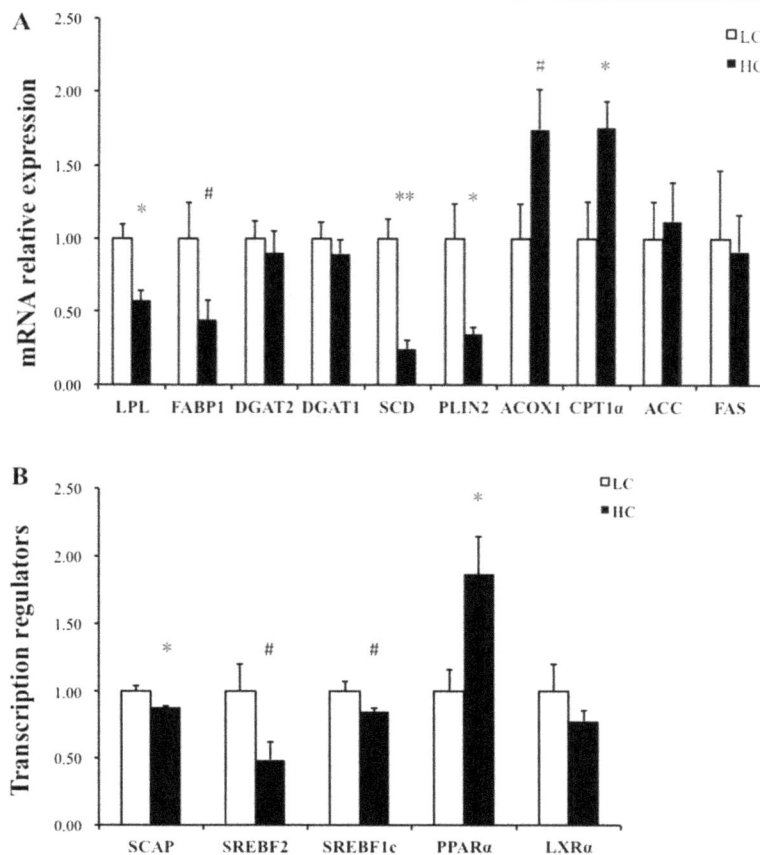

Figure 2 The hepatic gene expression profile analyzed via real-time PCR. Each value was normalized to the expression of GAPDH, and data were compared using Student's t-test between LC (n = 4) and HC (n = 4). **A.** The genes involved in desaturation, lipogenesis, fatty acid oxidation, TG synthesis and lipid droplet formation were measured in the liver tissue. The error bars indicate the standard error of the mean. * indicates $p < 0.05$; ** indicates $p < 0.01$; # indicates significance values between $0.05 < p < 0.1$. **B.** The genes involved in transcriptional regulation were measured in the liver tissue. The error bars indicate the standard error of the mean. * indicates $p < 0.05$; ** indicates $p < 0.01$; # indicates significance values between $0.05 < p < 0.1$.

of SCD in the liver was significantly down-regulated in the HC group compared to the LC group ($p < 0.05$).

Discussion

In this study, we showed that an altered fatty acid composition is induced by a HC diet. The reduced oleate and palmitoleate content may be associated with the down-regulated expression of SCD1 in the liver, which primarily resulted from the release of LPS during long-term HC feeding. These findings provide insights into the role of endogenous LPS on hepatic SCD1 expression in dairy cows and its relationship with fatty acid composition.

Previous studies have reported that SARA is characterized by declined feed intake, inflammation and depressed milk fat [12]. In our experiment, the duration of a rumen pH less than 5.6 lasted for 223 min/day in the cows fed a high-concentrate diet, meanwhile, a decrease in the milk yield (kg/d), milk fat (%) and milk fat yield

(kg/d) was observed in the HC group. Therefore, our results are consistent with other studies.

Our data demonstrated that the total VFA and lactic acid levels in the ruminal fluid were significantly increased in the HC group. The ratio of acetate to propionate was decreased in the HC group due to an increase in propionate. Early experiments have also presented a low ratio of acetate to propionate in dairy cows fed with easily fermentable carbohydrates [22]. A previous study showed an increased ratio of ruminal propionate to butyrate in repartitioned milk from fat to lactose and protein [23]. In our study, the increased proportion of propionate may be related to glycogenesis [24,25]. Because most volatile fatty acids emerge in the portal vein after absorption from the digestive tract [26], alterations in volatile fatty acid concentrations may influence the metabolism in the liver.

When gram-negative bacteria in the rumen are lysed at low pH values, LPS is released and translocated into

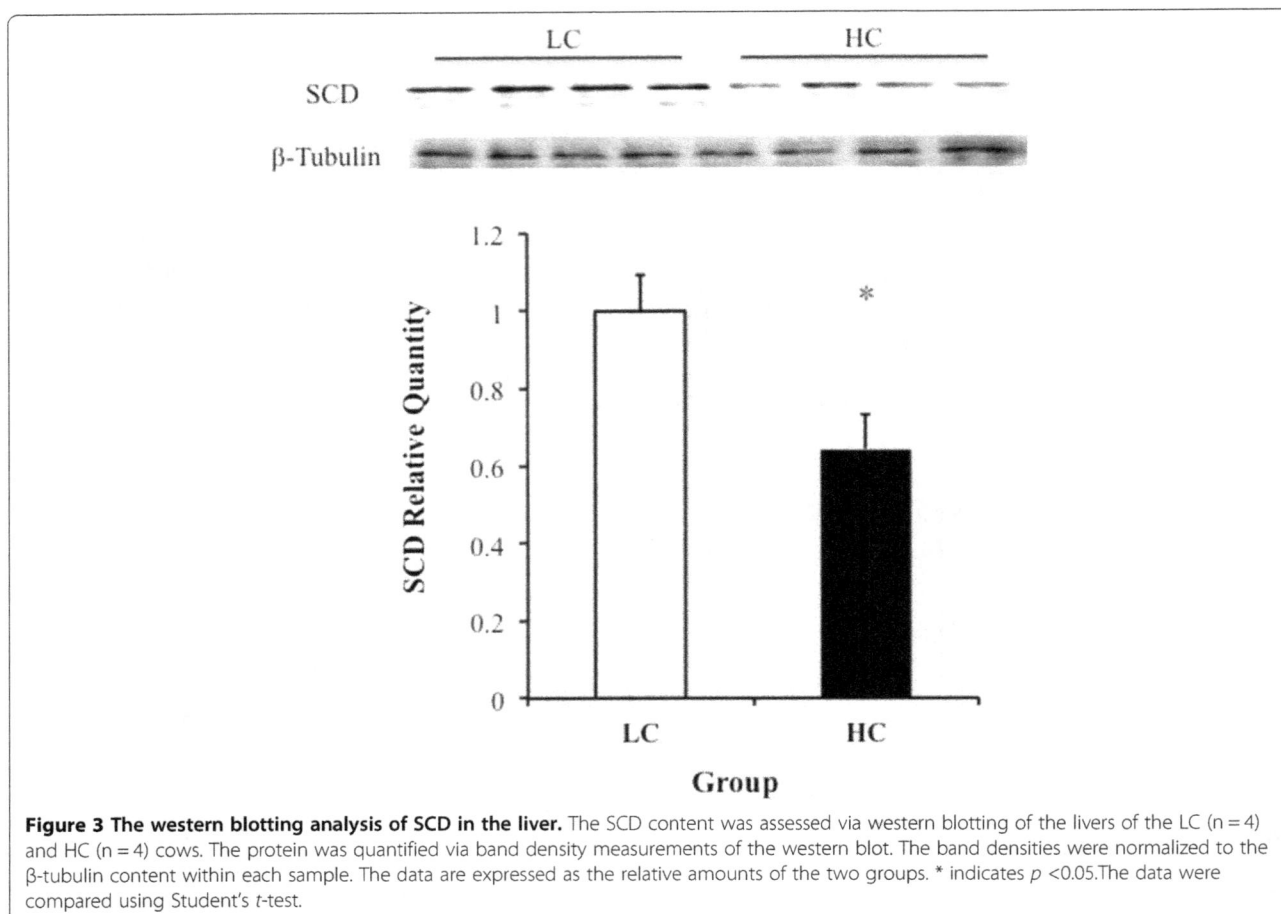

Figure 3 The western blotting analysis of SCD in the liver. The SCD content was assessed via western blotting of the livers of the LC (n = 4) and HC (n = 4) cows. The protein was quantified via band density measurements of the western blot. The band densities were normalized to the β-tubulin content within each sample. The data are expressed as the relative amounts of the two groups. * indicates p <0.05.The data were compared using Student's t-test.

the bloodstream, initiating an inflammatory response. In our experiment, the high endogenous LPS content may have triggered metabolic disorders in the digestive tract and liver. It has been documented that the liver has a strong ability to clear LPS [27-29]. A recent study showed that the LPS gene expression profile was altered in the liver of lactating goats fed a long-term high-concentrate diet, and the overall metabolism was shifted towards energy supply, in order to meet the higher energy expenditure demands for tissue anti-inflammation [30].

Our results indicated that SARA also influences plasma metabolites. Cholesterol in the plasma is negatively associated with the presence of LPS in the rumen [31,32], which explains our results of lower cholesterol concentrations in the plasma of the HC group. Among the hormones in peripheral plasma, insulin plays a crucial role in lipid metabolism, particularly in case of feeding cows with a high-concentrate diet. Decreased milk fat yield caused by SARA might have been because of an increased plasma insulin concentration and the ratio of insulin to glucagon [31,33,34], which has shown that high-concentrate diet resulted in greater plasma insulin

concentration in our experiment. Due to the higher ruminal propionate and plasma glucose, increased plasma insulin might promote energy expenditure in hepatic through lipolysis and glycolysis, rather than fatty acid synthesis and gluconeogenesis [35], which in turn repressed the expression of lipogenic enzymes, such as SCD1. NEFAs are primarily mobilized from stored TGs in the adipose tissue [36]. In our experiment, the increased propionate and glucose resulted in a decrease in the NEFA concentration in the plasma, which is attributed to their inhibitory effect on adipose tissue lipolysis [35,37,38]. A lower TG concentration was observed in the HC group, which could be explained by the reduced adipose lipolysis and the restriction of biohydrogenation at low rumen pHs [39]. The restricted biohydrogenation led to a decreased saturated FA content, particularly of C16:0 and C18:0, in the rumen.

The fatty acid profiles in the ruminal fluid and the hepatic vein plasma were altered in this study. Decreased saturated FA concentrations in the ruminal fluid reflects the inhibition of biohydrogenation at lower pH values in the rumen of cows fed a long-term high-concentrate diet.

A previous study demonstrated that the conversion of long-chain fatty acids to TGs and phospholipids (PLs) in the livers of dairy cows is dependent on adipose tissue lipolysis [40]. The decrease in the palmitic (C16:0), stearic (C18:0) and oleic (C18:1) content in the liver may be explained by the decreased NEFA levels released from the adipose tissue and the lower production in the rumen. Similarly, a decrease in C18:2n-6 is associated with decreased lipolysis in the adipose tissue [41]. A decrease of both C18:2n-6 and C20:4n-6 in the hepatic vein plasma was observed in the HC group. It was reported that arachidonic acid (C20:4n-6),which comes from the cell cytoplasm, could be synthesized by Δ^5desaturase from C20:3n-6, and the latter could be desaturated and elongated from C18:2n-6 in the endoplasmic reticulum [42]. In addition, α-linoleic acid (C18:3n-3) could be desaturated and elongated to C22:6n-3, which could explain the decrease in C22:6n-3 in the HC group. Decreased C18:3n-3 may cause an accumulation of TGs [43], due to its function of enhancing the stability of apolipoprotein B:100 [44]. Furthermore, *trans11* C18:1n is considered to bethe precursor of *trans10* C:18:1n, which is a known inhibitor of milk fat in dairy cows [37]. Therefore, its increased levels in the rumen are associated with milk fat depression.

Fatty acid binding protein 1 (FABP1) is related to fatty acid uptake, transport, and metabolism and the activation of PPARα via NEFAs [45]. In our study, the down-regulated expression of FABP1 was likely observed because of the low NEFA concentrations in the peripheral plasma. As increased levels of *trans11* C18:1n in the rumen of the HC group emerged in the portal vein, it may have activated the PPARα pathway, as was demonstrated in a previous in vitro study [46].

In the liver, the activation of carnitine palmitoyltransferase 1α (CPT1α) and acyl-CoA oxidase 1 (ACOX1) is regulated by PPARα [8]. In dairy cows, the above enzymes are responsible for regulating the entry of LCFAs into the mitochondria for oxidation [47,48]. Because of the increased energy demand to resist inflammation during induced SARA, the gene expression of the above enzymes was increased in the HC group, which is consistent with the expression of the transcription factor PPARα. Additionally, shorter-chain fatty acyl-CoA, which is produced via peroxisomal fatty acid β-oxidation, is subsequently channeled to be oxidized completely in the mitochondria [45]. Therefore, the up-regulated expression of CPT1α suggests that hepatic energy export is necessary during induced SARA.

It was reported that the expression of SREBF1c and FAS, which are involved in lipid synthesis, was down-regulated in SCD1 knockout mice [8]. In our study, the expression of the transcription factor SREBF1c was decreased in the HC group, similar to its activation-dependent ligand SCAP,

which could further explain the downregulation of SREBF2. In the liver, SREBF1c regulates the genes involved in fatty acid synthesis, while SREBF2 modulates the genes associated with cholesterol biosynthesis [49]. Therefore, the decreased cholesterol in the plasma could be regulated by SREBF2. SCD is a key lipogenic enzyme that regulates the synthesis of monounsaturated fatty acids, particularly oleate (C18:1) and palmitoleate (C16:1) [50]. The transcription of SCD is co-regulated by SREBF1c and PPARα [51,52]. The decreased C16:1 and C18:1n-9 content in the hepatic vein plasma indicated the downregulation of SCD in the dairy cows fed a high-concentrate diet. However, the *cis9,trans11*CLA content was unchanged because the process of *trans11*C18:1n desaturation to *cis9,trans11*CLA via SCD exists in most lipogenic and adipogenic tissues, except in the livers of rats and bovine [53,54]. Moreover, it is considered that the Δ^9 desaturation index poorly predicts the activity and/or expression of SCD [55]. Similar to SCD, the expression of perilipin 2 (PLIN2), which is involved in the intracellular accumulation of TGs and lipid droplet (LD) formation, was decreased in the HC group [56], which led to the attenuation of LD formation in the liver. Diacylglycerol acyltransferases (DGATs) plays key roles in the synthesis of TGs and very low-density lipoprotein (VLDL) secretion in the liver [57]. In our present study, the similar expression of DGAT1 and DGAT2 between the HC and LC group may be attributed to compensation of the down regulated SCD, which is partly due to a positive correlation between inflammation and fatty liver [58].

A previous study showed that the AMP-activated protein kinase (AMPK) signaling pathway is associated with the inhibition of SCD1 [59]. To some extent, this may contribute to the down regulation of SCD at the mRNA and protein levels. The unchanged mRNA expression of ACCα and FAS may not reflect the phosphorylation status of the enzymes. Therefore, further research is needed to elucidate the underlying mechanism.

Conclusions

In summary, lipid metabolism in the livers of dairy cows is influenced by long-term high-concentrate diet feeding. Lipopolysaccharide derived from the rumen down-regulates stearoyl-CoA desaturase 1 expression and alters fatty acid composition in the liver of dairy cows fed a high-concentrate diet. Our findings may shed light on the regulation of fatty acid metabolism and reprogramming in the livers of dairy cows fed high-concentrate diets.

Abbreviations
ACOX1: Acyl-CoA oxidase 1; CPT1: Carnitine palmitoyltransferase 1; DGAT: Diacylglycerol acyltransferase; FABP1: Fatty acid binding protein 1; FAME: Fatty acid methyl esters; LCFA: Long chain fatty acid; LPS: Lipopolysaccharide; LXR: Liver X receptor; PLIN2: Perilipin 2; PPARα: peroxisome proliferator-activated receptor α; SCAP: SREBP cleavage

activating protein; SCD: Stearoyl-CoA desaturase; SREBF: Sterol regulatory element binding transcription factor; VFA: Volatile fatty acid.

Competing interests
The authors declare that they have no financial, personal or professional interests that would have influenced the content of the paper or interfered with their objective assessment of the manuscript.

Authors' contributions
XS and TX: conceived and designed the experiments. TX, HT, GC, KZ and LX: performed the experiments. TX and XS: analyzed the data. TX and XS: drafted the manuscript. All authors read and approved the final manuscript.

Acknowledgements
This study was supported by the National Basic Research Program of China (2011CB100802), National Natural Science Foundation of China (31172371; 30371040), the Federal Ministry of Food, Agriculture and Consumer Protection of Germany and the Ministry of Agriculture of China (Grant No. 30/2008-2009), and the Priority Academic Program Development of Jinagsu Higher Education Institutions (PAPD).
The authors are grateful to Dr. Dirk Dannenberger and Dr. Karin Nuernberg, from the Leibniz Institute for Farm Animal Biology, Germany, for their valuable advice on fatty acid analysis via gas chromatography (GC).

References
1. Gozho GN, Plaizier JC, Krause DO, Kennedy AD, Wittenberg KM. Subacute ruminal acidosis induces ruminal lipopolysaccharide endotoxin release and triggers an inflammatory response. J Dairy Sci. 2005;88:1399–403.
2. Chen Y, Oba M, Guan LL. Variation of bacterial communities and expression of Toll-like receptor genes in the rumen of steers differing in susceptibility to subacute ruminal acidosis. Vet Microbiol. 2012;159(3–4):451–9.
3. Plaizier JC, Krause DO, Gozho GN, McBride BW. Subacute ruminal acidosis in dairy cows: the physiological causes, incidence and consequences. Vet J. 2008;176(1):21–31.
4. Emmanuel DG, Dunn SM, Ametaj BN. Feeding high proportions of barley grain stimulates an inflammatory response in dairy cows. J Dairy Sci. 2008;91(2):606–14.
5. Arisqueta L, Nunez-Garcia M, Ogando J, Garcia-Arcos I, Ochoa B, Aspichueta P, et al. Involvement of lipid droplets in hepatic responses to lipopolysaccharide treatment in mice. Biochem Biophys Acta. 2013;1831(8):1357–67.
6. Jiang QD, Li HP, Liu FJ, Wang XJ, Guo YJ, Wang LF, et al. Effects of lipopolysaccharide on the stearoyl-coenzyme A desaturase mRNA level in bovine primary hepatic cells. Genet Mol Res. 2014;13(2):2548–54.
7. Ntambi JM. Regulation of stearoyl-CoA desaturase by polyunsaturated fatty acids and cholesterol. J Lipid Res. 1999;40:1549–58.
8. Ntambi JM, Miyazaki M, Stoehr JP, Lan H, Kendziorski CM, Yandell BS, et al. Loss of stearoyl-CoA desaturase-1 function protects mice against adiposity. Proc Natl Acad Sci U S A. 2002;99(17):11482–6.
9. Feingold KR, Staprans I, Memon RA, Moser AH, Shigenaga JK, Doerrler W, et al. Endotoxin rapidly induces changes in lipid metabolism that produce hypertriglyceridemia: low doses stimulate hepatic triglyceride production while high doses inhibit clearance. J Lipid Res. 1992;33:1765–76.
10. Chen C, Shah YM, Morimura K, Krausz KW, Miyazaki M, Richardson TA, et al. Metabolomics reveals that hepatic stearoyl-CoA desaturase 1 downregulation exacerbates inflammation and acute colitis. Cell Metab. 2008;7(2):135–47.
11. Kleen JL, Hooijer GA, Rehage J, Noordhuizen JPTM. Subacute Ruminal Acidosis (SARA): a review. J Vet Med. 2003;50:406–14.
12. Khafipour E, Krause DO, Plaizier JC. A grain-based subacute ruminal acidosis challenge causes translocation of lipopolysaccharide and triggers inflammation. J Dairy Sci. 2009;92(3):1060–70.
13. Gaynor PJ, Waldo DR, Capuco AV, Erdman RA, Douglass LW, Teters BB. Milk fat depression, the glucogenic theory, and trans-C18:1 fatty acids. J Dairy Sci. 1995;78:2008–15.
14. Zebeli Q, Ametaj BN. Relationships between rumen lipopolysaccharide and mediators of inflammatory response with milk fat production and efficiency in dairy cows. J Dairy Sci. 2009;92(8):3800–9.
15. Graugnard DE, Moyes KM, Trevisi E, Khan MJ, Keisler D, Drackley JK, et al. Liver lipid content and inflammometabolic indices in peripartal dairy cows are altered in response to prepartal energy intake and postpartal intramammary inflammatory challenge. J Dairy Sci. 2013;96(2):918–35.
16. Hamada T, Omori S, Kameoka K, Horii S, Morimoto H. Direct determination of rumen volatile fatty acids by gas chromatography. J Dairy Sci. 1968;51:228–9.
17. Folch J, Lees M, Sloane Stanley GH. A simple method for the isolation and purification of total lipides from animal tissues. J Biol Chem. 1957;226:497–509.
18. Chouinard PY, Corneau L, Barbano DM, Metzger LE, Bauman DE. Conjugated linoleic acids alter milk fatty acid composition and inhibit milk fat secretion in dairy cows. J Nutr. 1999;129:1579–84.
19. Akbar H, Schmitt E, Ballou MA, Correa MN, Depeters EJ, Loor JJ. Dietary lipid during late-pregnancy and early-lactation to manipulate metabolic and inflammatory gene network expression in dairy cattle liver with a focus on PPARs. Gene Regul Syst Bio. 2013;7:103–23.
20. Bionaz M, Loor JJ. Gene networks driving bovine milk fat synthesis during the lactation cycle. BMC Genomics. 2008;9:366.
21. Joseph SJ, Robbins KR, Pavan E, Pratt SL, Duckett SK, Rekaya R. Effect of diet supplementation on the expression of bovine genes associated with fatty acid synthesis and metabolism. Bioinf Biol Insights. 2010;4:19–31.
22. Fairfield AM, Plaizier JC, Duffield TF, Lindinger MI, Bagg R, Dick P, et al. Effects of prepartum administration of a monensin controlled release capsule on rumen pH, feed intake, and milk production of transition dairy cows. J Dairy Sci. 2007;90:937–45.
23. Harri M, Pekka H. Effects of the ratio of ruminal propionate to butyrate on milk yield and blood metabolites in dairy cows. J Dairy Sci. 1996;79:851–61.
24. Blanch M, Calsamiglia S, DiLorenzo N, DiCostanzo A, Muetzel S, Wallace RJ. Physiological changes in rumen fermentation during acidosis induction and its control using a multivalent polyclonal antibody preparation in heifers. J Anim Sci. 2009;87(5):1722–30.
25. Penner GB, Taniguchi M, Guan LL, Beauchemin KA, Oba M. Effect of dietary forage to concentrate ratio on volatile fatty acid absorption and the expression of genes related to volatile fatty acid absorption and metabolism in ruminal tissue. J Dairy Sci. 2009;92(6):2767–81.
26. Bergman EN. Energy contributions of volatile fatty acids from the gastrointestinal tract in various species. Physiol Rev. 1990;70:567–90.
27. Buttenschoen K, Radermacher P, Bracht H. Endotoxin elimination in sepsis: physiology and therapeutic application. Langenbecks Arch Surg. 2010;395(6):597–605.
28. Deng M, Scott MJ, Loughran P, Gibson G, Sodhi C, Watkins S, et al. Lipopolysaccharide clearance, bacterial clearance, and systemic inflammatory responses are regulated by cell type-specific functions of TLR4 during sepsis. J Immunol. 2013;190(10):5152–60.
29. Vels L, Rontved CM, Bjerring M, Ingvartsen KL. Cytokine and acute phase protein gene expression in repeated liver biopsies of dairy cows with a lipopolysaccharide-induced mastitis. J Dairy Sci. 2009;92(3):922–34.
30. Dong H, Wang S, Jia Y, Ni Y, Zhang Y, Zhuang S, et al. Long-term effects of subacute ruminal acidosis (SARA) on milk quality and hepatic gene expression in lactating goats fed a high-concentrate diet. Plos One. 2013;8(12):e82850.
31. Zebeli Q, Dunn SM, Ametaj BN. Perturbations of plasma metabolites correlated with the rise of rumen endotoxin in dairy cows fed diets rich in easily degradable carbohydrates. J Dairy Sci. 2011;94(5):2374–82.
32. Bertok L. Bile acids in physico-chemical host defence. Pathophysiol. 2004;11(3):139–45.
33. Piccioli-Cappelli F, Loor JJ, Seal CJ, Minuti A, Trevisi E. Effect of dietary starch level and high rumen-undegradable protein on endocrine-metabolic status, milk yield, and milk composition in dairy cows during early and late lactation. J Dairy Sci. 2014;97(12):7788–803.
34. Waggoner JW, Löest CA, Turner JL, Mathis CP, Hallford DM. Effects of dietary protein and bacterial lipopolysaccharide infusion on nitrogen metabolism and hormonal responses of growing beef steers. J Anim Sci. 2009;87:3656–68.
35. Guo Y, Xu X, Zou Y, Yang Z, Li S, Cao Z. Changes in feed intake, nutrient digestion, plasma metabolites, and oxidative stress parameters in dairy cows with subacute ruminal acidosis and its regulation with pelleted beet pulp. J Anim Sci Biotechnol. 2013;4:31.

Lipopolysaccharide derived from the rumen down-regulates stearoyl-CoA desaturase 1 expression and...

139

36. Knegsel ATM, Brand H, Graat EAM, Dijkstra J, Jorritsma R, Decuypere E, et al. Dietary energy source in dairy cows in early lactation: metabolites and metabolic hormones. J Dairy Sci. 2007;90:1477–85.

37. Bauman DE, Griinari JM. Regulation and nutritional manipulation of milk fat: low-fat milk syndrome. Livest Sci. 2001;70:15–29.

38. Ametaj B, Bradford B, Bobe G, Nafikov R, Lu Y, Young J, et al. Strong relationships between mediators of the acute phase response and fatty liver in dairy cows. Can J Anim Sci. 2005;85:165–75.

39. Van Nevel CJ, Demeyer DI. Influence of pH on lipolysis and biohydrogenation of soybean oil by rumen contents in vitro. Reprod Nutr Dev. 1996;36:53–63.

40. Douglas GN, Rehage J, Beaulieu AD, Bahaa AO, Drackley JK. Prepartum nutrition alters fatty acid composition in plasma, adipose tissue, and liver lipids of periparturient dairy cows. J Dairy Sci. 2007;90:2941–59.

41. Rukkwamsuk T, Geelen MJH, Kruip TAM, Wensing T. Interrelation of fatty acid composition in adipose tissue, serum, and liver of dairy cows during the development of fatty liver postpartum. J Dairy Sci. 2000;83:52–9.

42. Ves-Losada A, Maté SM, Brenner RR. Incorporation and distribution of saturated and unsaturated fatty acids into nuclear lipids of hepatic cells. Lipids. 2001;36:273–82.

43. Mashek DG, Bertics SJ, Grummer RR. Metabolic fate of long-chain unsaturated fatty acids and their effects on palmitic acid metabolism and gluconeogenesis in bovine hepatocytes. J Dairy Sci. 2002;85:2283–9.

44. Wu X, Shang A, Jiang H, Ginsberg HN. Demonstration of biphasic effects of docosahexaenoic acid on apolipoprotein B secretion in HepG2 cells. Arterioscl Throm Vas. 1997;17:3347–55.

45. Loor JJ. Genomics of metabolic adaptations in the peripartal cow. Animal. 2010;4(07):1110–39.

46. Pawar A, Jump DB. Unsaturated fatty acid regulation of peroxisome proliferator-activated receptor alpha activity in rat primary hepatocytes. J Biol Chem. 2003;278(38):35931–9.

47. Dann HM, Drackley JK. Carnitine palmitoyltransferase I in liver of periparturient dairy cows: effects of prepartum intake, postpartum induction of ketosis, and periparturient disorders. J Dairy Sci. 2005;88:3851–9.

48. Vluggens A, Andreoletti P, Viswakarma N, Jia Y, Matsumoto K, Kulik W, et al. Reversal of mouse acyl-CoA oxidase 1 (ACOX1) null phenotype by human ACOX1b isoform. Lab Invest. 2010;90(5):696–708.

49. Bommer GT, MacDougald OA. Regulation of lipid homeostasis by the bifunctional SREBF2-miR33a locus. Cell Metab. 2011;13(3):241–7.

50. Hofacer R, Magrisso IJ, Jandacek R, Rider T, Tso P, Benoit SC, et al. Omega-3 fatty acid deficiency increases stearoyl-CoA desaturase expression and activity indices in rat liver: positive association with non-fasting plasma triglyceride levels. Prostag Leukotr Ess. 2012;86(1–2):71–7.

51. Biddinger SB, Almind K, Miyazaki M, Kokkotou E, Ntambi JM, Kahn CR. Effects of diet and genetic background on sterol regulatory element–binding protein-1c, stearoyl-CoA desaturase 1, and the development of the metabolic syndrome. Diabetes. 2004;54:1314–23.

52. Miyazaki M, Dobrzyn A, Sampath H, Lee SH, Man WC, Chu K, et al. Reduced adiposity and liver steatosis by stearoyl-CoA desaturase deficiency are independent of peroxisome proliferator-activated receptor-alpha. J Biol Chem. 2004;279(33):35017–24.

53. Shen X, Nuernberg K, Nuernberg G, Zhao R, Scollan N, Ender K, et al. Vaccenic acid and cis-9, trans-11 CLA in the rumen and different tissues of pasture- and concentrate-fed beef cattle. Lipids. 2007;42(12):1093–103.

54. Gruffat D, Torre ADL, Chardigny J-M, Durand D, Loreau O, Bauchart D. Vaccenic acid metabolism in the liver of rat and bovine. Lipids. 2005;40:295–301.

55. Invernizzi G, Thering BJ, McGuire MA, Savoini G, Loor JJ. Sustained upregulation of stearoyl-CoA desaturase in bovine mammary tissue with contrasting changes in milk fat synthesis and lipogenic gene networks caused by lipid supplements. Funct Integr Genomics. 2010;10(4):561–75.

56. Chang BH, Chan L. Regulation of triglyceride metabolism. III emerging role of lipid droplet protein ADFP in health and disease. Am J Physiol Gastrointest Liver Physiol. 2007;292(6):G1465–8.

57. Yamazaki T, Sasaki E, Kakinuma C, Yano T, Miura S, Ezaki O. Increased very low density lipoprotein secretion and gonadal fat mass in mice overexpressing liver DGAT1. J Biol Chem. 2005;280(22):21506–14.

58. Bradford BJ, Mamedova LK, Minton JE, Drouillard JS, Johnson BJ. Daily injection of tumor necrosis factor-{alpha} increases hepatic triglycerides and alters transcript abundance of metabolic genes in lactating dairy cattle. J Nutr. 2009;139(8):1451–6.

59. Dobrzyn P, Dobrzyn A, Miyazaki M, Cohen P, Asilmaz E, Hardie DG, et al. Stearoyl-CoA desaturase 1 deficiency increases fatty acid oxidation by activating AMP-activated protein kinase in liver. Natl Acad Sci USA. 2004;101(17):6409–14.

16

A bovine respiratory syncytial virus model with high clinical expression in calves with specific passive immunity

Krister Blodörn[1], Sara Hägglund[1], Dolores Gavier-Widen[2,3], Jean-François Eléouët[4], Sabine Riffault[4], John Pringle[1], Geraldine Taylor[5] and Jean François Valarcher[1,6*]

Abstract

Background: Bovine respiratory syncytial virus (BRSV) is a major cause of respiratory disease in cattle worldwide. Calves are particularly affected, even with low to moderate levels of BRSV-specific maternally derived antibodies (MDA). Available BRSV vaccines have suboptimal efficacy in calves with MDA, and published infection models in this target group are lacking in clinical expression. Here, we refine and characterize such a model.

Results: In a first experiment, 2 groups of 3 calves with low levels of MDA were experimentally inoculated by inhalation of aerosolized BRSV, either: the Snook strain, passaged in gnotobiotic calves (BRSV-Snk), or isolate no. 9402022 Denmark, passaged in cell culture (BRSV-Dk). All calves developed clinical signs of respiratory disease and shed high titers of virus, but BRSV-Snk induced more severe disease, which was then reproduced in a second experiment in 5 calves with moderate levels of MDA. These 5 calves shed high titers of virus and developed severe clinical signs of disease and extensive macroscopic lung lesions (mean+/−SD, 48.3+/−12.0% of lung), with a pulmonary influx of inflammatory cells, characterized by interferon gamma secretion and a marked effect on lung function.

Conclusions: We present a BRSV-infection model, with consistently high clinical expression in young calves with low to moderate levels of BRSV-specific MDA, that may prove useful in studies into disease pathogenesis, or evaluations of vaccines and antivirals. Additionally, refined tools to assess the outcome of BRSV infection are described, including passive measurement of lung function and a refined system to score clinical signs of disease. Using this cognate host calf model might also provide answers to elusive questions about human RSV (HRSV), a major cause of morbidity in children worldwide.

Keywords: Bovine respiratory syncytial virus, Experimental infection model, Calves, Maternal immunity, Aerosol

Background

Bovine respiratory syncytial virus (BRSV), a pneumovirus in the family *Paramyxoviridae*, is highly prevalent in cattle, with a significant economic impact as the most important viral cause of bovine respiratory disease (BRD) worldwide [1]. Despite the high seropositivity, BRSV outbreaks occur frequently, peaking during the winter months in temperate climates [2]. BRSV is thought to be transmitted by direct and indirect routes, and possibly by aerosol over short distances [3], but all the mechanisms of introduction and maintenance within herds are not clear.

Severe disease is usually observed in calves less than 1 year old, and in particular between 1–3 months in BRSV-endemic regions [4]. BRSV replication in the upper and lower airways causes cellular damage and dysfunction, and may lead to misdirected immune responses, which compound clinical signs of disease [5,6].

Most colostrum fed calves in endemic areas have BRSV-specific maternally derived antibodies (MDA) in serum, affording them limited protection from BRSV infection during the first weeks of life, but having a negative effect on the degree and duration of protection

* Correspondence: jean-francois.valarcher@slu.se
[1]Department of Clinical Sciences, Swedish University of Agricultural Sciences, Host Pathogen Interaction Group, Uppsala, Sweden
[6]Department of Virology, National Veterinary Institute, Immunology, and Parasitology, Uppsala, Sweden
Full list of author information is available at the end of the article

induced by vaccination [7]. The use of commercial vaccines in these animals has not always been fully satisfactory, and the development of a safe and effective BRSV vaccine, with a long duration of protection, therefore remains a high priority for the cattle industry [1]. Furthermore, following vaccination, exacerbated reaction to natural or experimental infection, although uncommon, has been described in calves [8,9], and resembles that previously observed in children immunized with an inactivated vaccine against the genetically and antigenically closely related pneumovirus, human RSV (HRSV) [10].

For these reasons, as well as to improve understanding of the pathogenic mechanisms during an acute infection, a clinically expressive BRSV model is needed to study BRSV pathogenesis, and to evaluate the protective efficacy of vaccine candidates and antivirals.

Several studies have attempted to reproduce field-like BRSV disease in young calves with varying levels of MDA, by administrating BRSV intranasally [11], intratracheally [12-14], or by a combination of intranasal and intratracheal route [14,15]. Some studies report severe clinical disease following experimental BRSV infection, but omit observed or methodological details that would allow interstudy comparison (e.g. rectal temperature [16]). Whereas most studies have failed to reproduce severe clinical signs of disease, despite using high titers of virus and repeated inoculations [17], studies utilizing inoculation by inhalation of aerosol have been those most successful [7,14,18-21], although this is not consistent [22]. Here, our objective was to improve and characterize a BRSV model in calves, by selecting one of two inocula, based on two different strains passaged in calves or in cell culture, and used by two different research groups, to obtain a model that would induce clinical signs comparable to those observed in the field. In addition, we describe a refined scoring system for clinical signs of disease, and objective tools that can be used to monitor and assess the effects of BRSV infection in calves.

Methods
Cells and viruses
The BRSV Snook strain was isolated in calf kidney cells [11], and then passaged three consecutive times in gnotobiotic calves by inoculation by respiratory route, and prepared from bronchoalveolar lavage (BAL), as previously described [13] (BRSV-Snk inoculum). BRSV isolate no. 9402022 Denmark [5] was isolated in fetal lung cells, passaged in bovine turbinate cells, and prepared as described previously [21] (passage 8, BRSV-Dk inoculum). Aliquots of the BRSV-Snk and BRSV-Dk inocula were titrated by plaque assay using calf kidney cells, as previously described [11]. Through inoculation of appropriate cell cultures and mycoplasmal or bacterial media, all cells and virus preparations were determined to be

free from bovine viral diarrhea virus and bacteria, including mycoplasma (data not shown).

Animals
The calves included were male, of Swedish Holstein or Swedish red and white breed, and originated from two conventional dairy herds, both free from bovine viral diarrhea virus. The herds were monitored for natural BRSV infections through monthly analysis of BRSV-specific IgG_1 (see section Detection of BRSV-specific antibodies) in bulk tank milk and in sera from calves, heifers and cows. Herd 1 was monitored from 17 days after the birth of the oldest calf, 1 day after the birth of the second oldest, and before the birth of the remaining calves in study 1. Herd 2, was monitored from 2 months before birth of the oldest calf to be challenged with BRSV in study 2.

For study 1, six calves (A1-3 and B1-3) were obtained from herd 1. These calves had low levels of BRSV-specific serum MDA on the day of challenge; mean $4.1 \pm 4.8\%$ COD of kit positive at a dilution of 1:25, where ≤10%COD positive is considered negative by the ELISA kit. In study 2, five calves (C1-5) were obtained from herd 2, all with moderate levels of BRSV-specific serum MDA; mean $49 \pm 30\%$ COD positive, or $\log_{10}$ titer 2.0 ± 0.2, defined as moderate. In addition, three calves (D1-3) were obtained from herd 1 to act as uninfected controls.

Challenge and experimental design
Groups of calves were housed in an animal facility, in separate rooms, with free access to clean water and roughage, and additional daily rations of concentrate. Each room had separate negative-pressure ventilation, physical bio-barriers and protective clothing for all staff. All calves were healthy on arrival, and no respiratory clinical signs were observed during one week of acclimation and quarantine. To minimize interference by bacterial co-infections, all calves were treated with antibiotics for five consecutive days (20 mg/kg/day procaine benzyl penicillin intramuscularly). On post-infection day (PID) 0, all calves were challenged by aerosol inhalation.

In study 1, calves were inoculated with either BRSV-Snk (calves A1-3; 9 ± 3 weeks old) or BRSV-Dk (calves B1-3; 9 ± 2 weeks old). Each dose of inoculum contained $10^{4.0}$ (BRSV-Snk) or $10^{4.4}$ (BRSV-Dk) pfu of BRSV, diluted in Dulbecco's modified Eagle medium (DMEM) to a final volume of 5 ml, and aerosolized using a compressor/nebulizer system (Super Dandy Inhaler, PARI, Germany), producing 67% of droplets with a diameter <5 μm, according to the manufacturer.

Inhalation was facilitated by a face mask designed for drug-inhalation in foals (Swevet Piab AB, Sweden). Following challenge, calves were clinically monitored and samples collected until PID 7, when they were euthanized.

In study 2, five calves (C1-5) were challenged with BRSV-Snk and monitored for seven days before euthanasia on PID 7, using the facilities and protocol described for study 1 (except where otherwise noted). In addition to these five calves (6 ± 3 weeks old), post-mortem (PM) BAL samples were collected and analyzed from three healthy calves (calves D1-3; 13 ± 4 weeks old), to act as controls for BAL samples from BRSV infected animals in study 2.

Euthanization was performed by an overdose of general anesthesia (5 mg/kg ketamine and 15 mg/kg pentobarbital sodium) followed by exsanguination.

Approval for both experiments were retained from the Ethical Committee of the district court of Uppsala, Sweden (Ref. no. C330/11). The ethical endpoint of both experiments, defined as the condition when animals would be euthanized prematurely, included: i) marked abdominal dyspnea or respiratory rate >100/min, in conjunction with severely depressed general state, or ii) anorexia for >24 h, or iii) rectal temperature >41°C for >36 h.

Clinical and pathological examination

Following challenge, daily clinical examinations were performed on each calf, and numerical values were determined for a set of predetermined parameters reflecting general state and respiratory disease (Table 1). Daily individual clinical scores were calculated by summing these numerical values multiplied by a coefficient for each parameter (Table 1). Coefficient weights reflect parameter association with disease severity in BRSV-infected calves less than 3 months of age, based on observations during natural BRSV-outbreaks [23]. Thus, general depression and reduced or absent appetite in BRSV-infected calves were considered moderate to severe signs of BRSV disease with high clinical impact and poor prognosis (coefficients of 4), abdominal dyspnea a moderate sign (coefficient of 3), and increased rectal temperature and respiratory rate, mild to moderate signs (coefficients of 2). The other recorded parameters have varying clinical specificity and severity, from mild to severe, but typically have little clinical impact, and may be very transient. These parameters were assigned a coefficient of 1 (Table 1). Individual accumulated clinical scores (ACS) were calculated as the area under daily clinical scores, using the Trapezoid method. At PM examination, lung lesions were evaluated, recorded and quantified, as previously described [24]. Tissue samples, preferentially from lesioned areas, were collected from each of the lobes in the right lung and trachea, and preserved in 5% paraformaldehyde.

Sampling

Serum was obtained from blood collected on PID −37, −15, 0 and 7, and stored at −20°C, until antibody analysis. Nasal secretions were collected and stored at −70°C, as previously described [21] using sterile cotton-tipped swabs daily from PID 0 to 7, and tampons on PID 0 and 6.

In study 1 endoscopic BAL in sedated calves was performed the day before challenge in all calves as previously described, including disinfection of the endoscope between each calf [23], except lungs were flushed with PBS with 120 µg/ml benzyl penicillin sodium. In both study 1 and study 2 PM BAL was performed in all calves as previously described [12], except lungs were flushed using PBS. BAL fluid was stored on ice after recovery. BAL cells in 10 ml BAL fluid were pelleted by centrifugation (200 × g, 10 min), and resuspended in either 350 µl RLT buffer (Qiagen, Sweden) or 1 ml DMEM with 20% fetal calf serum, and stored at −70°C. BAL supernatant was recovered from centrifugation and stored at −70°C. Bacterial culture was attempted by inoculating bovine blood agar plates with 1 ml of unprocessed BAL fluid.

Detection of BRSV-specific antibodies

BRSV-specific IgG$_1$ antibodies were analyzed using a commercial ELISA kit (SVANOVIR® BRSV-Ab ELISA, Svanova, Sweden), in accordance with the manufacturer's instructions, including calculations of corrected optic density (COD) and percent of kit positive control (%COD positive).

Detection and isolation of virus

BRSV-F gene RNA present in nasal secretions or in BAL cells corresponding to 10 ml of BAL, was quantified by RT-qPCR as previously described [21], and expressed as TCID$_{50}$ equivalent units to dilutions of a virus sample with known titer. Accumulated virus shed (AVS) was calculated as the area under individual curves of BRSV detected by RT-qPCR in nasal secretions from PID 0 to PID 7. Virus isolation was attempted by inoculating bovine turbinate cells with BAL and nasal secretion samples, as previously described [21]. Cultures of inoculated bovine turbinate cells were examined daily, and were considered positive if cytopathic effects appeared within seven days.

Histological analysis

Lung and trachea tissue samples were fixed in 10% buffered formalin, embedded in paraffin, sectioned and stained with hematoxylin and eosin (HE) and by immunohistochemistry (IHC) to detect BRSV antigen.

BRSV immunohistochemistry staining

For unmasking, sections were treated with heat-induced epitope retrieval (HIER). They were placed in HIER buffer (Target Retrieval Solution, pH = 6, DAKO, Sweden) and subjected to heat treatment in HIER Microwave at

Table 1 Parameters and coefficients used to calculate clinical scores in BRSV infected calves

Clinical parameter	Parameter coefficient	State description	Numerical value
General state	4	Normal	0
		Moves slowly, head down	1
		Lying down/staggers	2
		Recumbent	3
Appetite	4	Normal	0
		Reduced	1
		Absent	2
Abdominal dyspnea	3	Normal	0
		Slight (short, rapid)	1
		Moderate (labored)	2
		Severe (very labored, grunting)	3
Rectal temperature	2	<39.6°C	0
		<40.0°C	1
		<40.5°C	2
		<41.0°C	3
		≥41.0°C	4
Respiratory rate	2	<50/min	0
		<55/min	1
		<65/min	2
		<75/min	3
		≥75/min	4
Intensity of lung sounds	1	Normal	0
		Slightly enhanced	1
		Moderately enhanced	2
		Severely enhanced	3
Added respiratory sounds (wheezing or crackles)	1	Normal	0
		Slight	1
		Moderate	2
		Severe	3
Coughing	1	Absent	0
		Only provoked	1
		Spontaneous, infrequent	2
		Persistent	3
Nasal discharge	1	Normal	0
		Slight uni-/bilat. serous	1
		Moderate bilat. serous to purulent	2
		Copious bilat. purulent	3

During clinical examination, each clinical parameter was assigned a numerical value according to the appropriate state description for that parameter. A clinical score sum was then calculated, by multiplying each numerical value with the parameter coefficient.

750 W for 7 minutes followed by 350 W for 14 minutes and were allowed to stand for 20 min at room temperature. Endogenous peroxidase activity was blocked with 3% hydrogen peroxide for 20 min at room temperature. Unspecific antigen staining was blocked with 2% bovine serum albumin (Sigma-Aldrich, Sweden AB) for 20 min.

The slides were then incubated at room temperature for 45 min with mouse monoclonal antibody anti RSV (clone 5H5, 2G122, 5A6 and 1C3, NCL-RSV3, Novocastra, Leica Microsystems, Sweden) diluted 1:100 in diluents buffer (1% BSA/TBS pH = 7.6). The detection was conducted with the dextran polymer method (EnVisionTM/mouse,

DAKO, Sweden). The color was developed with diamino-benzidine substrate (DAB, DAKO, Sweden). Sections were counterstained with haematoxylin. Antibody-omission stained sections served as negative controls for each section. Appropriate positive and negative control sections were included in each run.

Scoring of histopathological severity of inflammation

The severity of histopathology was scored in each HE-stained section, from 0 (normal), 1 (mild), 2 (moderate) to 3 (severe). The extent and localization of BRSV-antigen was evaluated in IHC-stained sections. BAL cell type composition was determined by manual microscopic analysis of stained cytospin preparations of BAL fluid.

Detection of cytokines in BAL supernatant

To enhance the sensitivity of cytokine detection, BAL supernatant was concentrated 20X (BAL20X) by filtered (UFC900324, Amicon Ultra-15, 3 kDa, Merck Millipore, Sweden) centrifugation (swinging bucket rotor, 4000 × g, 25–30 min), to an equal final volume. Cytokines in BAL20X were analyzed using commercially available ELISA kits, and by following provided instructions for: interleukin 4 (IL-4; MCA5892KZZ Bovine Interleukin-4 ELISA, BioRad, Sweden), interleukin 6 (IL-6; ESS0029 Bovine IL-6 ELISA, Pierce, USA), interleukin 8 (IL-8; ABIN414016 Bovine IL-8 ELISA, Antibodies Online, Germany), tumor necrosis factor alpha (TNFα; VS0285B-002 Bovine TNFα ELISA, Divbio Science Europe, The Netherlands), and interferon gamma (IFNγ; MCA5638KZZ Bovine IFNγ ELISA, BioRad, Sweden). Cytokine concentration (ng/ml) in each sample of BAL supernatant was calculated using serial dilutions of supplied standards in each kit, and by correcting for the concentration factor of the BAL20X.

Measuring lung function

Lung function was passively measured before and after BRSV challenge, on PID 0 and 6, by the forced oscillation technique (EquineOsc Calf measurement head, EEMS, Harts, UK), using the same face mask described for aerosol inhalation. Values for resistance (R) and reactance (X)(kPa/L/s) were obtained at 3, 5, 7 and 10 Hz, as described by Reinhold and colleagues [25]. Each calf was tested at least twice on each day and the data sets with optimal coherence selected (coherence > 0.9; majority of data sets > 0.97). In the event of clear artifacts of breathing, such as cough or breath holding, the series were repeated. Daily calibration was performed using a 2.26 m long tube, with a 21 mm internal diameter.

Ranking of infected calves

To encompass the three major aspects of BRSV-infection clinical signs, lung pathology and virus replication, the six calves in study 1 (calves A1-3 and B1-3)

were ranked from least affected (1) to most affected (6) based on: accumulated clinical scores recorded from PID 0 to PID 7; degree of consolidative lesions in lungs on PID 7; and accumulated virus detected in nasal secretions from PID 0 to PID 7. Group rank sums were then calculated for each rank, and for all three ranks (total rank sum).

Statistical analysis

Where not otherwise stated, results are presented as group mean ± standard deviation (SD). For results presented as a percentage of a whole, SD is presented in percentage points (pp). Statistically significant differences were determined using either one-way ANOVA followed by Student's t-test, or pairwise t-test, or Kruskal–Wallis analysis followed by Wilcoxon test (JMP 10 for Mac, SAS Institute Inc.). Significance was assumed when p ≤ 0.05 and tendency when p ≤ 0.1.

Results

Study 1: Evaluation of clinical, pathological and virological expression of two virulent BRSV inocula in calves with low levels of MDA

Clinical signs following challenge

Following experimental infection, mild to severe clinical signs of respiratory disease were observed in all infected calves (Figure 1A). For all calves, upper respiratory signs, such as nasal discharge and coughing, as well as ocular discharge were observed on PID 3–5. In BRSV-Snk infected calves, these progressed to severe respiratory signs on PID7, whereas clinical signs were more moderate on PID 7 in calves infected with BRSV-Dk (Table 2).

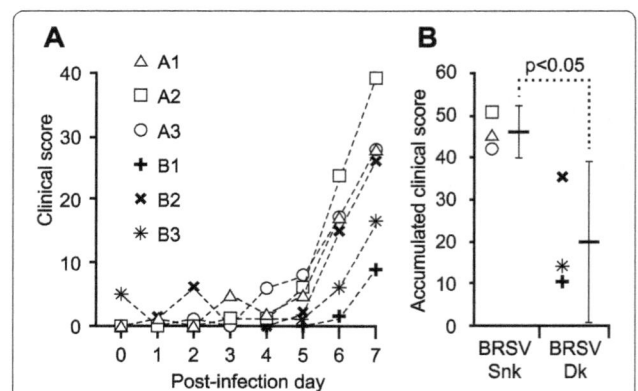

Figure 1 Daily and accumulated clinical score following aerosol challenge with either BRSV-Snk or BRSV-Dk. Six calves were experimentally infected with virulent BRSV, either passaged in vivo (BRSV-Snk, n = 3, calves A1-3), or in vitro (BRSV-Dk, n = 3, calves B1-3). Following infection on post-infection day (PID) 0, calves were monitored for seven days. Daily clinical scores (panel **A**) were calculated from observed clinical signs (see Tables 1 and 2). Accumulated clinical scores, from PID 0 to PID 7 (panel **B**), were calculated as the area under individual clinical score curves.

Table 2 Clinical scores in calves on day seven after experimental infection with BRSV

| Clinical sign | Group/Calf | | | | | |
| | BRSV-Snk | | | BRSV-Dk | | |
	A1	A2	A3	B1	B2	B3
General state	1	1	1	0	1	0
Appetite	1	1	1	0	0	0
Abdominal dyspnea	2	2	2	2	2	2
Temperature	0	4	0	0	1	2
Respiratory rate	3	3	3	1	3	0
Lung sounds intensity	2	3	3	0	2	1
Added lung sounds	0	3	2	0	2	1
Nasal discharge	1	2	1	1	1	1
Coughing	2	2	2	0	2	0
Clinical score	25	38	28	9	25	13

Six calves were experimentally infected with virulent BRSV, either passaged in vivo (BRSV-Snk, n = 3, calves A1-3), or in vitro (BRSV-Dk, n = 3, calves B1-3). Clinical signs were recorded daily for seven days, and scores calculated as described in Table 1.

Consequently, compared to BRSV-Dk infected calves, BRSV-Snk infected calves had significantly higher ($p \leq 0.05$) accumulated clinical scores (Figure 1B).

Macroscopic and histological lung pathology

BRSV-Snk infected calves tended to have more extensive consolidated lung lesions ($38.5 \pm 26.3\%$ of total lung tissue) on PID7, compared to calves infected with BRSV-Dk ($12.8 \pm 14.6\%$), but this difference was not statistically significant ($p = 0.23$; Figure 2A and C).

Histologically, lesions in the trachea in both groups of calves consisted of degeneration and necrosis of epithelium, and epithelial hyperplasia in some areas (Figure 2B:I and II show representative pictures from BRSV-Snk and BRSV-Dk infected animals, respectively). In the lungs, BRSV-Snk infected calves showed extensive moderate to severe bronchointerstitial pneumonia, as well as purulent bronchitis and bronchiolitis (Figure 2B:III; representative picture of lung, calf A2). BRSV-Dk infected calves showed similar but less severe histopathological changes in the lungs, ranging from mild to moderate (Figure 2B:IV; representative picture of lung, calf B3).

In summary, BRSV-Snk infected animals tended to have macroscopically more extensive, and histologically more severe lung lesions, compared to BRSV-Dk infected animals (Figure 2C), but with no discernible difference in the severity of histological inflammation in the trachea.

Inflammatory cells in bronchoalveolar lavage

Bronchoalveolar lavage was performed to collect BAL cells in all calves, once before infection (PID −1), and again on the day of euthanization (PID 7). Regardless of challenge inoculum, experimental infection altered the composition of BAL cell types (Figure 2D). Before infection, the predominant BAL cell type were macrophages ($63.0 \pm 26.0\%$ for BRSV-Snk and $69.0 \pm 10.1\%$ for BRSV-Dk), followed by neutrophils ($30.0 \pm 27.8\%$ for BRSV-Snk and $21.3 \pm 18.5\%$ for BRSV-Dk), whereas after infection, neutrophils were the predominant BAL cell type ($79.0 \pm 4.4\%$ for BRSV-Snk and $80.3 \pm 6.0\%$ for BRSV-Dk), followed by macrophages ($18.7 \pm 2.3\%$ for BRSV-Snk and $17.7 \pm 4.5\%$ for BRSV-Dk) (Figure 2D).

However, the total number of BAL cells was significantly increased only in BRSV-Snk infected calves following challenge ($6.9 \pm 2.0 \times 10^6$ cells/ml at PID 7), compared to before challenge ($1.0 \pm 0.2 \times 10^6$ cells/ml at PID −1; $p \leq 0.01$; pairwise t-test), and compared to BRSV-Dk infected calves before and after challenge ($1.1 \pm 0.2 \times 10^6$ cells/ml at PID −1; $0.8 \pm 0.7 \times 10^6$ cells/ml at PID 7; $p \leq 0.01$; pairwise t-test; Figure 2D).

Virology
RT-qPCR detection and isolation of BRSV in nasal secretion and BAL

BRSV RNA was detected by RT-qPCR in nasal secretions collected daily from PID 0 to PID 7, and in BAL collected on PID 7 (PM BAL). In addition, BRSV was isolated in the first passage in bovine turbinate cell culture, from all infected calves, in both nasal secretions from PID 6, and PM BAL fluid. Attempted bacterial culture from BAL fluid indicated no bacterial coinfection in the lungs of any of the calves. Two of the BRSV-Snk infected calves (A2 and A3) started shedding virus on PID 2, and shed high amounts of virus (A2 $\log_{10}$ AVS 19.3 TCID$_{50}$ equiv.; A3 $\log_{10}$ AVS 14.9 TCID$_{50}$ equiv.), both in nasal secretions and PM BAL, whereas the third BRSV-Snk infected calf (A1), shed substantially less virus ($\log_{10}$ AVS 3.6 TCID$_{50}$ equiv.) (Figure 3A-B).

Compared to the two high-shedding BRSV-Snk infected calves, calves infected with BRSV-Dk shed markedly less virus in nasal secretions (B1, B2 and B3 $\log_{10}$ AVS 3.5, 9.4 and 11.1 TCID$_{50}$ equiv., respectively), and had less viral RNA in BAL, although this was not statistically significant (Figure 3A-B).

BRSV immunostaining in lung and trachea sections

In IHC-stained sections of trachea very little or no BRSV antigen was detected in BRSV-Snk infected calves (Figure 3C:I is representative), whereas viral antigen was abundant in sections of trachea from BRSV-Dk infected calves (Figure 3C:II is representative). Conversely, whereas viral antigen was abundant in the lungs of 2/3 BRSV-Snk infected calves (Figure 3C:III is representative), very little or no BRSV antigen was detected in the lungs from BRSV-Dk infected calves (Figure 3C:IV is representative).

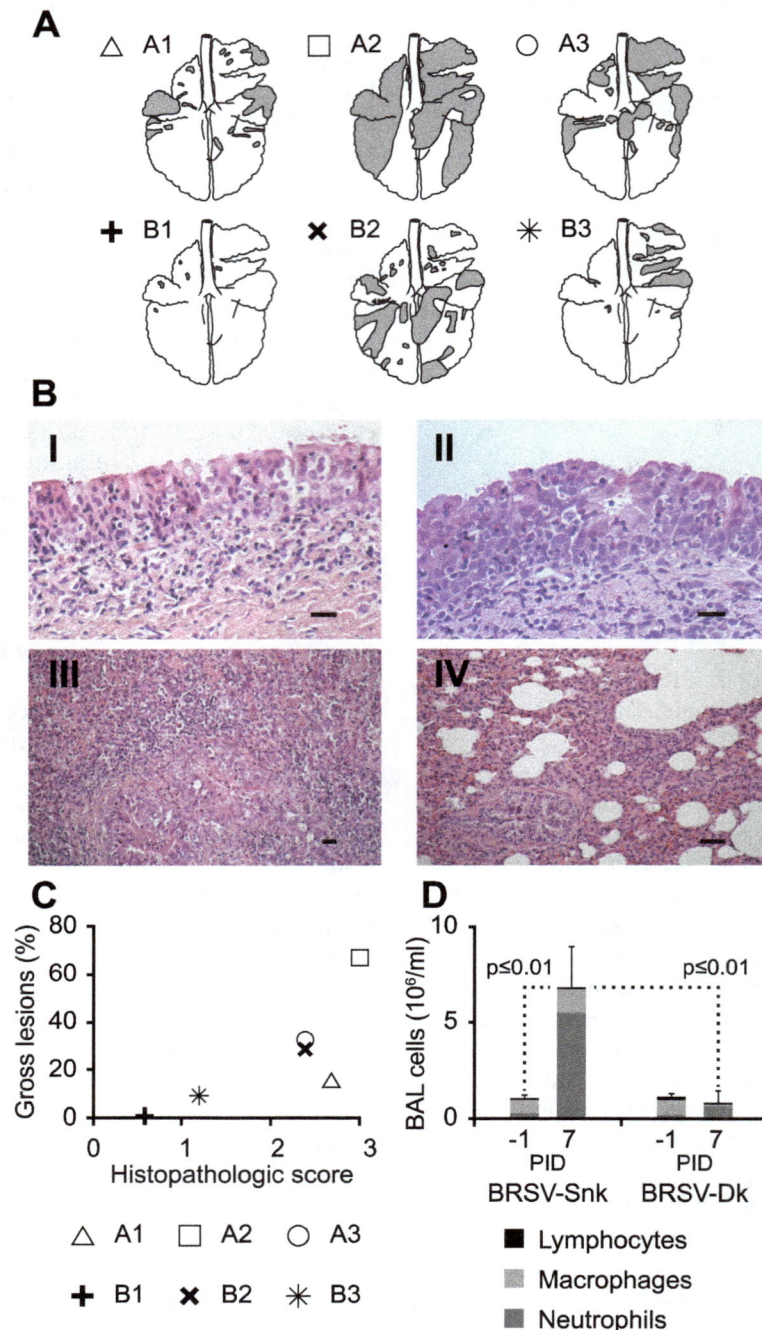

Figure 2 Pulmonary pathology and neutrophil influx in calves following aerosol challenge with either BRSV-Snk or BRSV-Dk. Calves were experimentally infected as described in Figure 1. Calves were euthanized seven days after infection and the macroscopic extent of lung lesions were documented (panel **A**). From each calf, trachea tissue and four lung tissue samples were collected for sectioning, staining and histopathological description and scoring of severity of inflammation (1–3). Panels **B**:I-IV show representative HE-stained sections from: (**B**:I) trachea from calf A2; (**B**:II) trachea from calf B3; (**B**:III) lung from calf A2; and (**B**:IV) lung from calf B3. Horizontal bars indicate 50 µm in panels **B**:I and **B**:II, and 100 µm in panels **B**:III and **B**:IV. Mean histopathological severity of inflammation per calf, is shown on the x-axis in panel **C**, along with the proportion (%) of macroscopic lung lesions per calf on the y-axis. Bronchoalveolar lavage (BAL) was performed on PID −1 and PID 7, and cell types in BAL samples enumerated (Panel **D**). Stacks represent the mean total number of cells in BAL per ml, with associated standard deviation, as well as the number of neutrophils, macrophages and lymphocytes in BAL per ml. The proportion of eosinophils were <1% in all samples.

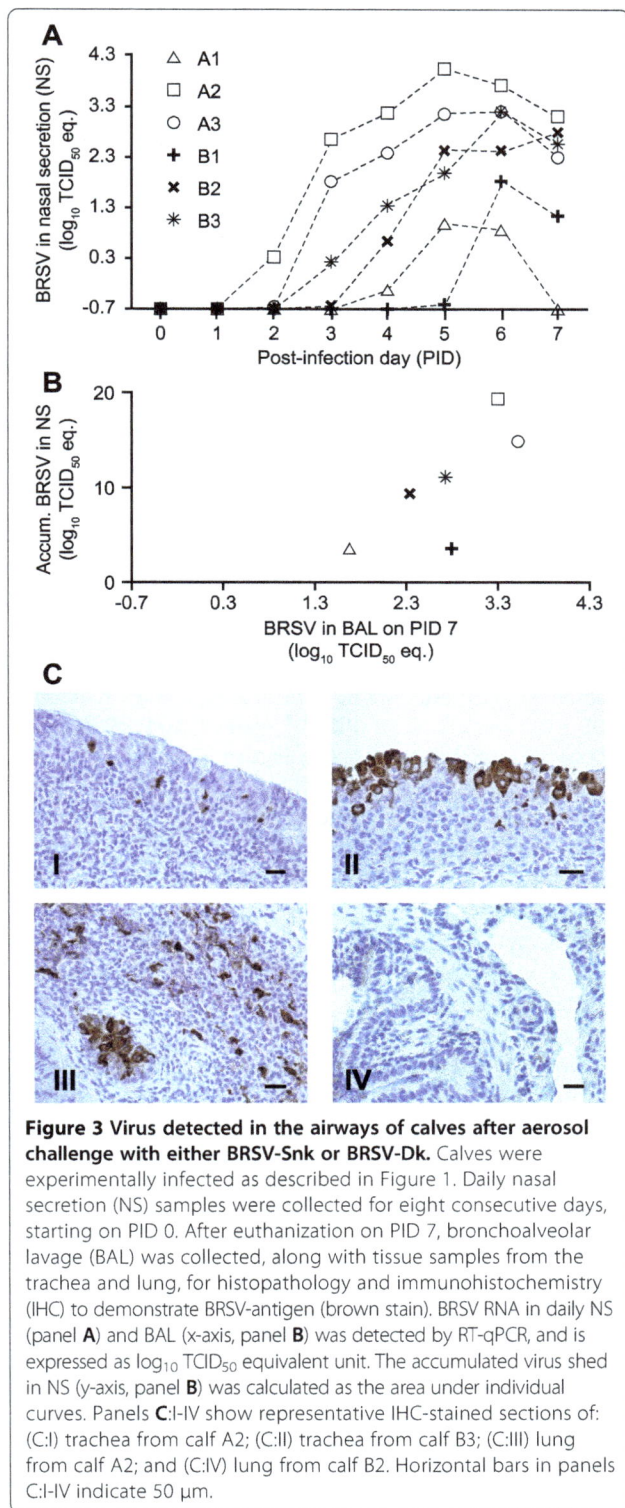

Figure 3 Virus detected in the airways of calves after aerosol challenge with either BRSV-Snk or BRSV-Dk. Calves were experimentally infected as described in Figure 1. Daily nasal secretion (NS) samples were collected for eight consecutive days, starting on PID 0. After euthanization on PID 7, bronchoalveolar lavage (BAL) was collected, along with tissue samples from the trachea and lung, for histopathology and immunohistochemistry (IHC) to demonstrate BRSV-antigen (brown stain). BRSV RNA in daily NS (panel **A**) and BAL (x-axis, panel **B**) was detected by RT-qPCR, and is expressed as $\log_{10}$ TCID$_{50}$ equivalent unit. The accumulated virus shed in NS (y-axis, panel **B**) was calculated as the area under individual curves. Panels **C**:I-IV show representative IHC-stained sections of: (C:I) trachea from calf A2; (C:II) trachea from calf B3; (C:III) lung from calf A2; and (C:IV) lung from calf B2. Horizontal bars in panels C:I-IV indicate 50 μm.

The third BRSV-Snk infected calf (A1) was negative for BRSV antigen by IHC, both in the trachea and in the lungs (data not shown).

Serum BRSV-specific antibodies

All calves, except A1, had low and consistently decreasing levels of BRSV-specific MDA, throughout the experiment (Figure 4). In contrast, the BRSV-Snk infected calf A1 (the oldest calf in study 1) seroconverted within 7 days after challenge, strongly suggesting that this calf had been previously primed against BRSV.

Animal ranking

When calves were ranked from least affected (1) to most affected (6) based on clinical score, degree of lung pathology and accumulated virus shed in nasal secretions, two of the BRSV-Snk infected calves (A2 and A3) consistently received the highest ranks (Figure 5A). Conversely, the calves infected with BRSV-Dk received low ranks, as they demonstrated less severe clinical signs, less lung pathology, and less virus shedding (Figure 5A). The BRSV-Snk infected calf that rapidly seroconverted following challenge (A1), received a high clinical rank, an intermediate lung pathology rank, and a low viral-shed rank (Figure 5A). Overall, the BRSV-Snk infected calves ranked significantly higher, compared to calves infected with BRSV-Dk (p ≤ 0.01; Figure 5B). Based on the overall ability of the BRSV-Snk inoculum to induce BRSV infection, it was chosen as the inoculum in study 2, to reproduce and characterize the model in calves with moderate levels of MDA.

Study 2: Reproduction of clinical signs, virology and pathology using aerosolized BRSV-Snk in calves with passive immunity

Based on the high level of clinical signs of disease observed in calves with low levels of MDA, following challenge with BRSV-Snk in study 1, an additional five calves (calves C1-5), which were all BRSV-naive and had moderate levels of BRSV-specific serum IgG$_1$ MDA were

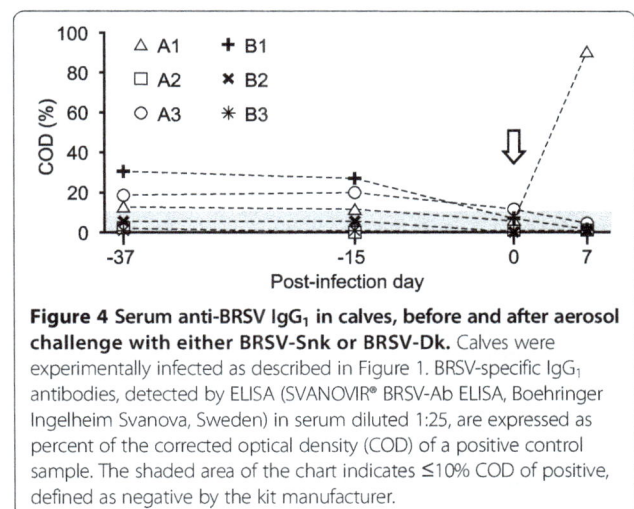

Figure 4 Serum anti-BRSV IgG$_1$ in calves, before and after aerosol challenge with either BRSV-Snk or BRSV-Dk. Calves were experimentally infected as described in Figure 1. BRSV-specific IgG$_1$ antibodies, detected by ELISA (SVANOVIR® BRSV-Ab ELISA, Boehringer Ingelheim Svanova, Sweden) in serum diluted 1:25, are expressed as percent of the corrected optical density (COD) of a positive control sample. The shaded area of the chart indicates ≤10% COD of positive, defined as negative by the kit manufacturer.

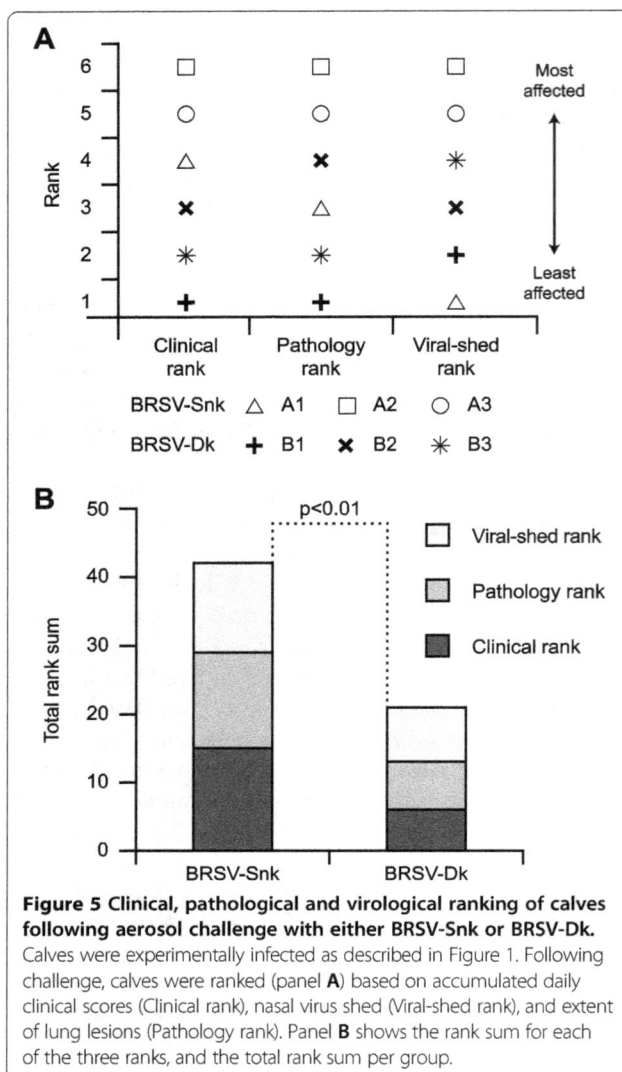

Figure 5 Clinical, pathological and virological ranking of calves following aerosol challenge with either BRSV-Snk or BRSV-Dk. Calves were experimentally infected as described in Figure 1. Following challenge, calves were ranked (panel **A**) based on accumulated daily clinical scores (Clinical rank), nasal virus shed (Viral-shed rank), and extent of lung lesions (Pathology rank). Panel **B** shows the rank sum for each of the three ranks, and the total rank sum per group.

challenged using the same inoculum and protocol as used in study 1.

Clinical signs, lung pathology and virology following challenge

Clinical signs of disease and lung pathology, as well as levels of viral RNA detected in the upper and lower airways in study 2, following challenge of calves C1-5, have been described in detail elsewhere [24]. The amplitude and kinetics of these parameters were in line with observations in BRSV-Snk infected calves in study 1 (Figure 6A-C). Briefly, all infected calves in study 2 developed clinical signs of upper respiratory disease starting on PID 3–5, which progressed to severe lower respiratory disease from PID 5 to PID 7 (Figure 6A). On PID 7, all five calves were moderately to severely depressed (recumbent, and staggering when prompted to rise), with reduced or absent appetite. Although both groups of BRSV-Snk infected calves in

study 1 and 2 shed high amounts of virus, as detected by RT-qPCR, calves in study 2 shed less accumulated virus in nasal secretions compared to those in study 1 ($\log_{10}$ 1.6 $TCID_{50}$ eq. difference in mean), but more in BAL fluid on PID 7 ($\log_{10}$ 2.1 $TCID_{50}$ eq. difference in mean). At postmortem, BRSV-Snk infected calves in study 2 had extensive consolidated lung lesions and histopathological changes on PID 7, similar in extent to those in study 1 ($38.5 \pm 26.3\%$ and $48.3 \pm 12.0\%$ of total lung area for study 1 and study 2, respectively; Figure 6C; mean histological score 2.7 ± 0.3 and 2.9 ± 0.1 for study 1 and study 2, respectively; Figure 6C).

Quantitative assessment of lung function

The impact of lower respiratory disease (as demonstrated by clinical signs of disease and lung pathology) on lung function in the five calves in study 2 was evaluated by the forced oscillation technique before and after challenge (on PID 0 and 6). Following challenge, infected animals demonstrated a tendency at 10 Hz measurements for increased airway resistance (0.17 ± 0.03 kPa/L/s on PID 0; 0.20 ± 0.06 kPa/L/s on PID 6; $p = 0.2$, pairwise t-test) and significantly decreased airway reactance (0.03 ± 0.03 kPa/L/s on PID 0; -0.02 ± 0.04 kPa/L/s on PID 6; $p \leq 0.05$, pairwise t-test; Figure 7).

Cytology and cytokine profile in BAL

Seven days after experimental BRSV infection, BAL was collected from all five infected calves in study 2, and in addition, from three uninfected calves. BAL cell types in cytospin preparations were analyzed by light microscopy (Figure 8A) and BAL supernatant was analyzed using ELISAs, specific to bovine inflammatory cytokines (Figure 8B-F).

Following infection, infected calves demonstrated a significant increase in inflammatory cells in BAL ($11.0 \pm 3.7 \times 10^6$ cells/ml), compared to uninfected controls ($1.1 \pm 0.2 \times 10^6$ cells/ml) ($p \leq 0.005$; Figure 8A). As observed in BRSV-Snk infected calves in study 1, this increase consisted mostly of neutrophils ($68.6 \pm 14.4\%$), followed by macrophages ($27.8 \pm 13.0\%$) and lymphocytes ($3.6 \pm 2.0\%$). Very few eosinophils were seen in the BAL of infected calves (<0.5%).

Cytokine analysis of BAL supernatant from infected calves demonstrated significantly higher levels of IFNγ ($p \leq 0.005$; Figure 8E) and a tendency for higher levels of IL-6 ($p = 0.08$; Figure 8C), compared to uninfected control calves. In contrast, levels of IL-4, IL-8 and TNFα in BAL, did not differ from those of uninfected controls, seven days after infection (Figure 8B,D and F).

Discussion

In the present paper, we describe an experimental model of BRSV infection with strong clinical and pathological

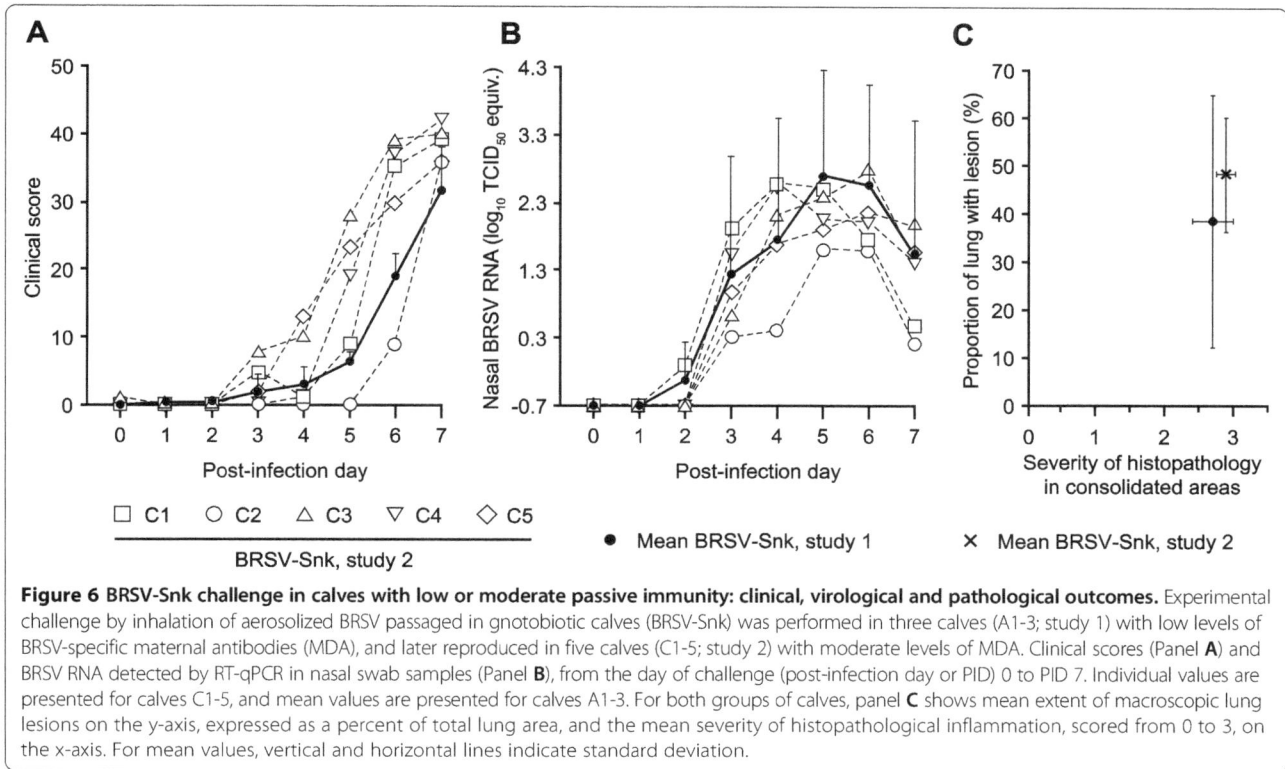

Figure 6 BRSV-Snk challenge in calves with low or moderate passive immunity: clinical, virological and pathological outcomes. Experimental challenge by inhalation of aerosolized BRSV passaged in gnotobiotic calves (BRSV-Snk) was performed in three calves (A1-3; study 1) with low levels of BRSV-specific maternal antibodies (MDA), and later reproduced in five calves (C1-5; study 2) with moderate levels of MDA. Clinical scores (Panel **A**) and BRSV RNA detected by RT-qPCR in nasal swab samples (Panel **B**), from the day of challenge (post-infection day or PID) 0 to PID 7. Individual values are presented for calves C1-5, and mean values are presented for calves A1-3. For both groups of calves, panel **C** shows mean extent of macroscopic lung lesions on the y-axis, expressed as a percent of total lung area, and the mean severity of histopathological inflammation, scored from 0 to 3, on the x-axis. For mean values, vertical and horizontal lines indicate standard deviation.

expression in calves with maternal antibodies. This model combines and refines elements from previously published studies, including aerosol inoculation, the use of inoculum passaged in gnotobiotic calves, and methods to monitor and quantify clinical, pathological and virological parameters [12,14,21]. We believe that this model can serve to enable a better evaluation of vaccine and

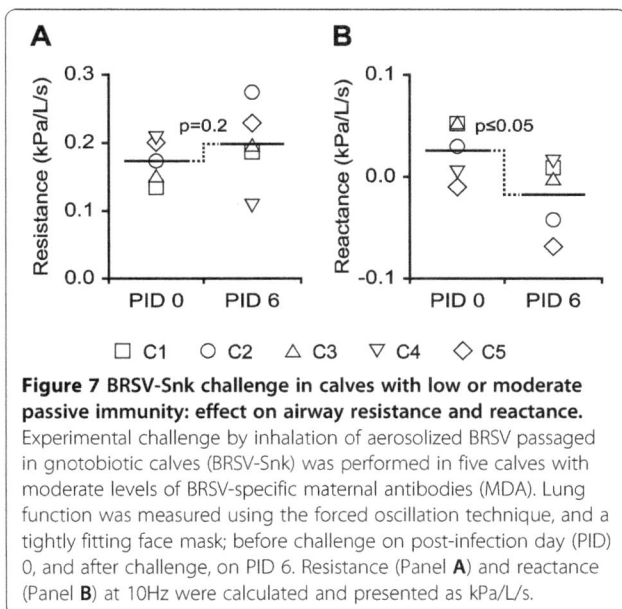

Figure 7 BRSV-Snk challenge in calves with low or moderate passive immunity: effect on airway resistance and reactance. Experimental challenge by inhalation of aerosolized BRSV passaged in gnotobiotic calves (BRSV-Snk) was performed in five calves with moderate levels of BRSV-specific maternal antibodies (MDA). Lung function was measured using the forced oscillation technique, and a tightly fitting face mask; before challenge on post-infection day (PID) 0, and after challenge, on PID 6. Resistance (Panel **A**) and reactance (Panel **B**) at 10Hz were calculated and presented as kPa/L/s.

antiviral safety and efficacy and further increase understanding of the pathogenesis of BRSV, and also of HRSV.

Regardless of the inoculum, all inoculated calves (n = 11), in both studies, developed manifest BRSV disease. The rapid seroconversion detected in calf A1 in study 1 indicated that, in contrast to the other calves, this BRSV-Snk-infected calf had been previously exposed to natural BRSV. This highlights that, to ascertain BRSV naiveté by seromonitoring in herds, seronegative sentinel animals need to be regularly monitored during the entire lifespan of calves to be included in experimental trials. This case also confirms earlier reports [26,27] that a sufficient amount of MDA can suppress detectable humoral immune responses, following BRSV infection in young calves, with the net effect of declining MDA detected by ELISA. However, although this previous priming appear to have provided some virological protection, compared to all other BRSV-Snk infected calves, calf A1 demonstrated severe clinical disease following BRSV infection, in the absence of any other detected pathogen, contrary to previously published reports [28,29]. In contrast, the moderate clinical signs, pathology and virus shed observed in calf B1 following BRSV-Dk challenge, may possibly be explained by favorable genetics, with more efficient innate and cellular responses. Any previous BRSV exposure of calf B1, even if virus replication was very limited, would have resulted in a rapid anamnestic humoral immune response upon reinfection, as seen in calf A1, and demonstrated elsewhere [24,30].

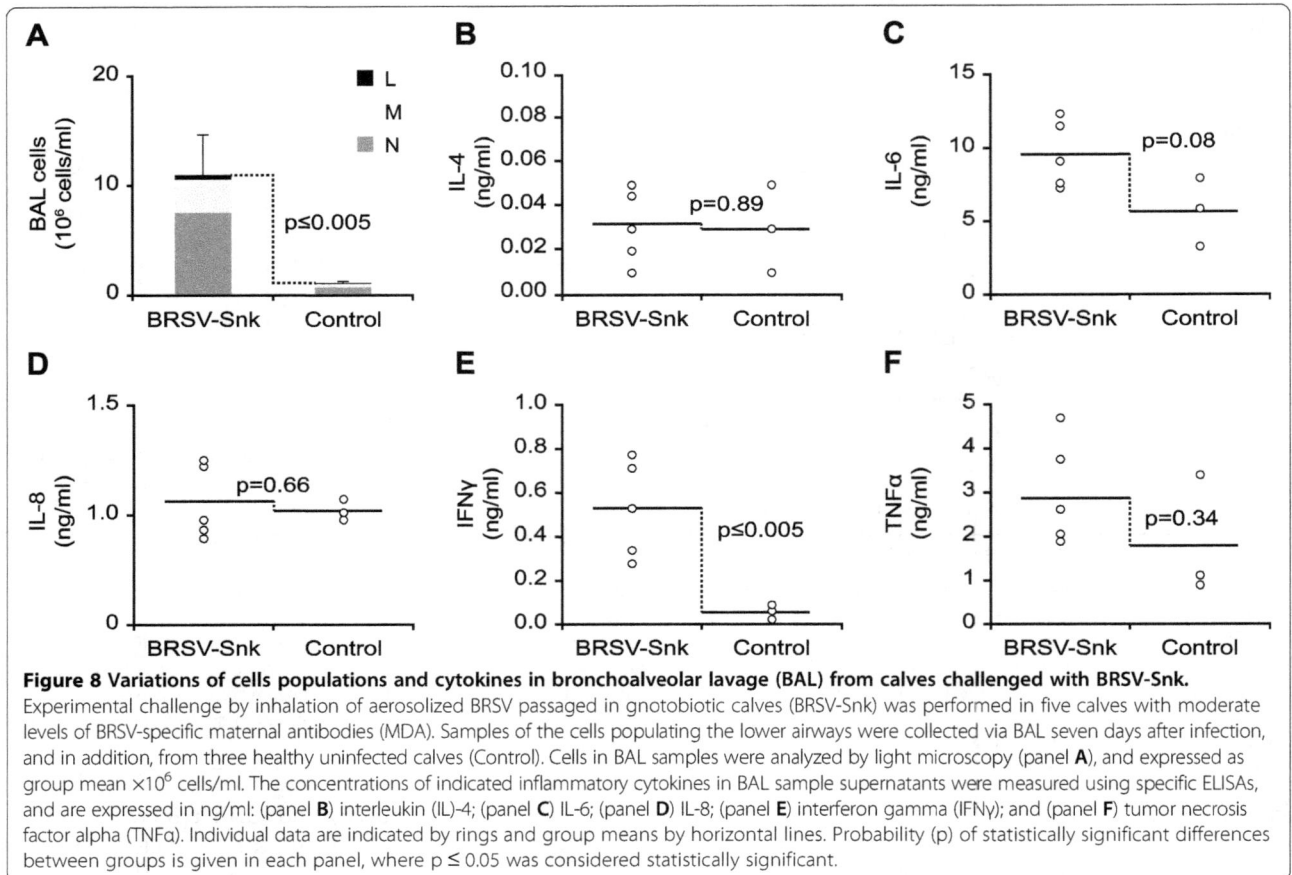

Figure 8 Variations of cells populations and cytokines in bronchoalveolar lavage (BAL) from calves challenged with BRSV-Snk.
Experimental challenge by inhalation of aerosolized BRSV passaged in gnotobiotic calves (BRSV-Snk) was performed in five calves with moderate levels of BRSV-specific maternal antibodies (MDA). Samples of the cells populating the lower airways were collected via BAL seven days after infection, and in addition, from three healthy uninfected calves (Control). Cells in BAL samples were analyzed by light microscopy (panel **A**), and expressed as group mean $\times 10^6$ cells/ml. The concentrations of indicated inflammatory cytokines in BAL sample supernatants were measured using specific ELISAs, and are expressed in ng/ml: (panel **B**) interleukin (IL)-4; (panel **C**) IL-6; (panel **D**) IL-8; (panel **E**) interferon gamma (IFNγ); and (panel **F**) tumor necrosis factor alpha (TNFα). Individual data are indicated by rings and group means by horizontal lines. Probability (p) of statistically significant differences between groups is given in each panel, where p ≤ 0.05 was considered statistically significant.

Immunohistochemical staining for BRSV antigen in study 1 showed a marked difference in localization of virus on PID 7, where two BRSV-Snk infected calves had large amounts of virus in the lungs and only small amounts of virus in the trachea, while the reverse was true for BRSV-Dk infected calves. This disparity in antigen localization on PID 7 might be due to delayed progression of viral replication in BRSV-Dk infected calves. This opens the possibility that BRSV-Dk infected calves might have developed more severe clinical signs, if the 7-day challenge model had been abandoned and the experiment had been prolonged. However, this would contradict previous observations using the BRSV-Dk inoculum, which indicate a peak of clinical signs on PID 6 [20]. Nonetheless, virus was isolated and high quantities of viral RNA were detected by RT-qPCR in samples from the upper and lower airways from all infected calves in both studies, including calves A1 and B1, although BRSV-Snk infected calves from both studies shed 10^3 times more virus in nasal secretions than BRSV-Dk infected calves.

Despite the differing data of calves A1 and B1, and although the number of animals in the first study was low

(n = 3 + 3), we concluded that BRSV-Snk infected calves tended to be more severely affected in the 7-day experimental infection model, compared to BRSV-Dk infected calves, when summarizing clinical, pathological and virological parameters (Figure 5B). Thus, results from study 1 were reproduced in study 2, using aerosol inoculation of the BRSV-Snk inoculum in an additional five BRSV-naive calves, with moderate levels of MDA.

Using a minimal amount of aerosolized inoculum ($10^{4.0}$ pfu for BRSV-Snk) to experimentally infect calves with and without MDA, the kinetics of severe naturally occurring BRSV infection in calves was recreated in this study [4,31]. On PID 7, most calves were severely affected, and all BRSV-Snk infected calves in study 2 were demonstrating depression, anorexia, pyrexia, tachypnea, abdominal dyspnea and wheezing lung sounds.

The high level of clinical expression in BRSV-Snk infected calves was mirrored by the great extent of macroscopic lung lesions and by the severity of histopathological changes in the lungs on PID 7. Manifest inflammation was further verified in BRSV-Snk infected calves in study 2, with significantly increased numbers of neutrophils, macrophages and lymphocytes in BAL, similar to that reported following natural BRSV infection in calves [32].

At the peak of clinical signs, 7 days post infection, the calves in study 2 also demonstrated an increase of IFNγ and minimal amounts of IL-4 in BAL supernatant, which agrees with previously reported responses to primary BRSV infection in calves [33]. Previous studies have shown that T lymphocytes migrating to the lung during BRSV infection are predominantly IFNγ producing CD8 + T cells [34,35], which have been shown to be important for BRSV clearance [12,36]. However, at least a proportion of the IFNγ detected in BAL supernatant in study 2, may also have been produced by NK cells, or alveolar macrophages, as have been shown in vitro with human alveolar macrophages [37]. Similar to that seen in calves, infants hospitalized with severe HRSV bronchiolitis, had an increased frequency of IFNγ producing CD8+ T cells, collected by nasal brush, compared to infants with milder upper respiratory tract infections [38]. Thus, IFNγ in BAL supernatant can serve as an objective measurement of disease severity, following experimental BRSV challenge.

Elevated levels of TNFα, IL-6 and IL-8 in BAL or serum have also been associated with clinical signs and pathology caused by BRSV infection in calves [33,39,40]. The lack of detectable increases in these cytokines in BAL supernatant on PID 7 in study 2 may have been due to suboptimal timing of BAL collection, as another study where 6 weeks old calves where infected with BRSV reported TNFα and IL-6 concentrations in BAL to peak on PID 9 and PID 3, respectively [41].

The patent pneumonia in the BRSV-Snk infected calves following infection in study 2, as demonstrated by clinical signs, lung pathology, and the inflammatory picture in BAL, also reduced the lung function of affected animals; with increased airway resistance, and decreased airway reactance, which is suggestive of bronchoconstriction and obstructive airway processes [25,42]. The objective measurement of lung function by the forced oscillation technique can be a useful tool in further quantifying the outcome of a BRSV challenge, and the efficacy of vaccine candidates, in calves. Optimization of materials (e.g. face mask and tubing) and methods (e.g. frequencies used) could further improve the analysis, and need to be investigated in a larger set of calves.

The relative potency of the BRSV-Snk inoculum might be due to loss of virulence in the BRSV-Dk inoculum, following passage in cell culture. This is supported by previously published studies, which demonstrated a higher level of clinical signs of respiratory disease in calves with MDA, using the same mode of inoculation and the same isolate as the BRSV-Dk inoculum, but with fewer passages in vitro [21], and by propagation in fetal lung cells [20]. Loss of virulence following in vitro passage has been reported in some studies for BRSV and HRSV [43,44], but

not in others [45,46], and likely depends on the type of cells and number of passages, and may be associated with alterations in protein expression and post-translational modifications. The BRSV-Snk inoculum, in contrast to the BRSV-Dk inoculum, had been passaged in gnotobiotic calves.

Apart from the inoculum, challenge by aerosol inhalation hinges on two principal factors: the quality of the aerosol, and the quantity inhaled by each animal. Limited experimental infection studies in calves, using similar aerosolization of BRSV in conjunction with intratracheal injection [47], indicate that virus is mainly deposited in the upper airways using this method, with subsequent progression of virus replication to the lower airways. However, other studies using inhaled aerosols show that droplets ≤5 μm in diameter (67% of droplets in the present study) can reach the alveoli in humans [48], and reach the whole lung when infecting steers with aerosolized foot-and-mouth disease virus [49], and more accurately reproduces the symptoms of natural infection, compared to large droplet intranasal administration, when human volunteers were infected with influenza [50]. Thus, more research on the kinetics of natural BRSV infection is needed, to complement experimental findings, and to further elucidate the relevance of the model with regard to BRSV pathogenesis.

To study the unmodified pathogenesis of BRSV, field-like clinical signs are essential, and to calculate relevant treatment effects in vaccine or antiviral trials, a minimum clinical expression is required, making the model presented herein highly relevant, in contrast to comparable models with less clinical signs [51-53], or comparable clinical expression, but less neutralizing MDA at the time of challenge [7]. This cognate host calf model might also provide further understanding about HRSV in infants [54-56], with particular usefulness in the study of RSV pathogenesis and pathological processes in the lower airways, where data from infants is limited [57], but also to evaluate candidate vaccines that utilize proteins conserved across BRSV and HRSV [24].

Conclusions

In conclusion, we have established a BRSV model with a severe clinical expression in calves with maternal antibodies at the time of challenge. We furthermore describe tools to evaluate disease severity: consistently, using a rigid and comprehensive clinical scoring system; and objectively, using a passive lung function test and IFNγ concentration in BAL, to complement established parameters, such as extent of lung lesions and virus shedding following challenge. These tools can be used in future BRSV research and vaccine development studies and this model could also be valuable for the understanding of HRSV.

Abbreviations

ACS: Accumulated clinical scores; AVS: Accumulated virus shed; BAL: Bronchoalveolar lavage; BRD: Bovine respiratory disease; BRSV: Bovine respiratory syncytial virus; BRSV-Dk: BRSV, isolate no. 9402022 Denmark; BRSV-Snk: BRSV, Snook strain; COD: Corrected optic density; DMEM: Dulbecco's modified Eagle medium; ELISA: Enzyme-linked immunosorbent assay; HE: Hematoxylin and eosin; HIER: Heat-induced epitope retrieval; HRSV: Human respiratory syncytial virus; IFNγ: Interferon γ; IHC: Immunohistochemistry; IL-4: Interleukin 4; IL-6: Interleukin 6; IL-8: Interleukin 8; MDA: [BRSV-specific] maternally derived antibodies; PID: Post-infection day; PM: Post-mortem; RNA: Ribonucleic acid; RT-qPCR: Real-time quantitative polymerase chain reaction; SD: Standard deviation; TCID50: 50% tissue culture infective dose; TNFα: Tumor necrosis factor alpha.

Competing interests

The authors declare that they have no competing interests.

Authors' contributions

Conceived and designed experiments: KB, SH, JFE, SR, JP, GT and JFV. Performed experiments: KB, SH, DGW, SR, JP, GT and JFV. Analyzed data: KB, SH, DGW, JFE, SR, JP, GT and JFV. Contributed reagents/materials/analysis tools: KB, SH, DGW, JP, GT and JFV. Wrote paper: KB, SH, DGW, JFE, SR, JP, GT and JFV. All authors read and approved the final manuscript.

Acknowledgements

This project was funded by the Swedish Research Council (Formas, Sweden), the Biotechnology and Biological Sciences Research Council (BBSRC, UK) and L'Agence Nationale de la Recherche (ANR, France), through the Emerging and Major Infectious Diseases of Livestock (EMIDA) project in the European Research Area Network (ERA-NET), grant no FP#87. We thank the technical staff at SVA for their care of experimental animals, Annika Rikberg, SLU, for her help with histological samples, Ewa Westergren, SVA, for the histological sections and immunohistochemistry, Prof. L. E. Larsen, DTU, Denmark for kindly sharing the BRSV isolate no. 9402022, and Dr. Mikael Andersson Franko (SLU) for providing feedback on statistical analysis.

Author details

[1]Department of Clinical Sciences, Swedish University of Agricultural Sciences, Host Pathogen Interaction Group, Uppsala, Sweden. [2]Department of Pathology and Wildlife Diseases, National Veterinary Institute, Uppsala, Sweden. [3]Department of Biomedical Sciences and Veterinary Public Health, Swedish University of Agricultural Sciences, Uppsala, Sweden. [4]INRA, Unité de Virologie et Immunologie Moléculaires, Jouy-en-Josas, France. [5]The Pirbright Institute, Pirbright, Surrey, UK. [6]Department of Virology, National Veterinary Institute, Immunology, and Parasitology, Uppsala, Sweden.

References

1. Meyer G, Deplanche M, Schelcher F. Human and bovine respiratory syncytial virus vaccine research and development. Comp Immunol Microbiol Infect Dis. 2008;31:191–225.
2. Stott EJ, Thomas LH, Collins AP, Crouch S, Jebbett J, Smith GS, et al. A survey of virus infections of the respiratory tract of cattle and their association with disease. J Hyg (Lond). 1980;85:257–70.
3. Hägglund S, Svensson C, Emanuelson U, Valarcher JF, Alenius S. Dynamics of virus infections involved in the bovine respiratory disease complex in Swedish dairy herds. Vet J Lond Engl 1997. 2006;172:320–8.
4. Verhoeff J, Van der Ban M, van Nieuwstadt AP. Bovine respiratory syncytial virus infections in young dairy cattle: clinical and haematological findings. Vet Rec. 1984;114:9–12.
5. Viuff B, Uttenthal A, Tegtmeier C, Alexandersen S. Sites of replication of bovine respiratory syncytial virus in naturally infected calves as determined by in situ hybridization. Vet Pathol. 1996;33:383–90.
6. Valarcher J-F, Taylor G. Bovine respiratory syncytial virus infection. Vet Res. 2007;38:153–80.
7. Ellis JA, Gow SP, Mahan S, Leyh R. Duration of immunity to experimental infection with bovine respiratory syncytial virus following intranasal vaccination of young passively immune calves. J Am Vet Med Assoc. 2013;243:1602–8.

8. Schreiber P, Matheise JP, Dessy F, Heimann M, Letesson JJ, Coppe P, et al. High mortality rate associated with bovine respiratory syncytial virus (BRSV) infection in Belgian white blue calves previously vaccinated with an inactivated BRSV vaccine. J Vet Med B Infect Dis Vet Public Health. 2000;47:535–50.
9. Antonis AFG, Schrijver RS, Daus F, Steverink PJGM, Stockhofe N, Hensen EJ, et al. Vaccine-induced immunopathology during bovine respiratory syncytial virus infection: exploring the parameters of pathogenesis. J Virol. 2003;77:12067–73.
10. Kim HW, Canchola JG, Brandt CD, Pyles G, Chanock RM, Jensen K, et al. Respiratory syncytial virus disease in infants despite prior administration of antigenic inactivated vaccine. Am J Epidemiol. 1969;89:422–34.
11. Thomas LH, Gourlay RN, Stott EJ, Howard CJ, Bridger JC. A search for new microorganisms in calf pneumonia by the inoculation of gnotobiotic calves. Res Vet Sci. 1982;33:170–82.
12. Taylor G, Thomas LH, Wyld SG, Furze J, Sopp P, Howard CJ. Role of T-lymphocyte subsets in recovery from respiratory syncytial virus infection in calves. J Virol. 1995;69:6658–64.
13. Valarcher J-F, Furze J, Wyld S, Cook R, Conzelmann K-K, Taylor G. Role of alpha/beta interferons in the attenuation and immunogenicity of recombinant bovine respiratory syncytial viruses lacking NS proteins. J Virol. 2003;77:8426–39.
14. Tjørnehøj K, Uttenthal A, Viuff B, Larsen LE, Røntved C, Rønsholt L. An experimental infection model for reproduction of calf pneumonia with bovine respiratory syncytial virus (BRSV) based on one combined exposure of calves. Res Vet Sci. 2003;74:55–65.
15. Bryson DG, McNulty MS, Logan EF, Cush PF. Respiratory syncytial virus pneumonia in young calves: clinical and pathologic findings. Am J Vet Res. 1983;44:1648–55.
16. Xue W, Ellis J, Mattick D, Smith L, Brady R, Trigo E. Immunogenicity of a modified-live virus vaccine against bovine viral diarrhea virus types 1 and 2, infectious bovine rhinotracheitis virus, bovine parainfluenza-3 virus, and bovine respiratory syncytial virus when administered intranasally in young calves. Vaccine. 2010;28:3784–92.
17. Belknap EB, Ciszewski DK, Baker JC. Experimental respiratory syncytial virus infection in calves and lambs. J Vet Diagn Investig Off Publ Am Assoc Vet Lab Diagn Inc. 1995;7:285–98.
18. Larsen LE, Tjørnehøj K, Viuff B, Jensen NE, Uttenthal A. Diagnosis of enzootic pneumonia in Danish cattle: reverse transcription-polymerase chain reaction assay for detection of bovine respiratory syncytial virus in naturally and experimentally infected cattle. J Vet Diagn Investig Off Publ Am Assoc Vet Lab Diagn Inc. 1999;11:416–22.
19. Woolums AR, Anderson ML, Gunther RA, Schelegle ES, LaRochelle DR, Singer RS, et al. Evaluation of severe disease induced by aerosol inoculation of calves with bovine respiratory syncytial virus. Am J Vet Res. 1999;60:473–80.
20. Hägglund S, Hu K-F, Larsen LE, Hakhverdyan M, Valarcher J-F, Taylor G, et al. Bovine respiratory syncytial virus ISCOMs–protection in the presence of maternal antibodies. Vaccine. 2004;23:646–55.
21. Hägglund S, Hu K, Vargmar K, Poré L, Olofson A-S, Blodörn K, et al. Bovine respiratory syncytial virus ISCOMs-Immunity, protection and safety in young conventional calves. Vaccine. 2011;29:8719–30.
22. Otto P, Elschner M, Reinhold P, Köhler H, Streckert HJ, Philippou S, et al. A model for respiratory syncytial virus (RSV) infection based on experimental aerosol exposure with bovine RSV in calves. Comp Immunol Microbiol Infect Dis. 1996;19:85–97.
23. Valarcher JF, Bourhy H, Gelfi J, Schelcher F. Evaluation of a nested reverse transcription-PCR assay based on the nucleoprotein gene for diagnosis of spontaneous and experimental bovine respiratory syncytial virus infections. J Clin Microbiol. 1999;37:1858–62.
24. Blodörn K, Hägglund S, Fix J, Dubuquoy C, Makabi-Panzu B, Thom M, et al. Vaccine safety and efficacy evaluation of a recombinant bovine respiratory syncytial virus (BRSV) with deletion of the SH gene and subunit vaccines based on recombinant human RSV proteins: N-nanorings, P and M2-1, in calves with maternal antibodies. PLoS One. 2014;9:e100392.
25. Reinhold P, Macleod D, Lekeux P. Comparative evaluation of impulse oscillometry and a monofrequency forced oscillation technique in clinically healthy calves undergoing bronchochallenges. Res Vet Sci. 1996;61:206–13.
26. Uttenthal A, Larsen LE, Philipsen JS, Tjørnehøj K, Viuff B, Nielsen KH, et al. Antibody dynamics in BRSV-infected Danish dairy herds as determined by isotype-specific immunoglobulins. Vet Microbiol. 2000;76:329–41.
27. Kimman TG, Westenbrink F, Straver PJ. Priming for local and systemic antibody memory responses to bovine respiratory syncytial virus: effect of

28. Baker JC, Ames TR, Markham RJ. Seroepizootiologic study of bovine respiratory syncytial virus in a dairy herd. Am J Vet Res. 1986;47:240–5.

29. Van der Poel WH, Brand A, Kramps JA, Van Oirschot JT. Respiratory syncytial virus infections in human beings and in cattle. J Infect. 1994;29:215–28.

30. Kimman TG, Westenbrink F, Schreuder BE, Straver PJ. Local and systemic antibody response to bovine respiratory syncytial virus infection and reinfection in calves with and without maternal antibodies. J Clin Microbiol. 1987;25:1097–106.

31. Bryson D. Necropsy findings associated with BRSV pneumonia. Vet Med. 1993;88:894–9.

32. Kimman TG, Zimmer GM, Straver PJ, de Leeuw PW. Diagnosis of bovine respiratory syncytial virus infections improved by virus detection in lung lavage samples. Am J Vet Res. 1986;47:143–7.

33. Grell SN, Tjørnehøj K, Larsen LE, Heegaard PMH. Marked induction of IL-6, haptoglobin and IFNgamma following experimental BRSV infection in young calves. Vet Immunol Immunopathol. 2005;103:235–45.

34. Mcinnes E, Sopp P, Howard CJ, Taylor G. Phenotypic analysis of local cellular responses in calves infected with bovine respiratory syncytial virus. Immunology. 1999;96:396–403.

35. Antonis AFG, Claassen EAW, Hensen EJ, de Groot RJ, de Groot-Mijnes JDF, Schrijver RS, et al. Kinetics of antiviral CD8 T cell responses during primary and post-vaccination secondary bovine respiratory syncytial virus infection. Vaccine. 2006;24:1551–61.

36. Thomas LH, Cook RS, Howard CJ, Gaddum RM, Taylor G. Influence of selective T-lymphocyte depletion on the lung pathology of gnotobiotic calves and the distribution of different T-lymphocyte subsets following challenge with bovine respiratory syncytial virus. Res Vet Sci. 1996;61:38–44.

37. Darwich L, Coma G, Peña R, Bellido R, Blanco EJJ, Este JA, et al. Secretion of interferon-gamma by human macrophages demonstrated at the single-cell level after costimulation with interleukin (IL)-12 plus IL-18. Immunology. 2009;126:386–93.

38. De Waal L, Koopman LP, van Benten IJ, Brandenburg AH, Mulder PGH, de Swart RL, et al. Moderate local and systemic respiratory syncytial virus-specific T-cell responses upon mild or subclinical RSV infection. J Med Virol. 2003;70:309–18.

39. Røntved CM, Tjørnehøj K, Viuff B, Larsen LE, Godson DL, Rønsholt L, et al. Increased pulmonary secretion of tumor necrosis factor-alpha in calves experimentally infected with bovine respiratory syncytial virus. Vet Immunol Immunopathol. 2000;76:199–214.

40. Grell SN, Riber U, Tjørnehøj K, Larsen LE, Heegaard PMH. Age-dependent differences in cytokine and antibody responses after experimental RSV infection in a bovine model. Vaccine. 2005;23:3412–23.

41. Antonis AFG, de Jong MC, van der Poel WHM, van der Most RG, Stockhofe-Zurwieden N, Kimman T, et al. Age-dependent differences in the pathogenesis of bovine respiratory syncytial virus infections related to the development of natural immunocompetence. J Gen Virol. 2010;91(Pt 10):2497–506.

42. Oostveen E, MacLeod D, Lorino H, Farré R, Hantos Z, Desager K, et al. The forced oscillation technique in clinical practice: methodology, recommendations and future developments. Eur Respir J. 2003;22:1026–41.

43. Deplanche M, Lemaire M, Mirandette C, Bonnet M, Schelcher F, Meyer G. In vivo evidence for quasispecies distributions in the bovine respiratory syncytial virus genome. J Gen Virol. 2007;88(Pt 4):1260–5.

44. Kwilas S, Liesman RM, Zhang L, Walsh E, Pickles RJ, Peeples ME. Respiratory syncytial virus grown in Vero cells contains a truncated attachment protein that alters its infectivity and dependence on glycosaminoglycans. J Virol. 2009;83:10710–8.

45. Furze JM, Roberts SR, Wertz GW, Taylor G. Antigenically distinct G glycoproteins of BRSV strains share a high degree of genetic homogeneity. Virology. 1997;231:48–58.

46. Larsen LE, Uttenthal A, Arctander P, Tjørnehøj K, Viuff B, Røntved C, et al. Serological and genetic characterisation of bovine respiratory syncytial virus (BRSV) indicates that Danish isolates belong to the intermediate subgroup: no evidence of a selective effect on the variability of G protein nucleotide sequence by prior cell culture adaption and passages in cell culture or calves. Vet Microbiol. 1998;62:265–79.

47. Viuff B, Tjørnehøj K, Larsen LE, Røntved CM, Uttenthal A, Rønsholt L, et al. Replication and clearance of respiratory syncytial virus: apoptosis is an important pathway of virus clearance after experimental infection with bovine respiratory syncytial virus. Am J Pathol. 2002;161:2195–207.

48. Knight V. Viruses as agents of airborne contagion. Ann N Y Acad Sci. 1980;353:147–56.

49. Pacheco JM, Arzt J, Rodriguez LL. Early events in the pathogenesis of foot-and-mouth disease in cattle after controlled aerosol exposure. Vet J Lond Engl 1997. 2010;183:46–53.

50. Tellier R. Review of aerosol transmission of influenza A virus. Emerg Infect Dis. 2006;12:1657–62.

51. Mohanty SB, Ingling AL, Lillie MG. Experimentally induced respiratory syncytial viral infection in calves. Am J Vet Res. 1975;36:417–9.

52. Riffault S, Meyer G, Deplanche M, Dubuquoy C, Durand G, Soulestin M, et al. A new subunit vaccine based on nucleoprotein nanoparticles confers partial clinical and virological protection in calves against bovine respiratory syncytial virus. Vaccine. 2010;28:3722–34.

53. Van der Sluijs MTW, Kuhn EM, Makoschey B. A single vaccination with an inactivated bovine respiratory syncytial virus vaccine primes the cellular immune response in calves with maternal antibody. BMC Vet Res. 2010;6:2.

54. Taylor G. Bovine model of respiratory syncytial virus infection. Curr Top Microbiol Immunol. 2013;372:327–45.

55. Levast B, Schulz S, Hurk S v DL d, Gerdts V. Animal models for neonatal diseases in humans. Vaccine. 2013;31:2489–99.

56. Domachowske JB, Bonville CA, Rosenberg HF. Animal models for studying respiratory syncytial virus infection and its long term effects on lung function. Pediatr Infect Dis J. 2004;23(11 Suppl):S228–34.

57. Borchers AT, Chang C, Gershwin ME, Gershwin LJ. Respiratory syncytial virus-a comprehensive review. Clin Rev Allergy Immunol. 2013;45:331–79.

17

Reducing microbial ureolytic activity in the rumen by immunization against urease therein

Shengguo Zhao[1,2], Jiaqi Wang[1,2*], Nan Zheng[1,2], Dengpan Bu[2], Peng Sun[2] and Zhongtang Yu[3]

Abstract

Background: Ureolytic activity of rumen bacteria leads to rapid urea conversion to ammonia in the rumen of dairy cows, resulting possible toxicity, excessive ammonia excretion to the environment, and poor nitrogen utilization. The present study investigated immunization of dairy cows against urease in the rumen as an approach to mitigate bacterial ureolytic activity therein.

Results: Most alpha subunit of rumen urease (UreC) proteins shared very similar amino acid sequences, which were also highly similar to that of *H. pylori*. Anti-urease titers in the serum and the saliva of the immunized cows were evaluated following repeated immunization with the UreC of *H. pylori* as the vaccine. After the fourth booster, the vaccinated cows had a significantly reduced urease activity (by 17%) in the rumen than the control cows that were mock immunized cows. The anti-urease antibody significantly reduced ureolysis and corresponding ammonia formation in rumen fluid *in vitro*. Western blotting revealed that the *H. pylori* UreC had high immunological homology with the UreC from rumen bacteria.

Conclusions: Vaccine developed based on UreC of *H. pylori* can be a useful approach to decrease bacterial ureolysis in the rumen.

Keywords: Immunization, Rumen, Urease, Ureolytic activity

Background

Ruminal microbial urease plays an important role in the nitrogen metabolism in ruminants such as cattle and sheep. The urea from diet or recycled from blood to rumen is hydrolyzed by urease to ammonia, the major source of nitrogen for many ruminal bacteria including several known cellulolytic bacteria [1]. The traditional recommendation for urea feeding is less than 1% of the concentrate portion of the diet, approximately 135 g/ cow daily [2]. Between 40 and 80% of the urea-N synthesized by the liver also return to the rumen and gut, where 35 to 55% of this N is used in microbial anabolism in both cattle and sheep [3]. However, the rate of urea hydrolysis (ureolysis) is about four fold greater than that of ammonia assimilation, resulting in ammonia accumulation, which can lead to toxicity, excessive ammonia excretion to the environment, and poor N utilization when diets contain a high urea content [2,4]. To alleviate this problem, different urease inhibitors have been evaluated to reduced ureolytic activity, including acetohydroxamic acid, phenyl phosphorodiamidate, N-(n-butyl) thiophosphoric triamide, boric acid, and bismuth compounds, to slow down production of ammonia in the rumen [5]. However, their efficacy decreases over time due to microbial adaptation [6], and some of these compounds pose potential risk animal and human health, precluding their use in production.

Recent studies have shown that immunization is a potential approach to mitigate methane emissions [7-9], lactic acidosis [10], and to decrease protozoal population [11] in the rumen. We hypothesize that immunization against rumen urease can be an effective approach to slow down ureolysis in the rumen. Bacterial urease consists of two (alpha and beta) or three (alpha, beta and gamma) structural subunits. The alpha subunit (UreC)

* Correspondence: jiaqiwang@vip.163.com
[1]Ministry of Agriculture Laboratory of Quality & Safety Risk Assessment for Dairy Products (Beijing), Institute of Animal Science, Chinese Academy of Agricultural Sciences, No. 2 Yuanyingyuan West Road, Beijing 100193, PR China
[2]State Key Laboratory of Animal Nutrition, Institute of Animal Science, Chinese Academy of Agricultural Sciences, No. 2 Yuanyingyuan West Road, Beijing 100193, PR China
Full list of author information is available at the end of the article

contains a urea binding site and a catalytic site. The *ureC* gene has been used as a gene marker to examine UreC diversity in bacterial communities because it is quite conserved among different bacterial species [12]. In one study, the UreC of jack bean urease has been tried as an antigen to immunize sheep to inhibit rumen ureolysis in sheep rumen [13]; however, no obvious anti-urease activity was achieved probably because of low immunological homology between jack bean urease and rumen bacterial urease. The objectives of the present study were to examine the diversity of UreC in the rumen, identify an antigen that has high immunological homology with rumen UreC, develop an anti-urease vaccine from bacterial UreC, and evaluate anti-urease immunization as an approach to decrease ruminal ureolysis.

Results

Diversity of rumen bacterial urease gene

The *ureC* diversity in the rumen was examined by cloning and sequencing of *ureC* genes using degenerate primers. In total, 317 *ureC* sequences were obtained from the microbial DNA of rumen digesta of Chinese Holstein cows. Phylogenetic analysis revealed five *ureC* clusters (Figure 1). Cluster I contained 203 (64% of total sequences) of the *ureC* sequences, and it was about 84% identical (based on amino acid sequence) to the *ureC* gene of *Helicobacter pylori* (*H. pylori*). Clusters IIa and IIb represented 29 (9%) and 42 (13%) of the *ureC* sequences, respectively, and both were closely related (98-100% aa sequence identity) to the *ureC* of *H. pylori*. Clusters III and IV, each of which contained a small number of *ureC* sequences, and cluster V, represent the rest of the *ureC* sequences, had no match with any known *ureC* sequences.

Immunological homology between purified rumen urease and *H. pylori* urease

Immunological homology between urease purified from the rumen and the *H. pylori* urease was evaluated using Western blotting. Urease protein with an activity of 542 U was purified from rumen bacteria by anion exchange chromatography. Western blotting of the purified urease using anti-urease serum from the cows immunized with overexpressed UreC of *H. pylori* identified the positive

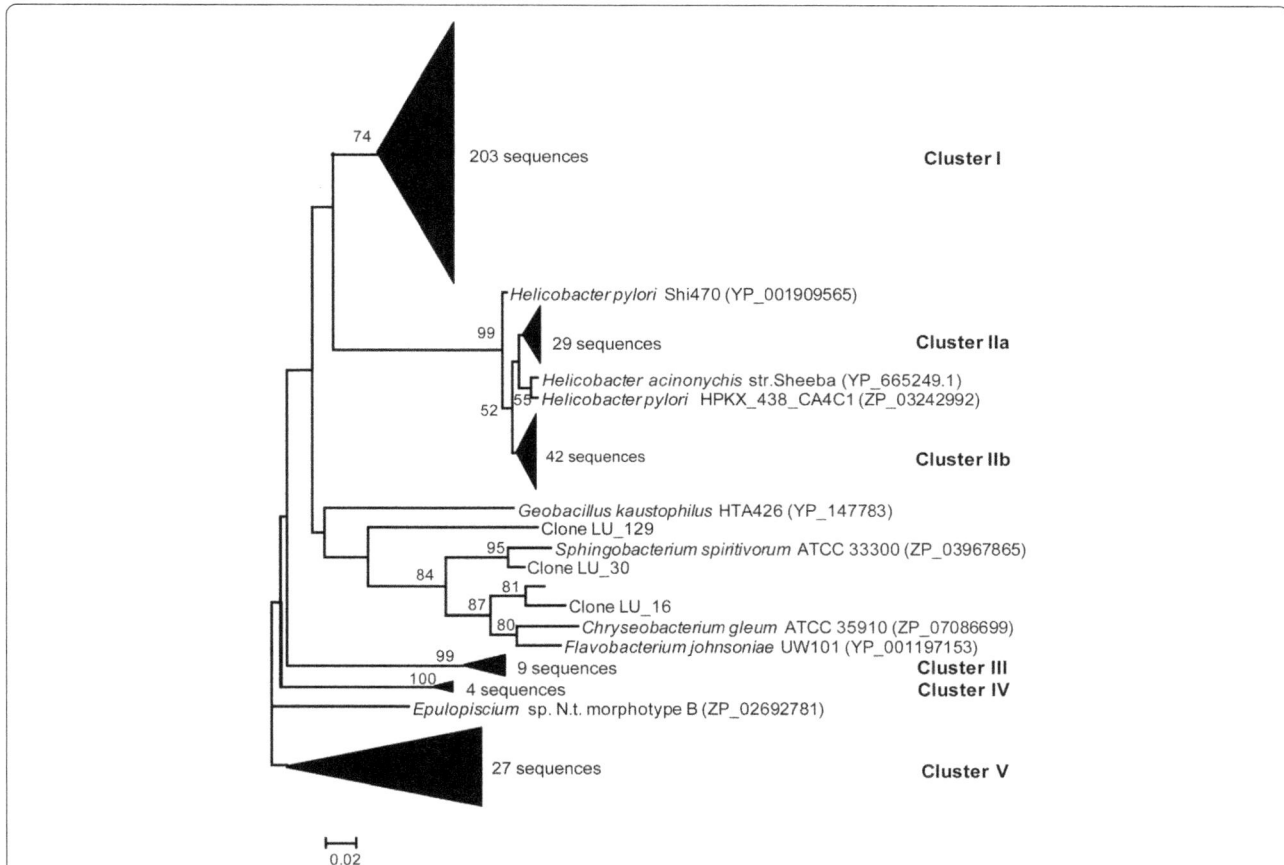

Figure 1 A neighbor-joining tree of the UreC sequences recovered from rumen digesta. The consensus tree was constructed from amino acid sequences inferred from the *ureC* sequences recovered from rumen and known bacterial species. Bootstrap values were calculated from 1,000 trees. Only bootstrapping values greater than 50% are shown.

band of expected molecular weight (Figure 2), indicating a high immunological homology between the overexpressed UreC of *H. pylori* and the urease purified from the rumen bacteria.

Vaccine and specific antibody titers

The above *ureC* diversity data showed that the majority (86%) of the UreC in the rumen share high homology (84-100% aa sequence identity) with the UreC of *H. pylori*. The urease of *H. pylori* also share high immunological homology with the urease of rumen bacteria. Therefore, *H. pylori* UreC was selected as the antigen to elicit immunization against urease in the rumen of dairy cows. Another reason to choose the UreC of *H. pylori* was the availability of full-length sequence of its *ureC* gene so that this UreC protein can be overexpressed in *E. coli*. The UreC of *H. pylori* was successfully expressed in *E.coli* BL21(DE3) following induction with IPTG. The molecular weight of the expressed UreC was about 66 kDa, consistent with the molecular mass predicted from the UreC sequence (see Additional file 1). About 20 mg purified UreC was obtained. The expressed UreC protein, together with Freund's adjuvant, was used as the vaccine to immunize the dairy cows.

After the immunization with *H. pylori* UreC, no apparent adverse effect was seen on health, milk production, or digestion of dry matter and crude protein (data not shown). Low titers of anti-urease antibody were detected in the serum and the saliva samples from the control group from day 0 (prior to mock immunization) to day 49 (Figure 3). Compared to the control group, the vaccinated group had higher (P < 0.01) serum titers of both IgG and IgA from day 7 onward, while higher (P < 0.01) saliva titers of IgG and IgA were noted from days 21 and

7 onward, respectively. The IgA titer peaked at day 35 in both the serum and the saliva, but the IgG titers peaked later at day 49. The variation of both IgA and IgG titers had similar trends in the serum and the saliva. The highest titers of both IgG and IgA in the serum were 13- and 20-fold greater, respectively, than those noted for the saliva.

Urease activity and rumen fermentation after immunization

The effect of immunization against urease was assessed by analyzing rumen fermentation characteristic and ureolysis in the rumen of the vaccinated cows. No significant difference in rumen urease activity was seen between the control and the vaccinated groups from days 0 to 35 (before the 3rd booster) (Figure 4A). At day 49 (two weeks after the third booster), however, urease activity in the vaccinated group was 17% lower (P < 0.01) than that in the control group. Rumen pH and volatile fatty acid (VFA) concentration were not affected by the immunization (see Additional file 2). After direct infusion of urea into the rumen at day 56, ammonia concentration in the rumen ascended during the first hour and then descended to the pre-infusion level (Figure 4B). Compared to the control group, the vaccinated group had lower (P < 0.01) ammonia concentration at 1 and 2 h post infusion, but not thereafter.

Inhibition of urea hydrolysis by anti-urease serum *in vitro*

The ability of anti-urease antibodies to decrease ureolysis by rumen microbes was evaluated using fresh rumen fluid *in vitro*. Compared to the control, the addition of serum anti-urease antibody from the vaccinated cows significantly reduced the rate of urea disappearance and corresponding ammonia formation (Figure 5). Urea was completely hydrolyzed within 4 h of the incubation in the absence of the anti-urease serum; however, urea disappearance was slowed down in the presence of the anti-urease serum. Concomitantly, increase in ammonia concentration was reduced within 12 h after the anti-urease serum addition.

Discussion

Most of the ureases in the rumen are produced by bacteria, but little is known about the diversity of the urease-producing bacteria because only 6.5% of the rumen bacteria have been cultured or characterized [14,15]. The urease genes carried by rumen ureolytic bacteria have not been systematically examined. In a study conducted in 1970's, Cook et al. [16] found that urease from rumen bacteria, such as *Staphylococcus* spp., was either intracellular or bound to the surface of the cell wall. The diversity of ureolytic bacteria and their urease gene have to be identified before highly effective urease vaccine can be developed. The present study is

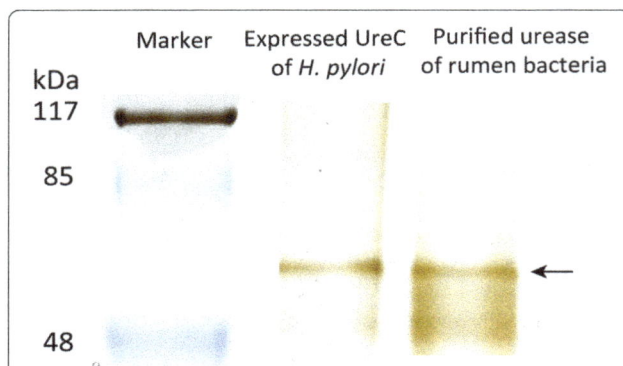

Figure 2 Western blot of urease purified from the rumen of dairy cows using anti-urease serum collected from cows immunized with overexpressed UreC of *H. pylori*. The UreC band was indicated by arrow.

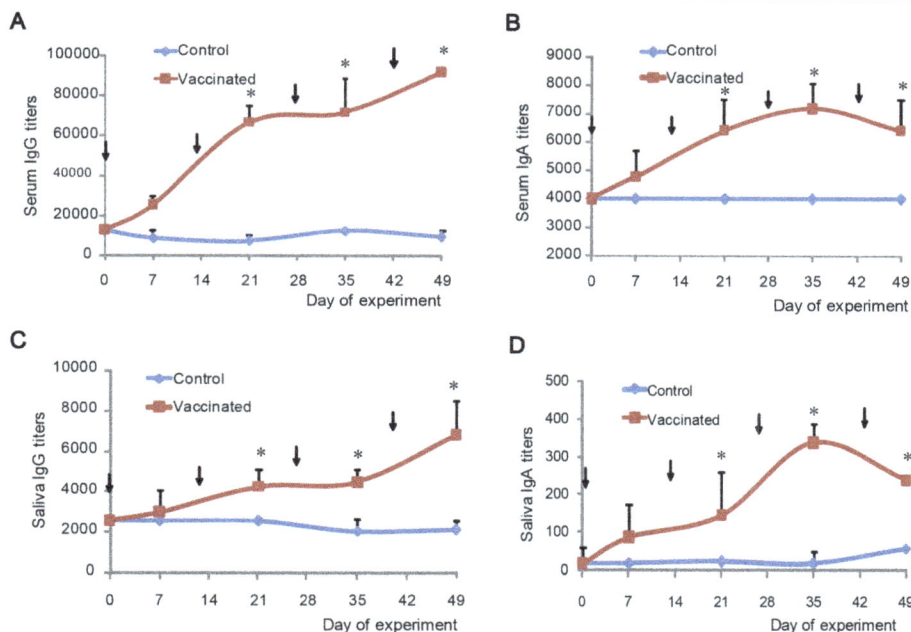

Figure 3 Titers of IgG (**A** and **C**) and IgA (**B** and **D**) in the serum (**A** and **B**) and the saliva (**C** and **D**) of cows. Arrow indicates days of vaccinations. Values are means (n = 4), with error bars representing standard deviation. The asterisks (*) indicate significant (P < 0.05) difference between the control group and the vaccinated group at the same days.

the first study that examined the diversity of *ureC* genes in the rumen of dairy cows using a cultivation-independent approach. About 86% of the recovered UreC sequences shared high sequence identity (84–100%) to that of *H. pylori*; however, interestingly, none of the recovered UreC sequences matched that previously recovered from any cultured rumen microbes. The UreC from *H. pylori* has been verified to have high immunogenicity in mice and human [17]. In the present study, overexpressed UreC of *H. pylori* was shown to be highly immunologically homologous to

rumen UreC of dairy cows. The observed inhibition to urease activity and corresponding decrease in ammonia accumulation suggest that specific antibodies against rumen bacterial urease were produced by the dairy cows vaccinated with the overexpressed UreC of *H. pylori*.

As demonstrated in the present study, urease vaccination did elicit a humoral immune response as indicated by the elevated serum and saliva specific antibody titers observed in the vaccinated cows but not in the control cows. Specific IgG and IgA titers in the serum and the saliva were further increased following booster immunization

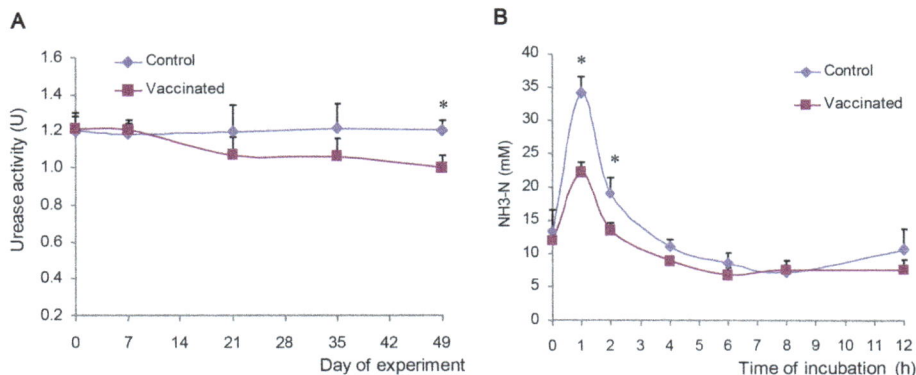

Figure 4 Urease activity in the rumen after immunization (**A**) and ammonia concentration variation after urea was infused into the rumen (**B**). Values are means (n = 4), with error bars representing standard deviation. The asterisks (*) indicate significant (P < 0.05) difference between the control group and the vaccinated group at the time points.

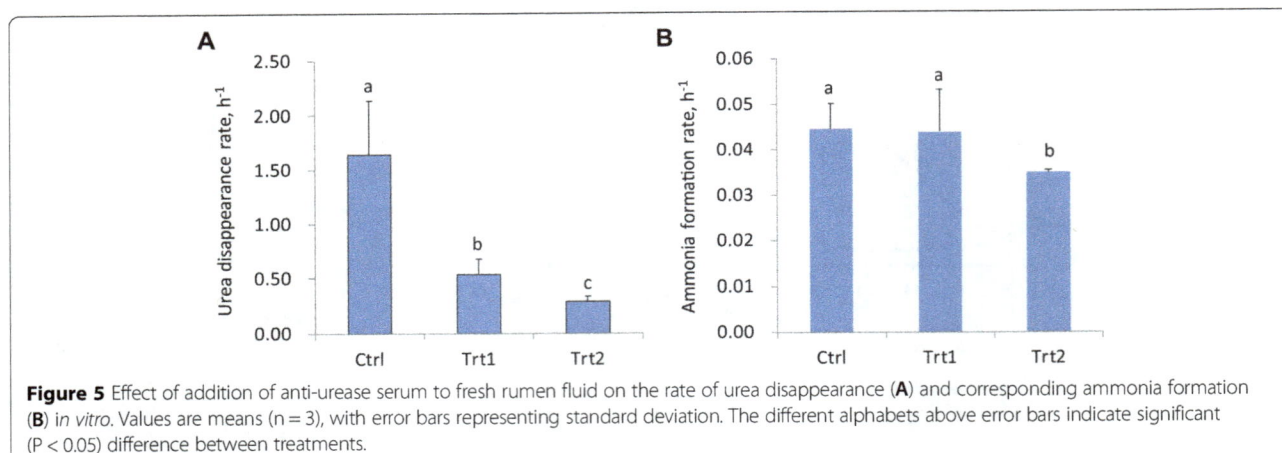

Figure 5 Effect of addition of anti-urease serum to fresh rumen fluid on the rate of urea disappearance (**A**) and corresponding ammonia formation (**B**) in vitro. Values are means (n = 3), with error bars representing standard deviation. The different alphabets above error bars indicate significant (P < 0.05) difference between treatments.

and peaked after the third and second booster immunization, respectively. The IgG and IgA titers in the serum had high positive correlation with those in the saliva. The specific IgG and IgA could flow into rumen fluid with saliva, because the liquid in the rumen is primarily (>70%) derived from saliva [18]. Although rumen contains proteolytic bacteria, no significant degradation of IgG molecules within the first 4 h of incubation in fresh rumen fluid [19,20]. As such, anti-urease antibodies produced by vaccination can persist long enough in the rumen to bind to urease and reduce ureolytic activity.

Immunization with jack bean urease failed to reduce urease activity or urea kinetics in sheep rumen [13] or produce antibody against the urease of *Helicobacter* in vaccinated mice [21]. This inability is probably attributed to a lack of immunological homology between bacterial urease and jack bean urease. The reduced urease activity by the bovine anti-urease antibody elicited by the UreC of *H. pylori*, both *in vitro* and *in vivo*, clearly indicates that the UreC of *H. pylori* has high immunological homology with rumen bacterial ureases, at least many of them, and can be used as an effective vaccine in cows. The Western blotting further confirmed the immunological homology between the rumen bacterial urease and the *H. pylori* urease. However, given the diverse UreC present in the rumen (Figure 1), a vaccine prepared from a combination of representatives of different rumen UreC clusters may be more effective than UreC of *H. pylori* or single rumen bacterial UreC. Future studies are also needed to identify ureolytic bacteria and their ureases so that anti-urease antibodies with greater efficacy might be developed.

Conclusions

The alpha subunit of *H. pylori* urease may serve as a vaccine to immunize cows to slow down ureolysis in the rumen. Combined representatives of rumen bacterial UreC may be an even more effective vaccine to improve

urea utilization efficiency without the adverse effects associated with chemical urease inhibitors.

Methods

Diversity of rumen bacterial urease gene

Rumen digesta samples were collected from four rumen-fistulated Chinese Holstein dairy cows before morning feeding. Total microbial DNA was extracted using the RBB + C method [22]. A degenerate primer set specific for the *ureC* gene (ureC forward:5′-TGGGCCTTAARMTH CAYGARGAYTGGG-3′, and ureC reverse:5′-GTGRTGR CAMACCATNANCATRTC-3′) [23] was used in PCR amplification of the UreC in the rumen samples. A 25 μL PCR reaction contained 2.5 μL PCR buffer (Invitrogen, Carlsbad, CA), 0.75 μL MgCl$_2$ (50 mM), 0.5 μL dNTP (10 mM), 1.5 μL each forward and reverse primer (10 μm), 0.3 μL Platinum Taq DNA polymerase (Invitrogen, Carlsbad, CA), 1 μL rumen microbial DNA (~100 ng μL^{-1}), and 16.95 μL sterile ddH$_2$O. The PCR cycling included 94°C for 5 min; 30 cycles of 94°C for 30 s, 50°C for 30 s, and 72°C for 30 s; 72°C for 15 min; and 10°C for 30 min. The expected PCR amplicons of about 324 bp were visualized on agarose (2%) gel and then purified using a Gel Purification Kit (Qiagen, Valencia, CA), cloned into the pMD19-T vector (TaKaRa, Dalian, LN, China), and then transformed into competent E.coli JM109 cells (TaKaRa, Dalian, LN). Random clones were sequenced with the T7 primer using a BigDye Terminator v3.1 cycle sequencing kit (Applied Biosystems, Inc., Foster, CA). All sequences were trimmed to remove the vector regions and low-quality ends using the PREGAP4 program of the STADEN software package [24]. The sequences were then compared to GenBank sequences using Blastx, and the most similar UreC sequences derived from known bacterial species were downloaded and combined with the UreC protein sequences recovered in this study. A phylogenetic tree was constructed from the combined UreC sequences using the MEGA software [25].

Expression and purification of urease alpha subunit (UreC)

The gene encoding the UreC of *H. pylori* was amplified from the genomic DNA of *H. pylori* UMAB41 using a forward primer (5′-AAAA*CATATG*AAAAAGATTAGCA GGAAAG-3′) with a *Nde*I cutting site (italic) and a reverse primer (5′-CCG*CTCGAG*CTACCGCGCCATCTTC CACCAG-3′) with a *Xho*I cutting site (italic). Following double digestion with *Nde*I and *Xho*I, the purified full-length gene was ligated into correspondingly double-digested pET-30a(+) (Novagen, Madison, WI). The recombinant plasmids were then transformed into competent *E. coli* BL21 (DE3) (Promega, Madison, WI). The transformants were grown until an OD_{600} of 0.6, and over expression of the cloned UreC was induced at 30°C by IPTG (1.0 mM). The *E. coli* cells were harvested by centrifugation, and total cell protein was isolated using the Bug-Buster® Protein Extraction Reagent (Novagen, Madison, WI). Purification of the overexpressed UreC was achieved using a Ni-NTA kit (Novagen, Madison, WI) per manufacturer's instructions. The UreC protein was analyzed by SDS-PAGE and visualized after staining with Coomassie Blue R-250. The UreC protein concentration was determined using the Bradford assay (Bio-Rad, Hercules, CA).

Purification of rumen urease and western blotting using UreC of *H. pylori*

Rumen fluid was collected fistulated dairy cows fed a total mixed ration (TMR) (see Additional file 3). The bacterial cells were isolated by gradient centrifugation and then disrupted by ultrasonication (300 W, 15 min). The cellular proteins were concentrated using ultrafiltration (50 kDa) and then a Hi Trap Capto Q ion exchange column (GE Healthcare, Little Chalfont, UK) that was pre-equilibrated with a Tris–HCl buffer (20 mm, pH 8.0). Gradient elution was used to separate urease protein using the same Tris–HCl buffer with a NaCl concentration ranging from 0 to 1 M at a flow rate of 1 mL min^{-1}. The fractions with positive urease activities were pooled and concentrated by lyophilization [26].

The urease protein was separated on SDS-PAGE and transferred to a nitrocellulose membrane (Sigma, St Louis, MO, USA) for immune blotting analysis. The membrane was blocked with 5% low-fat dry milk dissolved in TBS-T buffer for 1 h at room temperature and then stained overnight with the bovine anti-urease serum (1:1000). Following three washes for 10 min each in TBS-T buffer, the membrane was incubated in diluted (1:1000 diluted) horseradish peroxidase-conjugated sheep anti-bovine antibody (Bethyl Laboratories, Montgomery, TX) for 1 h at room temperature before incubation in 6 mL of chemiluminescence reagent (Sigma, St Louis, MO, USA) for 1 min. Positive immunostaining was determined based on the presence of a visible band corresponding to the expected UreC protein.

Immunization of dairy cows

Eight rumen-fistulated lactating Chinese Holstein dairy cows, with a body weight of 556 ± 19 kg, were randomly allocated to two treatment groups (n = 4), with one group (control) mock vaccinated with physiological saline containing the Freund's adjuvant only, while the other group (vaccinated) was vaccinated with the overexpressed UreC of *H. pylori*. Briefly, an UreC protein solution (0.4 mg mL^{-1} UreC protein) was combined with an equal volume of Freund's complete adjuvant. The mixture was emulsified, resulting in an UreC vaccine containing 0.2 mg mL^{-1} UreC protein. Each cow in the vaccinated group was injected subcutaneously on the neck and intramuscularly on the buttock [27] with 0.5 mL UreC vaccine at day 0. The injections were repeated at days 14, 28 and 42 as boosters, but with the Freund's complete adjuvant being replaced by Freund's incomplete adjuvant. The control group received the same injection procedures in parallel but with physiological saline containing Freund's adjuvant only. All cows were housed under identical conditions and fed the same TMR (see Additional file 3) thrice daily. The animals were strictly cared for following the standard protocols approved specifically for this study by the Institute of Animal Science, Chinese Academy of Agricultural Sciences, Beijing, China (Permit Number: RNL10/08).

Animal sample collection and analysis

At days 0, 7, 21, 35, and 49, samples of blood, saliva, and rumen fluid were collected about 2 h after morning feeding. Blood samples were collected from the caudal vein of each cow into evacuated tubes and centrifuged at 3000 × *g* for 10 min to separate the serum. Saliva samples were collected from the oral cavity of the cows using a suction tube and then centrifuged at 10000 × *g* for 15 min to collect the supernatant. Rumen fluid samples were collected through rumen fistula and filtered through four layers of cheesecloth. Subsamples of rumen fluid were also collected for analysis of urease activity. At day 56, 60 g urea was infused directly into the rumen of the cows of both groups through the rumen fistula after morning feeding. Rumen fluid was then collected at 0, 1, 2, 4, 6 and 8 h post infusion and analyzed for pH, ammonia concentration, and VFA profile.

The titers of specific anti-urease IgG and IgA in the serum and the saliva samples were determined using a modified ELISA protocol [28]. Briefly, the plates were coated with 100 μL well^{-1} UreC solution (40 μg mL^{-1}) and incubated overnight at 4°C. After washing, the plates were blocked with 150 μL well^{-1} of 1% (vol./vol.) chicken serum for 90 min at 37°C. An aliquot of 100 μL well^{-1} serially diluted serum (1:400 to 1:25600 for IgG, 1:500 to 1:32000 for IgA) and saliva (1:640 to 1:10240 for IgG, 1:20 to 1:640 for IgA) from either the vaccinated cows or the cows in the control group was added. Fetal calf serum was used as a negative control. The plates were incubated at 37°C for 2 h. Then, 100 μL donkey anti-bovine IgG or IgA alkaline phosphatase conjugate (Promega, Madison, WI) (1:10000 diluted) was added to each well and incubated at 37°C for 2 h. Following dilution to a final concentration of 1.5 mg mL^{-1} in a buffer containing 1 M diethanolamine and 0.5 mM MgCl$_2$, the substrate chromogen tetramethylbenzidine (100 μL) was added to each well. After incubation for 30 min at 37°C, the reaction was terminated by adding 50 μL of 2 N NaOH to each well. The absorbance was recorded at 405 nm using an ELISA plate-reader (Infinite F200; Tecan, Mannedorf Switzerland). The reaction was defined as positive when the absorbance exceeded twice that of the negative control. Antibody titers were expressed as the highest dilution that gave a positive reaction.

Urease activity was determined by measuring the amount of ammonia released from urea [29]. One unit of urease activity was defined as one μmol ammonia released per min per mL rumen fluid or mg microbial protein. Ammonia concentration was determined by the phenol-hypochlorite reaction as described by Weatherburn et al. [30]. Concentrations of VFA were analyzed by gas chromatography (model 6890, Series II; Hewlett Packard Co., Avondale, PA) as described by Mohammed et al. [31].

Evaluation of the anti-urease antibody on urea hydrolysis in rumen fluid in vitro

The TMR diet, which was the same as that fed to the cows, was weighed into serum bottles (0.25 g bottle^{-1}) containing 20 mL McDougall's buffer, 10 mL of strained fresh rumen fluid, and urea (final concentration of 1 g L^{-1}). To each bottle, bovine serum from either the control group or the vaccinated group was added. Two bovine serum concentrations from the vaccinated group was used in two treatments: Trt1 (IgG titer, 1:40000) and Trt2 (IgG titer, 1:80000). Three replicates were used both the control and the anti-urease serum treatments. The bottles were gassed with CO$_2$, sealed with rubber stoppers, and incubated in a 39°C shaking water bath. Subsamples were collected at 0, 1, 2, 4, 8 and 12 h post incubation, and the pH was measured immediately. Ammonia concentrations were determined colorimetrically as described above. Urea concentration was determined with the diacetyl monoxime method of Marsh et al. [32]. Rates of urea disappearance and concomitant ammonia N formation were computed as the slope of regression of the natural logarithm of urea and ammonia N concentration, respectively, over the course of the incubation.

Statistics

All data were subjected to analysis of variance using the MIXED procedure of SAS (version 9.0, SAS Institute Inc., Cary, NC). The REPEATED statement was used for variables measured over days (titers of IgA and IgG, and urease activity) or times (pH, VFA, NH3-N). Tukey multiple comparison test was used to separate the means when significant differences were indicated by the MIXED procedure. Differences were considered significant at $P < 0.05$.

Nucleotide sequence accession numbers

The *ureC* sequences obtained in this study were deposited in the GenBank database under accession numbers JQ611755 to JQ612071.

Additional files

Additional file 1: SDS-PAGE of UreC cloned from *H. pylori* and overexpressed in *E. coli*. Marker, protein molecular weight marker; lane 1, total protein after induction by IPTG; lane 2, total protein from uninduced *E. coli* cells; lane 3, protein after Ni-NTA purification.

Additional file 2: Rumen fermentation characteristics after immunization.

Additional file 3: Ingredient and chemical composition of the TMR diet.

Competing interests

The authors declare that they have no competing interests.

Authors' contributions

JW and DB conceived and designed the experiments. SZ performed the experiments, analyzed the data, and wrote the paper. PS and NZ determined Ig titers. ZY helped interpret data and revised the paper. All authors read and approved the final manuscript.

Acknowledgements

This work was supported by Natural Science Foundation of China (31430081), Basic Research Program (973) of China (2011CB100804), and Agricultural Science and Technology Innovation Program (ASTIP-IAS12).

Author details

[1]Ministry of Agriculture Laboratory of Quality & Safety Risk Assessment for Dairy Products (Beijing), Institute of Animal Science, Chinese Academy of Agricultural Sciences, No. 2 Yuanyingyuan West Road, Beijing 100193, PR China. [2]State Key Laboratory of Animal Nutrition, Institute of Animal Science, Chinese Academy of Agricultural Sciences, No. 2 Yuanyingyuan West Road, Beijing 100193, PR China. [3]Department of Animal Sciences, The Ohio State University, Columbus, OH 43210, USA.

References

1. Reynolds CK, Kristensen NB. Nitrogen recycling through the gut and the nitrogen economy of ruminants: an asynchronous symbiosis. J Anim Sci. 2008;86(14 Suppl):E293–305.
2. Kertz AF. Review: urea feeding to dairy cattle: a historical perspective and review. Prof Anim Sci. 2010;26(3):257–72.
3. Lapierre H, Lobley GE. Nitrogen recycling in the ruminant: a review. J Dairy Sci. 2001;84:E223–36.
4. Powell JM, Wattiaux MA, Broderick GA. Short communication: evaluation of milk urea nitrogen as a management tool to reduce ammonia emissions from dairy farms. J Dairy Sci. 2011;94(9):4690–4.
5. Krajewska B. Ureases I. Functional, catalytic and kinetic properties: a review. J Mol Catal B Enzym. 2009;59(1–3):9–21.
6. Ludden PA, Harmon DL, Huntington GB, Larson BT, Axe DE. Influence of the novel urease inhibitor N-(n-butyl) thiophosphoric triamide on ruminant

nitrogen metabolism: II. Ruminal nitrogen metabolism, diet digestibility, and nitrogen balance in lambs. J Anim Sci. 2000;78(1):188–98.

7. Wright ADG, Kennedy P, O'Neill CJ, Toovey AF, Popovski S, Rea SM, et al. Reducing methane emissions in sheep by immunization against rumen methanogens. Vaccine. 2004;22(29–30):3976–85.

8. Wedlock DN, Pedersen G, Denis M, Dey D, Janssen PH, Buddle BM. Development of a vaccine to mitigate greenhouse gas emissions in agriculture: vaccination of sheep with methanogen fractions induces antibodies that block methane production in vitro. N Z Vet J. 2010;58(1):29–36.

9. Williams YJ, Popovski S, Rea SM, Skillman LC, Toovey AF, Northwood KS, et al. A vaccine against rumen methanogens can alter the composition of archaeal populations. Appl Environ Microbiol. 2009;75(7):1860–6.

10. Herrera P, Kwon YM, Ricke SC. Ecology and pathogenicity of gastrointestinal *Streptococcus bovis*. Anaerobe. 2009;15(1–2):44–54.

11. Williams YJ, Rea SM, Popovski S, Pimm CL, Williams AJ, Toovey AF, et al. Reponses of sheep to a vaccination of entodinial or mixed rumen protozoal antigens to reduce rumen protozoal numbers. Brit J Nutr. 2008;99(1):100–9.

12. Mobley HLT, Island MD, Hausinger RP. Molecular biology of microbial ureases. Microbiol Rev. 1995;59(3):451–80.

13. Marini JC, Simpson KW, Gerold A, Van Amburgh ME. The effect of immunization with jackbean urease on antibody response and nitrogen recycling in mature sheep. Livest Prod Sci. 2003;81(2–3):283–92.

14. Wozny MA, Bryant MP, Holdeman LV, Moore WE. Urease assay and urease-producing species of anaerobes in the bovine rumen and human feces. Appl Environ Microbiol. 1977;33(5):1097–104.

15. Kim M, Morrison M, Yu Z. Status of the phylogenetic diversity census of ruminal microbiomes. FEMS Microbiol Ecol. 2011;76(1):49–63.

16. Cook AR. Urease activity in the rumen of sheep and the isolation of ureolytic bacteria. J Gen Microbiol. 1976;92(1):32–48.

17. Hatzifoti C, Roussel Y, Harris AG, Wren BW, Morrow JW, Bajaj-Elliott M. Mucosal immunization with a urease B DNA vaccine induces innate and cellular immune responses against *Helicobacter pylori*. Helicobacter. 2006;11(2):113–22.

18. Shu Q, Gill HS, Hennessy DW, Leng RA, Bird SH, Rowe JB. Immunisation against lactic acidosis in cattle. Res Vet Sci. 1999;67(1):65–71.

19. Gnanasampanthan G. Immune responses of sheep to rumen ciliates and the survival and activity of antibodies in the rumen fluid. Adelaide: University of Adelaide; 1993.

20. DiLorenzo N, Diez-Gonzalez F, DiCostanzo A. Effects of feeding polyclonal antibody preparations on ruminal bacterial populations and ruminal pH of steers fed high-grain diets. J Ani Sci. 2006;84(8):2178–85.

21. Chen MH, Lee A, Hazell SL, Hu PJ, Li YY. Lack of protection against gastric *Helicobacter* infection following immunization with jack bean urease: the rejection of a novel hypothesis. FEMS Microbiol Lett. 1994;116(3):245–50.

22. Yu Z, Morrison M. Improved extraction of PCR-quality community DNA from digesta and fecal samples. Biotechniques. 2004;36(5):808–12.

23. Reed KE. Restriction enzyme mapping of bacterial urease genes: using degenerate primers to expand experimental outcomes. Biochem Mol Biol Educ. 2001;29(6):239–44.

24. Bonfield JK, Whitwham A. Gap5–editing the billion fragment sequence assembly. Bioinformatics. 2010;26(14):1699–703.

25. Tamura K, Peterson D, Peterson N, Stecher G, Nei M, Kumar S. MEGA5: molecular evolutionary genetics analysis using maximum likelihood, evolutionary distance, and maximum parsimony methods. Mol Biol Evol. 2011;28(10):2731–9.

26. Zhao S, Wang J, Liu K, Li D, Yu P, Bu D. Isolation and identification of urease from the rumen content of Holstein cows by a culture-independent strategy. Xu Mu Shou Yi Xue Bao. 2010;41(6):692–6.

27. Shu Q, Bir SH, Gill HS, Duan E, Xu Y, Hiliard, et al. Antibody response in sheep following immunization with *Streptococcus bovis* in different adjuvants. Vet Res Commun. 2001;25(1):43–54.

28. Liu GL, Wang JQ, Bu DP, Cheng JB, Zhang CG, Wei HY, et al. Specific immune milk production of cows implanted with antigen-release devices. J Dairy Sci. 2009;92(1):100–8.

29. Moharrery A, Das TK. Correlation between microbial enzyme activities in the rumen fluid of sheep under different treatments. Reprod Nutr Dev. 2001;41(6):513–29.

30. Weatherburn M. Phenol-hypochlorite reaction for determination of ammonia. Anal Chem. 1967;39(8):971–4.

31. Mohammed N, Ajisaka N, Hara ZALK, Mikuni K, Hara K, Kanda S, et al. Effect of Japanese horseradish oil on methane production and ruminal fermentation *in vitro* and in steers. J Anim Sci. 2004;82(6):1839–46.

32. Marsh WH, Fingerhu B, Miller H. Automated and manual direct methods for determination of blood urea. Clin Chem. 1965;11(6):624–7.

18

Refinement and partial validation of the UNESP-Botucatu multidimensional composite pain scale for assessing postoperative pain in horses

Marilda Onghero Taffarel[1†], Stelio Pacca Loureiro Luna[2*†], Flavia Augusta de Oliveira[2], Guilherme Schiess Cardoso[2], Juliana de Moura Alonso[2], Jose Carlos Pantoja[2], Juliana Tabarelli Brondani[2], Emma Love[3], Polly Taylor[4], Kate White[5] and Joanna C Murrell[3]

Abstract

Background: Quantification of pain plays a vital role in the diagnosis and management of pain in animals. In order to refine and validate an acute pain scale for horses a prospective, randomized, blinded study was conducted. Twenty-four client owned adult horses were recruited and allocated to one of four following groups: anaesthesia only (GA); pre-emptive analgesia and anaesthesia (GAA,); anaesthesia, castration and postoperative analgesia (GC); or pre-emptive analgesia, anaesthesia and castration (GCA). One investigator, unaware of the treatment group, assessed all horses at time-points before and after intervention and completed the pain scale. Videos were also obtained at these time-points and were evaluated by a further four blinded evaluators who also completed the scale. The data were used to investigate the relevance, specificity, criterion validity and inter- and intra-observer reliability of each item on the pain scale, and to evaluate construct validity and responsiveness of the scale.

Results: Construct validity was demonstrated by the observed differences in scores between the groups, four hours after anaesthetic recovery and before administration of systemic analgesia in the GC group. Inter- and intra-observer reliability for the items was only satisfactory. Subsequently the pain scale was refined, based on results for relevance, specificity and total item correlation.

Conclusions: Scale refinement and exclusion of items that did not meet predefined requirements generated a selection of relevant pain behaviours in horses. After further validation for reliability, these may be used to evaluate pain under clinical and experimental conditions.

Keywords: Validity, Reliability, Responsiveness, Specificity, Sensitivity, Relevance, Horse, Pain

Background

Recognition of pain-related behaviours in animals is difficult due to inter-species and individual variation [1], yet it is universally acknowledged that improvements in pain assessment may facilitate diagnosis and analgesic treatment in horses. Previous studies have developed scales to assess equine orthopaedic [2] and abdominal pain [3-5]. However,

* Correspondence: stelio@fmvz.unesp.br
†Equal contributors
2Department of Veterinary Surgery and Anesthesiology, College of Veterinary Medicine and Animal Science, UNESP – Univ Estadual Paulista, Botucatu, SP 18618970, Brazil
Full list of author information is available at the end of the article

to our knowledge, there are no published studies investigating pain scales in horses undergoing soft tissue surgery or experiencing pain of a similar intensity to that associated with castration.

There are established psychometric methods for developing and refining structured questionnaires of abstract constructs such as acute pain in humans. This approach can be adopted for similar purposes in animals. Initially the items to be assessed must be collected and refined for inclusion in the questionnaire. Thereafter the scale must be scrutinized for both content and face validity and finally the scale must undergo reliability testing [6].

Furthermore the instrument should be responsive and be able to measure changes as a result of an intervention such as a painful event, or analgesic administration [2,7].

The aim of this study was to refine and validate a new acute pain scale for the assessment of mild or moderate pain in horses, and to evaluate its reliability.

Results

The GA group included four geldings and two mares (mean ± SD, 332 ± 48 kg and 9 ± 3 years old); the GAA group included three geldings and three mares (369 ± 68 kg and 10 ± 5 years old); the GC group comprised of six male horses (319 ± 48 kg and 4 ± 2 years old) and GCA also included six male horses (302 ± 27 kg and 4 ± 2 years old). Surgery and anaesthesia lasted approximately 45 minutes in all cases. Complete data were obtained from twenty horses. Four horses had missing data points; one horse (GA) at T4 and T6 and one horse (GCA) at T24 due to abdominal discomfort, which recovered after clinical treatment, one horse (GAA) at T24, due to technical problems with the camera and one horse (GC) at T24, due to postoperative haemorrhage.

Content validity of the items included in the scale are shown in Table 1. The score for each item, the relevance, specificity and item-total correlation are shown in Table 2. A refined pain scale was produced after exclusion of the categories that did not show at least one item with adequate relevance and specificity. Heart rate was the only physiological variable retained in the pain scale, as it was the only one that differed over time (Figure 1). Comparison of the total scores between groups and at the different assessment time points was performed to confirm construct validity. At T4, pain scores were greater in GC than in the other groups, and greater in GCA than in GAA. Even after the administration of analgesics at T6, GC scores were still greater than GA and GAA, and GCA scores were greater than in GAA. At the 24-hour time point (T24) the scores of GC and GCA were still greater than those horses in GAA. There were no differences with time in scores for GA and GAA. In GC the scores at T4 were greater than at T6 and both were greater than TC (prior to anaesthesia and or surgery) and T24. The scores of GCA were greater in T4 than TC and T24.

The percentage increase in pain score in GC between TC and T4 was 282%, and the scores decreased by 39% and 61% of T4 at T6 and T24 respectively (Table 3).

Results of the criterion validation of the scores assigned to each item of the scale (derived by comparing the different evaluators' scores to the standard evaluator's), showed moderate to excellent variability for "positioning in the stall", "appetite for hay" and "response to palpation of the groin". With the exception of one evaluator, reliability for the item "locomotion" ranged from moderate to excellent. The horses' response to opening the door and head movements showed moderate variability. "Appetite for concentrate/pelleted feed," "looking at the flank", "raising the hind limbs" and "tail movements" showed poor to moderate variability. Variability was also poor for the remaining items or otherwise the number of observations was low and therefore it was not possible to perform statistical analysis.

Results of the criterion validation investigated by item-total correlation are presented in Table 2. The convergent validity was confirmed by positive correlation between the refined scale and the numerical (0.87), visual analogue (0.86) and simple descriptive scales (0.88), (see Figure 2) which were also assessed [8].

The reproducibility of each item, defined by the ability to obtain the same results in repeated assessments by different evaluators [9], was evaluated by measurement of inter-observer reliability and data are shown in Table 1.

The repeatability of each item, investigated by intra-observer reliability, was moderate to excellent for "positioning in the stall" and "kicking at the abdomen", but ranged from poor to moderate for interactive behaviour, "lifting of hind limbs" and "penis protrusion". It was also moderate for "locomotion when the horse was led by the evaluator", "response to palpation" of the painful area (groin), "response to an auditory stimulus", "pawing at the floor" and "moving the tail".

There was no difference between groups in physiological parameters, except at time point T4 when heart rate was lower in GA than in GCA (P = 0.04). Heart rate was higher in GC and GCA at T4 and T6 compared to the other assessment time points. Item-total correlation was moderate for all physiological data.

After the refinement of the data based on the specificity, relevance and criterion validity, a modified acute pain scale was tested (Table 4).

Discussion

The pain scale demonstrated construct and content validity; however intra- and inter-observer reliability for the items were only satisfactory, suggesting that refinement and readjustment of the items was required.

Construct validity was demonstrated by the observed differences in scores between the groups at T4 [10]. The differences between GC, GA and GAA show that the scale is able to differentiate between horses with and without pain. Furthermore, in view of the fact that pain scores were different between GC and GCA, the scale was also able to identify different pain intensities. The ability of the scale to measure pain was confirmed by its responsiveness, seen in the change in GC scores between T4, T6 and T24 [2], and by the percentage change in pain scores after surgery and in response to analgesic administration [11].

In both groups that did not undergo surgery (GA, GAA) male and female horses were included, which may

Table 1 Variables, criteria, scores, content validity and reproducibility of the acute pain scale in horses

Variable		Criteria	Score	Content validity[1]	Reproducibility[2]					
					EV1 X EV2	EV1 X EV3	EV1 X EV4	EV2 X EV3	EV2 X EV4	EV3 X EV4
Posture	Positioning in the stall	The horse's head is at the outside door	0	0.7	0.6 (0.4-0.7)	0.6 (0.4-0.8)	0.6 (0.5-0.8)	0.7 (0.5-0.8)	0.5 (0.3-0.7)	0.6 (0.4-0.7)
		The horse is inside the stall, but looking at the outside door. Observing the environment	1	*	0.5 (0.3-0.7)	0.4 (0.2-0.6)	0.5 (0.3-0.7)	0.5 (0.3-0.7)	0.3 (0.1-0.6)	0.4 (0.2-0.6)
		The horse is eating	0	*	0.7 (0.4-1.0)	0.7 (0.5-1.0)	0.6 (0.3-0.9)	0.8 (0.6-1.0)	0.7 (0.4-1.0)	0.7 (0.4-1.0)
		The horse is not close to the outside stall door and does not look interested in the environment	2	1	0.9 (0.6-1.0)	0.6 (0.3-1.0)	0.7 (0.4-1.0)	0.7 (0.4-1.0)	0.8 (0.6-1.0)	0.8 (0.6-1.0)
	Head position	Above the withers or grazing	0	1	0.4 (0.1-0.7)	0.4 (0.1-0.7)	0.5 (0.2-0.7)	0.6 (0.3-1.0)	0.6 (0.2-0.9)	0.8 (0.6-1.0)
		At the level of the withers	1	*	0.3 (0-0.7)	0.3 (0-0.6)	0.3 (0-0.6)	0.5 (0.1-1.0)	0.3 (−0.2-0.7)	0.5 (−0.1-1.0)
		Below the withers but not eating	2	1	NE	NE	NE	1.0 (1.0-1.0)	0.7 (0.04-1.0)	0.7 (0.04-1.0)
Interactive behaviour	Response to opening the door	The horse moves towards the door or is already positioned at the outside door	0	0.7	0.7 (0.6-0.9)	0.7 (0.5-0.9)	0.4 (0.2-0.6)	0.7 (0.6-0.9)	0.4 (0.2-0.6)	0.5 (0.3-0.8)
		The horse looks at the door, but does not move towards the door	1	0.7	0.6 (0.04-0.8)	0.5 (0.2-0.7)	0.3 (0.1-0.6)	0.6 (0.4-0.8)	0.3 (0.1-0.6)	0.5 (0.2-0.7)
		The horse does not respond to opening the door	2	0.7	0.4 (0-0.8)	0 (0-0)	0.5 (0.0-0.9)	0.3 (−0.2-0.8)	0.2 (−0.2-0.7)	0 (0-0)
	Response to approach and presence of the observer	Moves towards or looks to the observer	0	0.7	0.2 (0.1-0.3)	0.3 (0.1-0.4)	0 (0-0.1)	0.5 (0.3-0.7)	0 (−0.1-0.2)	0.1 (−0.1-0.3)
		Moves away from the observer	1	0.7	0.1 (−0.2-0.4)	0.2 (−0.2-0.6)	0 (0-0)	0 (0-0)	0 (0-0)	0 (0-0)
		Does not move	2	0.7	0.2 (0-0.3)	0.2 (0-0.4)	0.1 (0-0.1)	0.5 (0.2-0.7)	0.1 (−0.1-0.3)	0.1 (0-0.4)
Appetite	Appetite for hay	The horse eats hay	0	0.7	0.2 (−0.2-0.6)	0.7 (0-1.0)	0.7 (0-1.0)	0.3 (−0.1-0.7)	0.3 (−0.1-0.7)	1.0 (1.0-1.0)
		The horse does not eat hay	1	0.7	0.3 (−0.2-0.7)	0.7 (0-1.0)	0.7 (0-1.0)	0.3 (−0.1-0.8)	0.3 (−0.1-0.8)	1.0 (1.0-1.0)
	Response to concentrate food	Moves to the food and eats	0	0.7	−0.2 (−0.3- −0.1)	0.4 (0-0.7)	0.3 (0-0.6)	0.2 (0.1-0.5)	−0.1 (−0.2- −0.1)	0.4 (0-0.7)
		Hesitates to move towards the food, but eats	1	0.7	−0.1 (−0.2- −0.1)	0.6 (0.2-0.9)	0.4 (0.1-0.8)	0.2 (−0.1-0.5)	−0.1 (−0.2- −0.1)	0.4 (0-0.7)
		Shows no interest in food, not eating	2	0.7	NE	NE	NE	NE	NE	NE
Activity	Locomotion	The horse moves freely alone	0	0.7	0.1 (0-0.2)	0.5 (0.3-0.8)	0.3 (0.1-0.6)	0.1 (0-0.2)	0.1 (0-0.2)	0.3 (0.1-0.6)
		The horse does not move, or is reluctant to move	1	1	0.1 (0-0.3)	0.5 (0.3-0.8)	0.5 (0.2-0.8)	0.1 (0-0.2)	0.1 (0-0.3)	0.5 (0.2-0.9)
		The horse is agitated, restless	2	1	NE	NE	NE	NE	0.1 (−0.2-0.5)	NE
	Locomotion when led by the evaluator	The horse moves freely when led	0	0.7	0 (−0.2-0.1)	0.3 (0-0.7)	0.7 (0.4-1.0)	0.1 (0-0.3)	0.1 (0-0.2)	0.6 (0.3-1.0)
		The horse does not move, or is reluctant to move when led	1	1	0.1 (0-0.2)	0.5 (0.1-0.9)	0.8 (0.5-1.0)	0.1 (0-0.3)	0.1 (0-0.2)	0.6 (0.3-1.0)
		The horse is agitated, restless	2	1	NE	NE	NE	NE	NE	NE

Table 1 Variables, criteria, scores, content validity and reproducibility of the acute pain scale in horses (Continued)

Variable		Criteria	Score	Content validity[1]	Reproducibility[2]					
					EV1 X EV2	EV1 X EV3	EV1 X EV4	EV2 X EV3	EV2 X EV4	EV3 X EV4
Palpation	Response to palpation of the painful area (approximately 3 cm besides the surgical wound)	No response or change in relation to pre-procedure palpation response of the surgical wound	0	1	0.5 (0.3-0.6)	0.7 (0.5-0.8)	0.7 (0.5-0.8)	0.7 (0.5-0.8)	0.6 (0.5-0.3)	0.7 (0.6-0.9)
		Mild reaction to palpation of the surgical wound	1	1	0.3 (0.1-0.5)	0.5 (0.3-0.7)	0.6 (0.5-0.8)	0.4 (0.3-0.6)	0.3 (0.1-0.5)	0.4 (0.2-0.6)
		Violent reaction to palpation of the surgical wound	2	1	0.3 (0-0.6)	0.4 (0.2-0.7)	0.6 (0.3-0.9)	0.6 (0.4-0.8)	0.4 (0.1-0.7)	0.5 (0.2-0.7)
Interactive behaviour	Response to an auditory stimulus (clap hands)	Moves and/or pays attention with ears or head movements	0	*	0.3 (0.1-0.5)	0.4 (0.1-0.6)	0.3 (0-0.5)	0.4 (0.1-0.6)	0.5 (0.2-0.7)	0.6 (0.4-0.8)
		Calm, no response	1	*	0.4 (0.2-0.7)	0.5 (0.3-0.8)	0.4 (0.1-0.6)	0.4 (0.1-0.6)	0.5 (0.2-0.7)	0.6 (0.4-0.8)
		No response to auditory stimulus due to prostration	2	*	NE	NE	NE	NE	NE	NE
Miscellaneous behaviours	Looking at the flank	The horse does not look at the flank	0	0.7	0.4 (0.2-0.7)	0.3 (0.1-0.5)	0.4 (0.2-0.7)	0.5 (0.3-0.7)	0.5 (0.3-0.7)	0.6 (0.4-0.7)
		The horse looks at the flank	1	0.7	0.4 (0.2-0.7)	0.3 (0.1-0.5)	0.4 (0.2-0.7)	0.5 (0.3-0.7)	0.5 (0.3-0.7)	0.6 (0.4-0.8)
	Kicking at the abdomen	The horse does not kick the abdomen	0	0.7	0 (0-0)	0.1 (-0.1-0.4)	0.3 (0-0.7)	0 (-0.1-0)	0 (0-0)	0.3 (0-0.6)
		The horse kicks at the abdomen	1	0.7	NE	0.2 (0-0.5)	0.5 (0-0.9)	NE	NE	0.3 (0-0.6)
	Lifting hind limbs	No lifting of hind limbs	0	*	0.5 (0.3-0.7)	0.5 (0.4-0.7)	0.6 (0.4-0.8)	0.4 (0.2-0.6)	0.5 (0.3-0.7)	0.6 (0.4-0.8)
		Lifting hind limbs	1	*	0.3 (0.1-0.5)	0.4 (0.2-0.5)	0.5 (0.3-0.7)	0.2 (0-0.4)	0.3 (0.1-0.5)	0.6 (0.4-0.8)
		Lifting hind limbs and extending the head	2	*	0.2 (0-0.5)	0 (0-0)	0 (0-0)	0 (0-0)	0.1 (-0.1-0.3)	0 (0-0)
	Head movement	Head straight ahead most of the time	0	*	0.1 (0-0.2)	0.1 (-0.2-0.4)	0.6 (0.3-0.9)	0 (-0.1-0.2)	0.2 (0-0.4)	0.4 (0-0.7)
		Lateral and/or vertical occasional head movements	1	*	0 (-0.1-0.1)	0 (-0.1-0)	0.5 (0.2-0.8)	0 (-0.1-0.2)	0.1 (0-0.3)	0.3 (0-0.7)
		Lateral and/or vertical continuous head movements	2	*	0 (0-0)	NE	NE	NE	NE	NE
	Pawing on the floor (fore limbs)	Quietly standing, no pawing	0	0.7	0.2 (0-0.5)	0.2 (0-0.4)	0.2 (0-0.5)	0.3 (0-0.5)	0.5 (0.2-0.7)	0.7 (0.5-0.9)
		Pawing	1	1	0.3 (0-0.6)	0.2 (0-0.4)	0.2 (0-0.5)	0.4 (0.1-0.7)	0.5 (0.2-0.7)	0.7 (0.5-0.9)
	Others	Moving the tail sharply and repeatedly	1	*	0.1 (-0.1-0.2)	0.3 (0.1-0.4)	0.1 (-0.1-0.4)	0.2 (0-0.4)	0.2 (0-0.4)	0.4 (0.3-0.6)
		Moving the tail sharply and repeatedly and lifting the hind limbs	2	*	0.4 (0.1-0.7)	0.4 (0.2-0.6)	0.4 (0.1-0.7)	0.3 (0.1-0.5)	0.5 (0.2-0.8)	0.5 (0.3-0.7)
		Partial penis protrusion	1	*	0.4 (0.1-0.5)	0 (-0.2-0.2)	0.1 (-0.1-0.4)	0.2 (0-0.5)	0.1 (-0.1-0.3)	0.3 (0-0.5)
		Penis protrusion	0	*	0.4 (0.2-0.6)	0.2 (0-0.4)	0.5 (0.2-0.7)	0.4 (0.1-0.7)	0.5 (0.3-0.8)	0.7 (0.5-0.9)

[1]Content validity obtained by the arithmetic mean of the scores given by the three evaluators for each item of the scale [20].
[2]Inter-observer reproducibility was tested with the Kappa coefficient comparing video analysis among observers. > 0.7 - Excellent; 0.4 to 0.7 - moderate; <0.4 - poor reliability [21].
EV – Evaluator. NE – not evaluated as there were not sufficient data for statistical analysis (the behaviour was either very infrequent or not observed). * Item included after content validation.

Table 2 Relevance, specificity and item-total correlation of each item and categories of the scale in horses submitted to castration or only anaesthesia

Variable	Criteria	Specificity (%)[1]	Relevance (confidence interval)[2]			Item-total correlation[3]
			GA x GC	GAA X GC	GCA x GC	
Positioning in the stall	**The horse's head is at the outside door**	78.3	18.6 (4.4-78.9)*	48.3 (10.0-233.1)*	0.1 (0-0.4)	0.4
	The horse is inside the stall, but looking at the outside door, observing the environment	19.5	0.6 (0.2-2.0)	0.1 (0.0-0.7)	1.9 (0.6-6.16)	
	The horse is eating	0.9	NE	NE	NE	
	The horse is not close to the outside stall door and does not look interested in the environment	0.9	NE	NE	NE	
Head position	Above the withers or grazing	95.0	NE	NE	NE	0.2
	At the level of the withers	3.3	NE	NE	NE	
	Below the withers but not eating	0.0	NE	NE	NE	
Response to opening the door	The horse moves towards the door or is already positioned at the outside door	15.8	1.0 (0.2-3.7)	1.5 (0.4-6.0)	1.9 (0.6-6.5)	0.3
	The horse looks at the door, but does not move towards the door	15.8	0.7 (0.2-3.3)	0.3 (0-1.7)	0.5 (0.1-1.7)	
	The horse does not respond to opening the door	1.7	NE	NE	NE	
Response to approach and presence of the observer	Moves towards or looks to the observer	84.7	0.3 (0.1-1.5)	0.2 (0.1-0.9)	1.4 (0.3-6.1)	0.2
	Moves away from the observer	2.5	NE	NE	NE	
	Does not move	12.7	3.8 (0.8-18.8)	4.6 (1.0-21.2)*	0.7 (0.1-3.7)	
Appetite for hay	The horse eats hay	99.1	NE	NE	NE	0.2
	The horse does not eat hay	0.8	NE	NE	NE	
Response to concentrate food	Moves to the food and eats	90.7	NE	NE	NE	0.2
	Hesitates to move towards the food, but eats	8.0	NE	NE	NE	
	Shows no interest in food, not eating	0	NE	NE	NE	
Locomotion	**The horse moves freely alone**	84.2	47.6 (4.9-464.0)*	5.8 (1.6-21.3)*	0.2 (0-0.6)	0.4
	The horse does not move, or is reluctant to move	10.0	0 (0-0.2)	0.2 (0.1-0.7)	6.2 (1.6-23.2)*	
	The horse is agitated, restless	5.8	NE	NE	NE	
Locomotion when led by the evaluator	**The horse moves freely when led**	86.5	108.2 (4.4- >999.9)*	68.1 (4.9-946.5)*	0 (<0.001-0.1)	0.4
	The horse does not move, or is reluctant to move when led	12.2	NE	NE	NE	
	The horse is agitated, restless	0.0	NE	NE	NE	

Table 2 Relevance, specificity and item-total correlation of each item and categories of the scale in horses submitted to castration or only anaesthesia (Continued)

Variable	Criteria	Specificity (%)[1]	Relevance (confidence interval)[2]			Item-total correlation[3]
			GA x GC	GAA X GC	GCA x GC	
Response to palpation of the painful area (approximately 3 cm besides the wound)	No response or change in relation to pre-procedure palpation response of the surgical wound	57.1	4.1 (1.1-15.)*	18.8 (4.6-76.0)*	0.3 (0.1-1.1)*	0.4
	Mild reaction to palpation of the surgical wound	29.4	0.1 (0-0.5)	0.1 (0-0.5)	1.9 (0.6-5.9)*	
	Violent reaction to palpation of the surgical wound	13.4	2.1 (0.6-7.8)*	0.1 (0-1.3)*	1.7 (0.4-7.5)*	
Response to an auditory stimulus (clap hands)	Moves and/or pays attention with ears or head movements	80.0	6.8 (0.5-84.0)	4.9 (0.7-33.6)	0.5 (0.1-2.0)	0.3
	Calm, no response	18.6	NE	NE	NE	
	No response to auditory stimulus due to prostration	0.0	NE	NE	NE	
Looking at the flank	The horse does not look at the flank	84.6	46.7 (9.9-219.0)*	128.9 (21.2-782.7)*	0.1 (0-0.3)*	0.4
	The horse looks at the flank	15.4	0 (0-0.1)	0 (0-0)	11.7 (3.1-43.7)*	
Kicking at the abdomen	The horse does not kick the abdomen	95.8	NE	NE	NE	0.3
	The horse kicks at the abdomen	2.5	NE	NE	NE	
Lifting hind limbs	No lifting of hind limbs	74.6	18.0 (3.9-81.9)*	96.5 (16.4-566.4)*	0.1 (0-0.4)	0.6
	Lifting hind limbs	22.0	0.2 (0.1-0.8)	0 (0-0.2)	4.6 (1.3-16.1)*	
	Lifting one of the hind limbs and extending the head	3.4	NE	NE	NE	
Head movement	Head straight ahead most of the time	87.1	91.2 (10.1-822.7)*	32.4 (6.7-155.7)*	0.1 (0-0.3)	0.4
	Lateral and/or vertical occasional head movements	12.1	NE	NE	NE	
	Lateral and/or vertical continuous head movements	0.9	NE	NE	NE	
Pawing on the floor (fore limbs)	Quietly standing, no pawing	89.7	17.5 (3.6-84.9)*	38.9 (6.6-230.1)*	0.1 (0-0.5)	0.4
	Pawing	9.4	0.1 (0-0.4)	0 (0-0.2)	4.1 (1.12-14.1)*	
Others	Moving the tail sharply and repeatedly	21.7	0.9 (0.2-3.5)	0.5 (0.1-2.1)	1.8 (0.5-6.7)	0.5
	Moving the tail sharply and repeatedly and lifting the hind limbs	9.2	0 (0-0.2)	0 (0-0)	2.4 (0.9-6.9)	
	Partial penis protrusion	23.2	2.3 (0.4-12.5)	8.5 (1.6-4.2)	0.4 (0-2.0)	0.2
	Penis protrusion	47.4	NE	NE	NE	
			GA x GC	GAA x GC	GCA x GC	
Heart rate		-	-	-	-	0.6
Respiratory rate		-	-	-	-	0.5
Systolic blood pressure		-	-	-	-	0.4
Digestive sounds		-	-	-	-	0.3

The categories written in bold letters were used for the sum of the total score. NE – not evaluated as there were not sufficient data for statistical analysis (the behaviour was either infrequently or not observed). GA – Anaesthesia only (n = 6). GAA – Pre-emptive analgesia followed by anaesthesia (n = 6). GC – Anaesthesia, castration and postoperative analgesia administered four hours after surgery (n = 6). GCA – Pre-emptive analgesia, followed by anaesthesia and castration (n = 6).

[1]The specificity of each item was evaluated by investigating if that particular behaviour was present or not at TC, moment without pain, in all observations from all evaluators, in all animals from all groups. Specificity was classified as excellent (0–4.9%), good (5–14.9%), moderate (15–29.9%), or nonspecific (≥30%).

[2]Relevance was tested based on the possibility of distinguishing the behaviour in T4 in GC compared to the other groups. The item was considered relevant when that item differentiated GC from the other three groups, or when GC was different from animals without pain (GA and GAA). The item was considered irrelevant when there were no differences between GC and the other groups. Asterisks (*) indicate differences between groups.

[3]Criterion validity for item-total correlation with Pearson correlation test (weak < 0.30; moderate 0.31 – 0.60; strong 0.61 – 0.9; very strong 0.91 -1.0) [8].

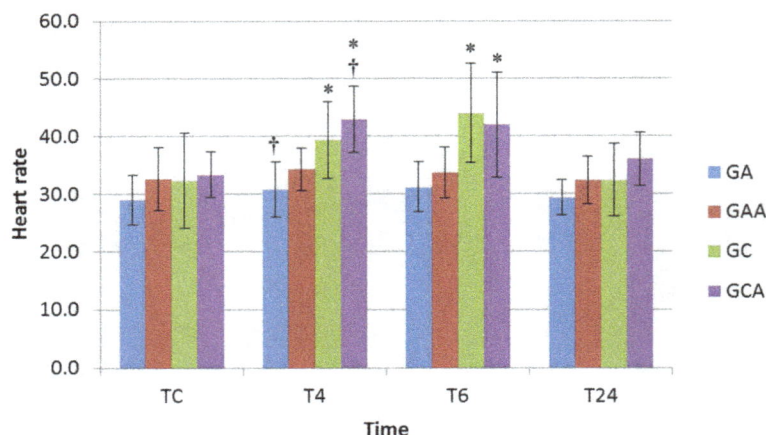

Figure 1 Heart rate before and after anaesthesia (GA), analgesia and anaesthesia (GAA), analgesia, anaesthesia and castration (GCA) and anaesthesia, castration and analgesia (GC) in horses. *Statistically significant difference between assessment time points within each group. † Significant difference between GA and GCA.

have been a limitation of the study; since the scale was based on assessment of behaviour, sex differences in behaviour may produce differences in scores between groups at TC. However, this did not occur and scores in the different sexes were similar. The absence of a difference between groups before surgery and/or anaesthesia provides an alternative means to confirm construct validity of the pain scale. Response to stress may mimic pain behaviour, and since it might be predicted that stallions would be more agitated prior to surgery, the lack of a difference between treatment groups in baseline scores shows that the construct validity of the scale was not compromised [6].

Another aspect that may have confused the interpretation of pain behaviours, especially in relation to assessments requiring the evaluator to interact with the horse, was the time allowed for each horse to acclimatise to the

stable, and to the investigator who interacted with the horses. Variability in the degree of this initial interaction between each horse and the investigator was expected. However, in order to limit this, one of the inclusion criteria for the study was that the horse must be halter trained and used to interacting with people.

Another limitation of the study is that the pain model used here (castration) probably results in only mild to moderate pain. Therefore the scale should also be tested under conditions considered to cause more severe pain and be validated under these circumstances as well.

To date there are no validated pain scales that measure mild to moderate soft tissue pain in horses and so criterion validity was evaluated by the contrast in variability between the standard evaluator and the other evaluators [7,11]. The total scores from the pain scale were correlated with three other classical scales used to measure clinical pain in animals and a strong positive correlation was evident [8]. Although these scales are also not validated, they are frequently used to evaluate pain [12] and lameness in horses [13,14]. Correlation with such classical scales has also been used previously to validate pain scales in horses for measurement of visceral pain [3,4].

The discrepancy in variability between the evaluators and the standard evaluator for each item of the scale suggests poor criterion validity. However, another possible explanation would be the limited training of the evaluators, combined with the complexity and large number of items that comprise the scale. The blinded evaluators were chosen because of their experience in pain-related studies in numerous other species, including horses. Furthermore, the item-total correlation, which denotes the importance of each item, showed that

Table 3 Median (minimal and maximal value) pain scores in horses undergoing castration or anaesthesia only

Treatment Moment	GA	GAA	GC	GCA
TC	3 (0–11)	2 (0–11)	4 (0–11)^C	4 (0–10)^B
T4	5 (1–14)^{bc}	5 (2–14)^c	14 (7–25)^{aA}	11 (3–16)^{bA}
T6	4 (1–6)^{bc}	4 (1–7)^c	10.5 (5–16)^{aB}	6.5 (1–19)^{abAB}
T24	3 (0–8)^{ab}	2 (0–7)^b	8 (1–14)^{aC}	6.5 (2–13)^{aB}

GA – Anaesthesia only (n = 6). GAA – Pre-emptive analgesia followed by anaesthesia (n = 6). GC – Anaesthesia, castration and postoperative analgesia administered four hours after surgery (n = 6). GCA – Pre-emptive analgesia, followed by anaesthesia and castration (n = 6). TC - before surgery and/or anaesthesia, T4 - maximum score of pain until 4 hours after anaesthetic recovery, T6 - six hours after anaesthetic recovery, T24 - 24 hours after anaesthetic recovery. Different small letters indicate differences between groups (rows – a > b > c); different capital letters indicate differences between time points in the same group (columns – A > B > C).

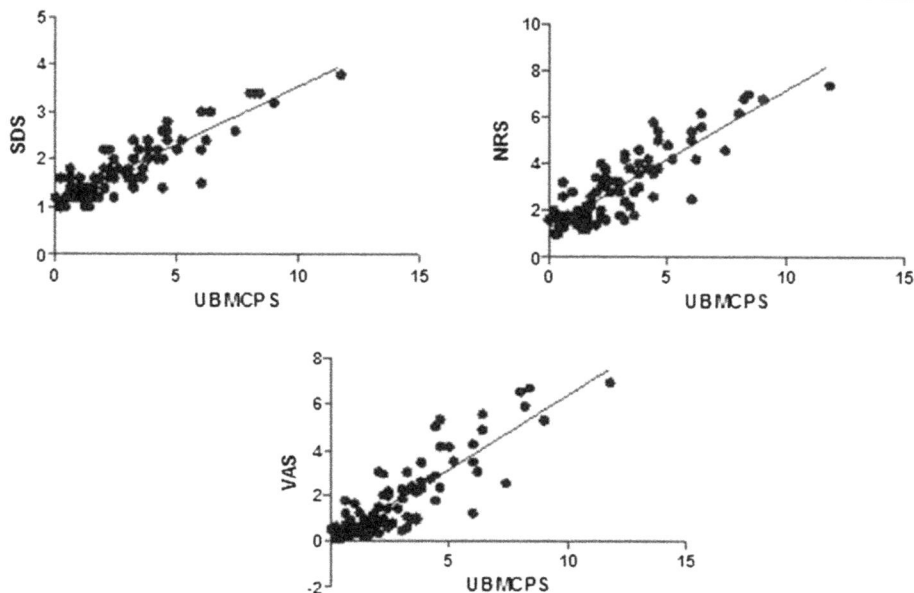

Figure 2 Pearson correlation between the UNESP-Botucatu Multidimensional Composite Pain Scale (UBMCPS) and the Simple Descriptive Scale (SDS – r = 0.88, P < 0.0001). Numerical Rate Scale (NRS – r = 0.87, P < 0.0001) and Visual Analogical Scale (VAS – r = 0.86, P < 0.0001).

most provided moderate correlation. Hence the very large number of items evaluated within the initial scale is likely to have reduced the overall criterion validity.

The variation in intra and inter-observer reliability for each item on the scale may suggest a low reliability of the proposed instrument under study. However, the process of pain scale validation does not occur in one step but is iterative, so after excluding items showing no specificity and relevance, the instrument should be re-evaluated using the same validity criteria [2,5,7]. The poor reproducibility for some items, such as "Response to approach" and "presence of the observer", may be related to failure of observation, due to the difficulty in observing the videos, a fact that might be resolved when observations are performed *in situ*. Otherwise the presence of the observer may also modify the animals' behaviour.

The scale items that gave the best relevance, specificity and total-item correlation results were retained in the scale after the refinement. However, despite the lack of relevance and low inter-observer reliability, the behaviour "kicking the abdomen" was retained in the scale as this is considered to be a classical abdominal pain related behaviour [12,15]. Although the inclusion of physiological parameters is questioned by some authors [3], these items are usually included in tools to assess acute pain in horses [2,5], as well as in other species [7] and provide a multidimensional character to the scale. Heart rate was retained after refinement as this was the only parameter that varied with time, it is easy to

evaluate and has historical importance in the assessment of pain [12]. In view of the fact that heart rate increased above 25% of pre-operative values (TC) in animals undergoing surgery (GC and GCA) at T4 and T6, overall changes in heart rate above 25% were considered relevant as an indicator of post-operative pain and were therefore included.

As noted in a study that described the behaviours of horses undergoing arthroscopic surgery and laparotomy [16], horses without pain were more likely to position themselves at the front of the stable compared to other positions in the box. Behaviours such as "head position" and "response to auditory stimuli" were excluded due to their variability and since they might be unduly influenced by environmental stimuli.

Behaviours related to the interaction with the observer showed similar relevance and specificity to those reported when using an orthopaedic pain scale [2] and similar item-total correlation to animals undergoing laparotomy [5]. However this behaviour may also be influenced by the type of management with which the animal is familiar [17]. In our study, locomotion was also useful to detect pain after soft tissue surgery, as animals in pain tend to be reluctant to move, reflecting the findings of altered locomotion in horses after orthopaedic surgery [13,14]. However this contrasts with results from other studies in which increased locomotion was associated with pain [2,3], indicating that it is the change in locomotion that is a useful characteristic to evaluate during pain assessment in horses.

Table 4 Refined acute pain scale in horses submitted to castration after the refinement of the data based on the specificity, relevance and criterion validity

Variable	Criteria	Score
Positioning in the stall	The horse's head is at the outside door	0
	The horse is inside the stall, but looking at the outside door, observing the environment	1
	The horse is eating	0
	The horse is not close to the outside stall door and does not look interested in the environment	2
Locomotion	The horse moves freely alone	0
	The horse does not move, or is reluctant to move	1
	The horse is agitated, restless	2
Locomotion when led by the evaluator	The horse moves freely when led	0
	The horse does not move, or is reluctant to move when led	1
	The horse is agitated, restless	2
Response to palpation of the painful area (approximately 3 cm besides the wound)	No response or change in relation to pre-procedure palpation response of the surgical wound	0
	Mild reaction to palpation of the surgical wound	1
	Violent reaction to palpation of the surgical wound	2
Looking at the flank	The horse does not look at the flank	0
	The horse looks at the flank	1
Kicking at the abdomen	The horse does not kick the abdomen	0
	The horse kicks at the abdomen	1
Lifting hind limbs	No lifting of hind limbs	0
	Lifting hind limbs	1
	Lifting hind limbs and extending the head	2
Head movement	Head straight ahead most of the time	0
	Lateral and/or vertical occasional head movements	1
	Lateral and/or vertical continuous head movements	2
Pawing on the floor (fore limbs)	Quietly standing, no pawing	0
	Pawing	1
Heart rate (compared to initial values)	25-50% increase	1
	>50% increase	2

Although palpation of the surgical site showed low item-total correlation in this study, specificity ranged from moderate to good and this item was relevant. In a previous study, horses undergoing laparotomy showed a high incidence of avoidance responses [5]. In our study, the reaction response was probably related to the inflammation caused by surgical incision. However, it is common for horses not to tolerate palpation of the inguinal area. Furthermore, in those cases where this behaviour was evaluated on the video, there may have been misinterpretation. Although the two cameras were placed in diagonally opposite positions in the stable to try to avoid blind spots, it was difficult to observe the animal when it was positioned close to the wall directly beneath one of the cameras. Under some of these circumstances it was

not possible to visualize the pelvic limbs during palpation of the groin.

This is the first study to identify the behaviour of lifting the pelvic limb as a pain-related behaviour in the horse, indicated by the relevance and moderate specificity and item-total correlation. This item was included in the scale after validation of content and before construct validation because it was a behaviour observed by the evaluator *in situ* during assessment of the GC group.

Since there is now a considerable body of work describing the development of tools for pain assessment, it was possible to evaluate the relevance, specificity and reliability of various pain behaviours previously described as relevant in horses. The low repeatability and reproducibility of some behaviours may indicate that their interpretation is influenced by the experience of the evaluator, and therefore they are imprecise. Although the reliability of the total score of the refined scale was not investigated, the sensitive and specific items of the behaviours and categories may be used to compose a refined scale for future validation, ideally under clinical conditions.

It should also be noted that during the initial part of the scale, the observer was not present in the box. I It is therefore difficult to accurately ascertain how much the evaluator's presence might interfere with the pain assessment. Consequently, whenever possible horses should be observed using a remote monitoring system. Although the time necessary for pain assessment has not been determined, after 700 hours of video analysis, we empirically suggest a time frame of 5 minutes would be sufficient for observation of pain-related relevant behaviours in the horse.

Conclusions

In conclusion, this is, to our knowledge, the first study to refine and validate a pain scale for assessing acute, mild clinical pain in horses undergoing castration. The proposed new scale showed construct validity and responsiveness, and differentiated between horses with and without pain as reported previously in horses undergoing moderate and severe pain intensity, like orthopaedic and abdominal pain. Reliability of the initial items included in the scale was variable, suggesting the need for refinement of the scale; this led to selection of items that showed relevance, specificity, and item-total correlation. Refinement of the scale, and exclusion of items that did not meet the predefined validity requirements, provided a simple version for evaluation of postoperative pain after soft tissue surgery in horses that may be further tested under clinical and experimental conditions.

Methods

The Institutional Animal Scientific Use Ethical Committee approved the study (protocol number 186/2009) and written informed consent was obtained from the owners before their horses were recruited to the study.

The acute pain scale was developed using previously published data [2,12] and by observing approximately 700 hours of videos before and after castration. Based on these data the behaviours of animals with or without pain were identified. Content validation review was based on evaluation of each item of the scale as relevant (1), irrelevant (−1) or not known (0) by three experienced equine veterinarians. The arithmetic mean was calculated for each item and those with values greater than or equal to 0.5 [8] were included in the scale. The scale composed 62 items with scores ranging from 0 to 3 and total score of 40 points (Table 1). Physiological parameters were also evaluated in addition to the items described in Table 1. Heart and respiratory rates and non-invasive systolic arterial blood pressure were evaluated according to the following criteria when compared to the initial (baseline) values: 0 – less than 10%; 1 – between 11 and 30%; 2 - between 31 and 50% and 3 – above 50% increase when compared to initial values. Intestinal sounds were evaluated as 0 – normal; 1 - decreased gut sounds; 2 – increase gut sounds or no gut sounds.

Construct validity was examined by contrast group analysis, comparing animals with or without pain. Twenty-four client owned adult horses confirmed as healthy following clinical and laboratory assessment were recruited and randomly (Excel®)[a] allocated to one of four following groups: anaesthesia only (GA); pre-emptive analgesia and anaesthesia (GAA); anaesthesia, castration and postoperative analgesia (GC); or pre-emptive analgesia, anaesthesia and castration (GCA). The same experienced surgeon performed all castrations. All animals were housed in individual stables and allowed to acclimatize for at least 36 hours before any behavioural data were collected. Only well-handled horses were recruited to the study. The sample size was determined using an expected mean pain score difference between the groups of 4.0, with a standard deviation of 3.0, based on pilot studies, with a test power of 90% and 5% level of significance.

All horses were sedated with 0.5 mg/kg xylazine IM (Sedomin®)[b], followed by induction of anaesthesia with 100 mg/kg of 10% guaiphenesin (Eter Gliceril Guaicol®)[c] and 5.0 mg/kg of thiopentone IV (Thiopentax®)[d]. After orotracheal intubation, anaesthesia was maintained with isoflurane (Isoforine®)[d] in oxygen. Ventilation was controlled (Mallard Medical®)[e]. Pre-emptive (GAA and GCA) or postoperative (GC) analgesia consisted of the administration of 0.2 mg/kg morphine (Dimorf®)[d] IM, 10 mg/kg dipyrone (metamizol) (Finador®)[f] IM and 1.1 mg/kg flunixin meglumine (Desflan®)[f] IV. Local anaesthesia was provided with 10 ml of 2% lidocaine with adrenaline (Lidocaina®)[d] injected into each spermatic cord before surgery in GCA. After recovery from anaesthesia the animals were transferred back to the observation stable, which was equipped with two video cameras (1.3 megapixels) placed in opposite corners at a height of 2 meters. The cameras provided colour images and were equipped with an infrared device to enable image capture under low light conditions. Video recording commenced immediately before anaesthesia and for 24 hours afterwards. Over this 24 hour period an investigator also assessed the animals directly by entering the stable and assessing pain in a standardised manner at the following time points: TC (before surgery and/or anaesthesia); T4 (four hours after anaesthetic recovery, before administration of systemic analgesia in the GC group); T6 (six hours after anaesthetic recovery) and T24 (24 hours after anaesthetic recovery). After the investigator entered the stable, the horse was approached and offered pelleted food in a small container. Pain assessments were then performed and after these were completed, the horse's heart rate and intestinal motility [18] were assessed by auscultation, respiratory rate by observation of thoracic wall movements and systolic arterial blood pressure by the Doppler technique (Parks Medical 812®)[g] with the probe and cuff positioned over the coccygeal artery. Following analysis of all of the video data, four 3 to 4 minute videos were generated for each animal at time points TC, T4, T6 and T24. These included footage recorded one hour before the presence of the investigator and during the time that the investigator was present in the stable undertaking the pain assessment. The duration of the video clips was sufficient for the included behaviours to be expressed by the horses.

The investigator (standard evaluator) and four experienced equine clinicians (evaluators) watched the videos on two different occasions at intervals of at least two weeks. The order of the videos was changed for the second assessment. The evaluators were blinded with respect both to treatment group (GA, GAA, GC, GCA) and to the assessment time point (TC-T24). The evaluators used the acute pain scale to assess pain in the horses, without any scores assigned to any item on the scale. The scores were subsequently included for statistical evaluation. The following instructions were given to the evaluators prior to watching each sequence of videos. 1) After watching each video clip answer the following questions according to your clinical experience fill in the numerical pain scale (1: without pain to 10: worst possible pain), followed by the simple descriptive scale (1: without pain to 4: severe pain) and then the visual analogue pain scale (0: without pain to 100 mm: worst possible pain); 2) Subsequently fill in the proposed pain scale choosing the descriptor level within each item that best represents what was observed; 3) If you are unsure at any time about what behaviours were shown in the video, the video may be replayed. Specific behaviours such as looking at the flank and lifting of hind limbs were considered after the behaviour had been observed once or several times.

Statistical analysis

For content validity, only values equal to or greater than 0.5, obtained by the arithmetic mean of the scores given by the three evaluators for each item, were accepted and included in the pain scale [19].

The specificity of each item (defined by the ability of the test to correctly identify patients that were exhibiting pain behaviours calculated by the ratio between the true negatives and the sum of the true negatives and false positives), was evaluated by investigating if that particular behaviour was present or not at TC in all

observations from all evaluators, in all animals from all groups. When a given behaviour was present in animals after surgery and likely feeling pain, but was not expressed or infrequently expressed in horses free of pain (TC), that behaviour was considered relevant to differentiate a horse with or without pain and therefore would be considered having high specificity. Specificity was classified as excellent (0–4.9%), good (5–14.9%), moderate (15–29.9%), or nonspecific (≥30%) [2].

The relevance of each item, i.e. the chance of observing a particular behaviour at T4 (when the most intense pain was expected) [2] was estimated by odds ratio using a logistic regression model for each item. An item was considered relevant when there was difference between GC *versus* GCA, GA and GAA, or when GC was different from GA and GAA, and irrelevant when there were no differences between GC and the other groups.

The total score of the refined scale was obtained by summing only the scores of the categories that showed items with relevance, specificity and item-total correlation. Categories that did not fulfil the above criteria were excluded from the sum of the total score of the refined scale (Table 4). Only the physiological variables showing changes over time were included in the sum of the total score of the refined scale.

The comparison of total scores between treatments was performed using the Kruskal-Wallis test and the difference between the scores over time in each group using the Friedman test. Construct validity was assessed by comparing the total score of the refined scale at the assessment time point where the animals were expected to have the most intense pain (T4 in GC and GCA) against the other time points (TC, T6, T24). Responsiveness was based on the percentage of change in pain score before and after administration of analgesia in groups GC [7,11], and by observing the difference between the groups in pain scores at time point T4 [2].

To investigate the criteria validity of each item, the Kappa coefficient was used to estimate the reliability of the score of the item between each evaluator and the standard evaluator, generating four kappa values; the values of each comparison were classified and grouped when reliability was similar [7,20]. The Pearson's correlation coefficient was used to estimate the correlation between each variable (Table 2) against the total score of the proposed scale. In addition the correlation between the scores of the proposed scale and numerical, simple descriptive and VAS scale correlations was tested to investigate the convergent validity.

Intra- and inter-observer reliability for each item of the scale were assessed by use of the Kappa coefficient to compare differences in scores assigned on the first and second occasion that each video was watched by each evaluator, and by comparing scores assigned to the same video between different evaluators. Physiological data were investigated by repeated measures modelling evaluated for distribution and the gastrointestinal sounds were evaluated using the Wilcoxon test.

Statistical analyses were conducted with SAS version 9.3 [21] and differences were considered significant when p < 0.05.

Endnotes

[a]Microsoft, EUA.

[b]Konig, Buenos Aires, Argentina.

[c]L.P.S. Agrofarma, Mogi Mirim, São Paulo, Brazil.

[d]Cristália, Lindóia, São Paulo, Brazil.

[e]Mallard Medical Skypark Drive Redding, CA, USA.

[f]Ourofino, Cravinhos, São Paulo, Brazil.

[g]Parks Medical Eletronics, Las Vegas, Nevada, USA.

Abbreviations
GA: Group anaesthesia only; GAA: Group pre-emptive analgesia and anaesthesia; GC: Group anaesthesia, castration and post-operative analgesia; GCA: Group pre-emptive analgesia, anaesthesia and castration; TC: moment before surgery and/or anaesthesia; T4: moment four hours after anaesthetic recovery before administration of systemic analgesia in the GC group; T6: moment six hours after anaesthetic recovery; T24: moment 24 hours after anaesthetic recovery; IM: intramuscular; IV: intravenous.

Competing interests
The authors declare that they have no competing interests.

Authors' contributions
Experimental design and planning: MOT, SPLL, FAO, GSC, JMA, JCM, JTB, PT, KW, EL. Statistical analysis: JCP, MOT, SPLL. Drafting of the manuscript: MOT, SPLL, JCM. All authors read and approved the manuscript.

Authors' information
MOT (DVM, PhD); SPLL (DVM, PhD, DipECVAA); FAO (DVM, PhD); GSC (DVM, PhD), JMA (DVM, Msci); JCP (DVM, PhD); JTB (DMV, PhD); EL (BVMS, PhD, DVA DipECVAA MRCVS FHEA); PT (MAVet, MB, PhD, DipECVAA); KW (MA, VetMB, DVA, DipECVA); JCM (BVSc, PhD, DipECVAA, MRCVS).

Acknowledgements
São Paulo Research Foundation (FAPESP) for financial support (Process 2010/00786-6 and 2010/08967-0).

Author details
[1]Veterinary Medicine Department, Universidade Estadual de Maringá, Estrada da Paca s/n, Umuarama, Brazil. [2]Department of Veterinary Surgery and Anesthesiology, College of Veterinary Medicine and Animal Science, UNESP – Univ Estadual Paulista, Botucatu, SP 18618970, Brazil. [3]School of Veterinary Science, Langford House, Langford, UK. [4]Taylor Monroe, Ely, Cambridgeshire, UK. [5]School of Veterinary Medicine and Science, University of Nottingham, Nottingham, UK.

References
1. Flecknell P. Analgesia from a veterinary perspective. Br J Anaesth. 2008;101 (1):121–4.
2. Bussieres G, Jacques C, Lainay O, Beauchamp G, Leblond A, Cadore JL, et al. Development of a composite orthopaedic pain scale in horses. Res Vet Sci. 2008;85(2):294–306.
3. Sutton GA, Dahan R, Turner D, Paltiel O. A behaviour-based pain scale for horses with acute colic: Scale construction. Vet J. 2013;196(3):394–401.
4. Sutton GA, Paltiel O, Soffer M, Turner D. Validation of two behaviour-based pain scales for horses with acute colic. Vet J. 2013;197(3):646–50.
5. Graubner C, Gerber V, Doherr M, Spadavecchia C. Clinical application and reliability of a post abdominal surgery pain assessment scale (PASPAS) in horses. Vet J. 2011;188(2):178–83.
6. DeVon HA, Block ME, Moyle-Wright P, Ernst DM, Hayden SJ, Lazzara DJ, et al. A psychometric toolbox for testing validity and reliability. J Nurs Scholarsh. 2007;39(2):155–64.
7. Brondani JT, Mama KR, Luna SP, Wright BD, Niyom S, Ambrosio J, et al. Validation of the English version of the UNESP-Botucatu multidimensional composite pain scale for assessing postoperative pain in cats. BMC Vet Res. 2013;9:143.
8. Callegari-Jacques SM. Bioestatística: princípios e aplicações. Porto Alegre: Artmed; 2003.
9. de Vet HCW, Bouter LM, Bezemer PD, Beurskens AJHM. Reproducibility and responsiveness of evaluative outcome measures. Int J Technol Assess Health Care. 2001;17(04):479–87.
10. Cronbach LJ, Meehl PE. Construct validity in psychological tests. Psychol Bull. 1955;52(4):22.
11. Brondani JT, Luna SPL, Minto BW, Santos BPR, Beier SL, Matsubara LM, et al. Validity and responsiveness of a multidimensional composite scale to assess postoperative pain in cats. Arquivo Brasileiro de Medicina Veterinária e Zootecnia. 2012;64:1529–38.
12. Ashley FH, Waterman-Pearson AE, Whay HR. Behavioural assessment of pain in horses and donkeys: application to clinical practice and future studies. Equine Vet J. 2005;37:565–75.
13. Viñuela-Fernández I, Jones E, Chase-Topping ME, Price J. Comparison of subjective scoring systems used to evaluate equine laminitis. Vet J. 2011;188(2):171–7.
14. Hewetson M, Christley RM, Hunt ID, Voute LC. Investigations of the reliability of observational gait analysis for the assessment of lameness in horses. Vet Record. 2006;158(25):852–8.
15. Pritchett LC, Ulibarri C, Roberts MC, Schneider RK, Sellon DC. Identification of potential physiological and behavioral indicators of postoperative pain in horses after exploratory celiotomy for colic. Appl Animal Behav Sci. 2003;80(1):31–43.
16. Price J, Catriona S, Welsh EM, Waran. Preliminary evaluation of a behaviour-based system for assessment of post-operative pain in horses following arthroscopic surgery. J Vet Anaesthesia Analgesia. 2003;30(3):124–37.
17. Short CE. Fundamentals of pain perception in animals. Appl Animal Behav Sci. 1998;59(1):125–33.
18. Queiroz-Neto A, Carregaro AB, Zamur G, Harkins JD, Tobin T, Mataqueiro MI, et al. Effect of amitraz and xylazine on some physiological variables of horses. Arquivo Brasileiro de Medicina Veterinária e Zootecnia. 2000;52:27–32.
19. Suraseranivongse S, Santawat U, Kraiprasit K, Petcharatana S, Prakkamodom S, Muntraporn N. Cross-validation of a composite pain scale for preschool children within 24 hours of surgery. Br J Anaesth. 2001;87(3):400–5.
20. Fleiss JL. The measurement of interrater agreement. In: Fleiss JL, editor. Statistical methods for rates and proportions. 2nd ed. New York: John Wiley & Sons Inc; 1981. p. 212–36.
21. Institute S: SAS Institute Inc. In. Edited by Documentation SHa, 9.3 edn. Cary, NC, USA; 2011.

19

Detection of the neuropathogenic variant of equine herpesvirus 1 associated with abortions in mares in Poland

Karol Stasiak, Jerzy Rola[*], Gabor Ploszay, Wojciech Socha and Jan F Zmudzinski

Abstract

Background: The incidence of reported cases of equine herpesvirus myeloencephalopathy (EHM) caused by infection with neuropathogenic strains of equine herpesvirus 1 (EHV-1) has markedly increased over the last decade in many Western countries. The purpose of this study was to estimate the prevalence of the neuropathogenic (*G2254*) and non-neuropathogenic (*A2254*) variants of EHV-1 among isolates associated with abortions in Polish stud farms.

Results: The results of polymerase chain reaction-restriction fragment length polymorphism (PCR-RFLP) and sequencing were consistent, and showed that two out of 64 abortions (3.1%) were induced by the neuropathogenic genotype *G2254*. All remaining 18 EHV-1 positive abortion cases (28.1%) were caused by the non-neuropathogenic genotype *A2254*.

Conclusions: Most of the abortions in mares in Poland from 1999 to 2012 were associated with non-neuropathogenic strains of EHV-1. However, the presented data indicate that the neuropathogenic genotype of the virus is also present in Polish stud farms. Such a presence suggests that the future emergence of EHM in Poland is probable.

Keywords: EHV-1, ORF30, Neuropathogenic genotype, Abortion

Background

Equine herpesvirus 1 (EHV-1) is a double-stranded DNA virus that occurs worldwide in all breeds of horses [1,2]. Infections caused by EHV-1 are important as clinical outbreaks of the disease still occur, despite preventive and control measures being taken [3,4]. Exposure to EHV-1 can cause upper respiratory tract infection in foals and young horses. In pregnant mares, the virus can be transferred across the uteroplacental barrier and infect the fetus, which can lead to late-gestation abortion. EHV-1 can also migrate with infected blood leukocytes to the central nervous system and replicate in endothelial cells of arterioles in the spinal cord and brain, causing vasculitis and thrombosis [5]; this syndrome is known as equine herpesvirus myeloencephalopathy (EHM). Previous research has shown that the neuropathogenicity of EHV-1 strains is strongly associated with a single point mutation in the open reading frame

(ORF) 30 of the gene encoding viral DNA polymerase [6-8]. This mutation is a single nucleotide adenine to guanine substitution at nucleotide 2,254, corresponding to an asparagine to aspartic acid substitution. Additionally, two other studies revealed that another nucleotide substitution at nucleotide 2,258 of ORF30 could possibly be associated with neuropathogenicity [6,9].

Although the clinical form of EHM is less frequently observed than the other types of EHV-1 infection, it can cause serious economic losses in breeding horses and have a very negative impact on the functioning of veterinary hospitals, riding schools, and racetracks [4,3,10,11]. Moreover, recent data from the United States of America (US) showed that neuropathogenic strains of EHV-1 could become an important causative agent of abortions in mares even in the absence of actual clinical signs of EHM or respiratory disease [9].

In Poland, EHV-1 abortion outbreaks in mares have been reported several times since the early 1950s [12-15]. However, there are no data on the occurrence of neuropathogenic EHV-1 strains in Poland. The purpose of this study was to determine the prevalence of

---
* Correspondence: jrola@piwet.pulawy.pl
Department of Virology, National Veterinary Research Institute, Al.
Partyzantow 57, 24-100 Pulawy, Poland

the neuropathogenic genotype of ORF30 among the strains of EHV-1 isolated from abortion cases in Poland.

Methods

Samples

We tested tissue samples (lung, liver, spleen, heart, kidney, and placenta, if delivered) from 64 aborted fetuses that were delivered to the Department of Virology of the National Veterinary Research Institute in Pulawy between 1999 and 2012. The whole fetuses or fetal organs came from horse studs located in different regions of Poland. None of the animals had been vaccinated against EHV-1, and none of the studs had a history of respiratory and neurological disease. Necropsy reports revealed that all 64 abortions occurred during the third trimester of pregnancy. A variety of macroscopic lesions were observed in most cases, including a large amount of pleural fluid, hepatic necrosis, and pulmonary oedema. No histological investigation was done. Organ samples from aborted fetuses were stored at $-70°C$ until further processing.

Two grams of each tissue sample was used for preparation of 10% (w/v) suspension in Eagle's Minimum Essential Medium (Sigma-Aldrich), supplemented with 1% antibiotic solution (Antibiotic Antimycotic Solution 100x, Sigma-Aldrich) using ULTRA-TURRAX® homogenizer. Tissue homogenates were centrifuged at 1,700 x g for 10 min, and then supernatants from the same fetus were pooled together and stored at $-70°C$ until testing.

DNA extraction

DNA was extracted from every pool of tissue supernatant using a phenol-chloroform-isoamyl alcohol mixture.

PCR testing

The DNA obtained from tissue homogenates was tested for the presence of EHV-1 and EHV-4 using primers for glycoprotein B previously described by Kirisawa et al. (EHV1/4 Forward: 5'-CTT GTG AGA TCT AAC CGC AC-3'[1477-1496/1468-1487], EHV-1 Reverse: 5'-GCG TTA TAG CTA TCA CGT CC-3'[1936–1917], EHV-4 Reverse: 5'-CCT GCA TAA TGA CAG CAG TG-3'[2410–2391]) [16].

Virus isolation

EHV-1 was isolated in 25-cm^2 tissue culture flasks containing monolayers of RK13 cells. Flasks were inoculated and checked daily for appearance of cytopathic effect (CPE). CPE-positive flasks were frozen and stored at $-70°C$.

Polymerase chain reaction-restriction fragment length polymorphism (PCR-RFLP)

PCR-RFLP neuropathogenic/non-neuropathogenic discrimination testing was performed on EHV-1-positive

samples. PCR amplification of a 380-bp fragment of ORF30 was based on a modified protocol described by Allen [17]. A 25-μl reaction mix was prepared for PCR containing 0.05 U/μl AccuTaq LA DNA Polymerase, 200 μM of deoxynucleotide triphosphate mix, 1 × PCR buffer, 400 nM of the primer ORF30-Forward (5'-GTG GAC GGT ACC CCG GAC-3'[2005–2022]) and ORF30-Reverse (5'-GTG GGG ATT CGC GCC CTC ACC-3'[2384–2364]) and 2.5 μl DNA template, suspended in RNAse-DNAse-free water. The reaction was run in a Biometra Thermocycler (Biometra, Germany) under the following conditions: initial denaturation at 94°C for 3 min, followed by 35 cycles of denaturation at 94°C for 30 s, annealing at 60°C for 1 min, and elongation at 72°C for 30 s.

PCR products were digested with *Sal*I enzyme [recognition site: 5'...G↓TCGAC...3'] (EURx, Poland). Digestion was performed in a 50-μl reaction mixture containing 10 μl of PCR product, 5 μl 10x Buffer High, 0.5 μl 100x BSA (EURx), and 1 μl *Sal*I enzyme, suspended in nuclease free water. Digestion was run at 37°C for 2 h in a thermocycler. Products were visualized by electrophoresis on 1.5%

Table 1 Polish ORF30 genotype of EHV-1 isolates by PCR-RFLP

Strain designation[a]	Genotype at position 2254	Region[b]
PL/1999/I	A 2254	LU
PL/1999/II	A 2254	MA
PL/2001/I	A 2254	LU
PL/2002/I	A 2254	MA
PL/2003/I	A 2254	WP
PL/2004/I	A 2254	LU
PL/2004/II	A 2254	PM
PL/2005/I	A 2254	WM
PL/2006/I	A 2254	MP
PL/2006/II	A 2254	LU
PL/2007/I	A 2254	MA
PL/2008/I	A 2254	DS
PL/2009/I	A 2254	SL
PL/2009/II	G 2254	LU
PL/2010/I	A 2254	MA
PL/2010/II	G 2254	SL
PL/2010/III	A 2254	LU
PL/2011/I	A 2254	MP
PL/2012/I	A 2254	MA
PL/2012/II	A 2254	LU

[a]Based on the year of isolation.
[b]Voivodship SL-Silesian; MA-Masovian; WM-Warmian-Masurian. LU-Lublin; MP-Lesser Poland; PM-Pomeranian; DS-Lower Silesian. WP-Greater Poland. The regions are described in detail at: http://en.wikipedia.org/wiki/Voivodeships_of_Poland.

agarose gel. DNA from two EHV-1 strains was used as a positive control: Ab4 (neuropathogenic strain) and V592 (non-neuropathogenic strain).

Sequencing

All positive samples were confirmed by sequencing the 380-bp ORF30 fragment using the Sanger method at the Institute of Biochemistry and Biophysics Polish Academy of Science (Warsaw, Poland). Nucleotide sequences were assembled and aligned using Molecular Evolutionary Genetics Analysis (MEGA) version 5.0.5. The nucleotide sequences reported in this study were submitted to GenBank under the accession numbers KR080374-KR080393.

Results

PCR analysis using Kirisawa's PCR primers showed that 20 pooled samples were EHV-1 positive, but no samples were EHV-4 positive. Virus isolation was successful in all PCR positive samples, with a clearly visible CPE developing within 3–5 days after inoculation of cells (Table 1).

Amplification using ORF30-specific PCR and further digestion of PCR products with *Sal*I enzyme showed that two of the 20 EHV-1 positive isolates were the neuropathogenic variant *G2254* (10% of EHV-1 positive isolates, and 3.1% of total abortion cases), whereas 18 were the non-neuropathogenic variant *A2254* (90% of EHV-1 positive isolates, and 28.1% of all abortion cases).

Comparative nucleotide sequence analysis of the 380-bp fragment gene encoding the catalytic subunit (ORF30) of the viral DNA polymerase confirmed the presence of guanine at nucleotide position 2,254 in two isolates. The other EHV-1 isolates encoded adenine at the position 2,254 and were classified as non-neuropathogenic variants. No nucleotide substitution was found at position 2,258. The consensus alignment indicated that partial ORF30 sequences were identical to the sequences of appropriate reference strains of EHV-1: Ab4 (neuropathogenic) and V592 (non-neuropathogenic) (Figure 1).

Discussion

There have been no previous reports of EHM outbreaks in Poland, and no potentially neuropathogenic variants of EHV-1 have previously been identified [18]. We have shown, for the first time, that the neuropathogenic genotype of EHV-1 circulates in the horse population in Poland. There was a clear predominance of the non-neuropathogenic (90% of EHV-1 positive cases) over the neuropathogenic EHV-1 genotype (10% of EHV-1 positive cases) as a causative agent of abortions in Polish stud farms. This proportion is similar to the results of recent studies in which abortion was associated with the neuropathogenic variant of EHV-1 in 0.9% of abortion cases in Japan [19], 7% in Argentina [20], 8.9% in Central Kentucky of the US [9], 10.6% in Germany [21], and 25.9% in France [22].

In contrast to a few abortion outbreaks in Argentina and Germany that were associated with neurological signs in mares, there were no clinical signs indicating EHM in any case of aborted fetuses tested in this study. These results are not unusual as previous studies have proved that although the presence of the

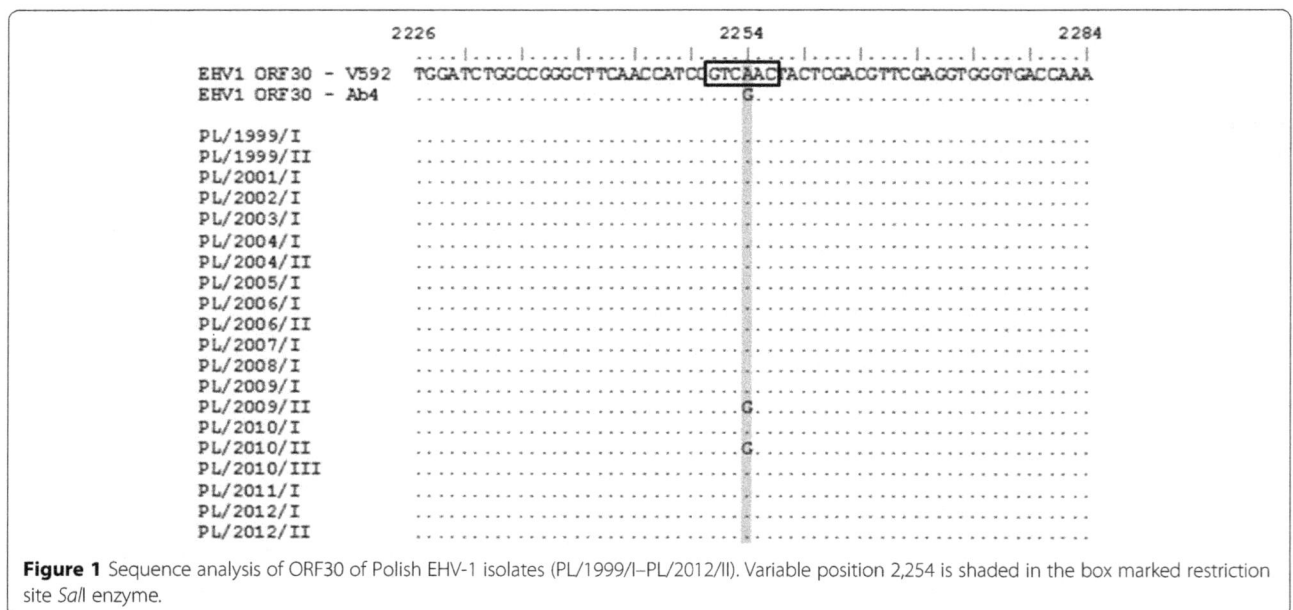

Figure 1 Sequence analysis of ORF30 of Polish EHV-1 isolates (PL/1999/I–PL/2012/II). Variable position 2,254 is shaded in the box marked restriction site *Sal*I enzyme.

neuropathogenic strain is a factor fostering an increase in EHM cases, it is not the only factor that determines the appearance of neurological disease in infected horses [23,24]. For example, a German study found that only two out of seven abortion cases caused by neuropathogenic EHV-1 strains were associated with EHM signs in pregnant mares [21]. Some studies have associated EHM with the presence of another substitution (adenine to cytosine) in ORF30 at the 2,258 position [9,21]; however, this was not detected in our study.

The EHV-1 isolates possessing a nucleotide substitution from A to G at the 2,254 position were detected in two distant provinces of Poland, hence it is unlikely that the abortions were caused by the same strain of the virus. As this study concentrated on abortion cases, only a fraction of the total EHV-1 infections in Poland were analyzed, whereas a previous study by Pronost et al. showed that the G2254 genotype could also be associated with respiratory disease [22]. It is also possible that some of our cases were caused by mixed infection with two viral strains. Allen et al. described the occurrence of dual infections in the Thoroughbred broodmare population, with both neuropathogenic and non-neuropathogenic strains involved [25]. A similar situation took place in the case of horses infected after natural exposure at a racetrack in California [26]. Unfortunately, the diagnostic techniques used in our study were not able to detect simultaneous infection with both genotypes.

Finally, it cannot be excluded that EHM cases may have already appeared in Poland, but were either not reported or not identified properly by veterinarians. Even if this assumption is wrong, the fact that the G2254 ORF30 variant of EHV-1 is present in the horse population means that the risk of EHM outbreaks in Poland should be taken into consideration.

Conclusion

The presented data demonstrate that the neuropathogenic genotype of EHV-1 is present in Polish stud farms. Of the 20 EHV-1 abortion isolates, the vast majority belonged to the non-neuropathogenic marker A2254 (18 out of 20 isolates, which was 90%), with only two out of the 20 isolates (10%) identified as the neuropathogenic genotype G2254. However, the presence of neuropathogenic EHV-1 strains in Polish studs suggests that the emergence of EHM cases in Poland is probable.

Availability of supporting data

The data sets supporting the results of this article are included within the article.

Competing interests

The authors declare that they have no competing interests.

Authors' contributions

JR designed the study, isolated viral strains, and prepared the manuscript. KS, WS, and GP carried out the laboratory work, molecular genetic studies, sequence analysis, and manuscript preparation. JFZ reviewed the manuscript. All authors read and approved the final manuscript.

Acknowledgments
The authors thank Elwira Orlowska and Malgorzata Glowacka for their technical assistance.

References

1. Paillot R, Case R, Ross J, Newton R, Nugent J. Equine herpes virus-1: virus, immunity and vaccines. Open Vet Sci J. 2008;2:68–91.
2. Harless W, Pusterla N. Equine herpesvirus 1 and 4 respiratory disease in the horse. Clin Tech Equine Pract. 2006;5:197–202.
3. Friday PA, Scarratt WK, Elvinger F, Timoney PJ, Bonda A. Ataxia and paresis with equine herpesvirus type 1 infection in a herd of riding school horses. J Vet Intern Med. 2000;14:197–201.
4. Henninger RW, Reed SM, Saville WJ, Allen GP, Hass GF, Kohn CW, et al. Outbreak of neurologic disease caused by equine herpesvirus-1 at a university equestrian center. J Vet Intern Med. 2007;21:157–65.
5. Edington N, Bridges CG, Patel JR. Endothelial cell infection and thrombosis in paralysis caused by equid herpesvirus-1: equine stroke. Arch Virol. 1986;90:111–24.
6. Nugent J, Birch-Machin I, Smith KC, Mumford JA, Swann Z, Newton JR, et al. Analysis of equid herpesvirus 1 strain variation reveals a point mutation of the DNA polymerase strongly associated with neuropathogenic versus nonneuropathogenic disease outbreaks. J Virol. 2006;80:4047–60.
7. Goodman LB, Loregian A, Perkins GA, Nugent J, Buckles EL, Mercorelli B, et al. A point mutation in a herpesvirus polymerase determines neuropathogenicity. PLoS Pathog. 2007;3:1583–92.
8. Perkins GA, Goodman LB, Tsujimura K, Van de Walle GR, Kim SG, Dubovi EJ, et al. Investigation of the prevalence of neurologic equine herpes virus type 1 (EHV-1) in a 23-year retrospective analysis (1984–2007). Vet Microbiol. 2009;139:375–8.
9. Smith KL, Allen GP, Branscum AJ, Cook RF, Vickers ML, Timoney PJ, et al. The increased prevalence of neuropathogenic strains of EHV-1 in equine abortions. Vet Microbiol. 2010;141:5–11.
10. van Maanen C, Sloet Van Oldruitenborgh Oosterbaan M, Damen EA, Derksen AGP. Neurological disease associated with EHV-1 infection in a riding school: clinical and virological characteristics. Equine Vet J. 2001;33:191–6.
11. Pronost S, Legrand L, Pitel PH, Wegge B, Lissens J, Freymuth F, et al. Outbreak of equine herpesvirus myeloencephalopathy in France: a clinical and molecular investigation. Tran Emer Dis. 2012;59:256–63.
12. Bazanow B, Jackulak N, Florek M, Staronowicz Z. Equid herpesvirus- associated abortion in Poland between 1977–2010. J Equine Vet Sci. 2011;32:747–51.
13. Frymus T, Kita J, Woyciechowska S, Ganowicz M. Foetal and neonatal foal losses on equine herpesvirus type 1 (EHV-1) infected farms before and after EHV-1 vaccination was introduced. Pol Arch Weter. 1986;26:7–14.
14. Rola J, Zmudzinski J. Equine herpesvirus type 1 (EHV-1) a cause of mare's abortions in Poland. Med Weter. 1997;53:268–9.
15. Woyciechowska S. Adaptacja krajowego wirusa zakaźnego ronienia klaczy, szczep Rac-Heraldia do chomików syryjskich. Med Dosw Mikrobiol. 1960;XII 3:255–63.
16. Kirisawa R, Endo A, Iwai H, Kawakami Y. Detection and identification of herpesvirus-1 and −4 by polymerase chain reaction. Vet Microbiol. 1993;36:57–67.
17. Allen GP. Antemortem detection of latent infection with neuropathogenic strains of equine herpesvirus-1 in horses. Am J Vet Res. 2006;67:1401–5.
18. Ploszay G, Rola J, Zmudzinski JF. Neurologic form of equine herpesvirus 1 infection as a new emerging infectious disease of horses. Med Weter. 2012;68:65–128.
19. Tsujimura K, Oyama T, Katayama Y, Muranaka M, Bannai H, Nemoto M, et al. Prevalence of equine herpesvirus type 1 strains of neuropathogenic genotype in a major breeding area of Japan. J Vet Med Sci. 2011;73:1663–7.

20. Vissani MA, Becerra ML, Olguin Perglione C, Tordoya MS, Mino S, Barrandeguy M. Neuropathogenic and non - neuropathogenic genotypes of Equid Herpesvirus type 1 in Argentina. Vet Microbiol. 2009;139:361–4.

21. Fritsche AK, Borchers K. Detection of neuropathogenic strains of Equid Herpesvirus 1 (EHV1) associated with abortions in Germany. Vet Microbiol. 2011;147:176–80.

22. Pronost S, Leon A, Legrand L, Fortier C, Miszczak F, Freymuth F, et al. Neuropathogenic and non - neuropathogenic variants of equine herpesvirus 1 in France. Vet Microbiol. 2010;145:329–33.

23. Allen GP. Risk factors for development of neurologic disease after experimental exposure to equine herpesvirus-1 in horses. Am J Vet Res. 2008;69:1595–600.

24. Pronost S, Cook RF, Fortier G, Timoney PJ, Balasuriya UBR. Relationship between equine herpesvirus-1 myeloencephalopathy and viral genotype. Equine Vet J. 2010;42:672–4.

25. Allen GP, Bolin DC, Bryant U, Carter CN, Giles RC, Harrison LR, et al. Prevalence of latent, neuropathogenic equine herpesvirus-1 in the Thoroughbred broodmare population of central Kentucky. Equine Vet J. 2008;40:105–10.

26. Pusterla N, Wilson WD, Mapes S, Finno C, Isbell D, Arthur RM, et al. Characterization of viral loads, strain and state of equine herpesvirus-1 using real- time PCR in horses following natural exposure at a racetrack in California. Vet J. 2009;179:230–9.

20

Local and systemic effect of transfection-reagent formulated DNA vectors on equine melanoma

Kathrin Mählmann[1], Karsten Feige[1], Christiane Juhls[2], Anne Endmann[2], Hans-Joachim Schuberth[3], Detlef Oswald[2], Mareu Hellige[1], Marcus Doherr[4] and Jessika-MV Cavalleri[1]*

Abstract

Background: Equine melanoma has a high incidence in grey horses. Xenogenic DNA vaccination may represent a promising therapeutic approach against equine melanoma as it successfully induced an immunological response in other species suffering from melanoma and in healthy horses. In a clinical study, twenty-seven, grey, melanoma-bearing, horses were assigned to three groups (n = 9) and vaccinated on days 1, 22, and 78 with DNA vectors encoding for equine (eq) IL-12 and IL-18 alone or in combination with either human glycoprotein (hgp) 100 or human tyrosinase (htyr). Horses were vaccinated intramuscularly, and one selected melanoma was locally treated by intradermal peritumoral injection. Prior to each injection and on day 120, the sizes of up to nine melanoma lesions per horse were measured by caliper and ultrasound. Specific serum antibodies against hgp100 and htyr were measured using cell based flow-cytometric assays. An Analysis of Variance (ANOVA) for repeated measurements was performed to identify statistically significant influences on the relative tumor volume. For post-hoc testing a Tukey-Kramer Multiple-Comparison Test was performed to compare the relative volumes on the different examination days. An ANOVA for repeated measurements was performed to analyse changes in body temperature over time. A one-way ANOVA was used to evaluate differences in body temperature between the groups. A p–value < 0.05 was considered significant for all statistical tests applied.

Results: In all groups, the relative tumor volume decreased significantly to 79.1 ± 26.91% by day 120 (p < 0.0001, Tukey-Kramer Multiple-Comparison Test). Affiliation to treatment group, local treatment and examination modality had no significant influence on the results (ANOVA for repeated measurements). Neither a cellular nor a humoral immune response directed against htyr or hgp100 was detected. Horses had an increased body temperature on the day after vaccination.

Conclusions: This is the first clinical report on a systemic effect against equine melanoma following treatment with DNA vectors encoding eqIL12 and eqIL18 and formulated with a transfection reagent. Addition of DNA vectors encoding hgp100 respectively htyr did not potentiate this effect.

Keywords: Horse, Melanoma, Interleukin, Glycoprotein 100, Tyrosinase, DNA vaccine

Background

Equine melanoma, a tumor of pigment producing cells, is the most common skin tumor in aging grey horses with a prevalence of up to 95% [1].

So far, conventional therapies such as surgical excision [2], cryosurgery [2], radiotherapy [3], or chemotherapy with cisplatin [4] or cimetidine [5] have not been curative in advanced cases. Obviously, there is need for innovative approaches to treat equine melanoma lesions of later stages.

Xenogenic DNA vaccination against the melanoma differentiation antigens glycoprotein (gp) 100 [6-9] and tyrosinase (tyr) [10-13] have been shown to overcome auto-tolerance and to elicit an immune response in mice, dogs, and humans [10-16] and a clinical antitumoral effect in mice and dogs [10-12,14,16].

In clinically healthy horses, specific antibodies at relatively low levels and a variable cellular immune response were elicited upon vaccination with a plasmid encoding the human tyrosinase (htyr) [17]. There are no reports about the immunogenicity of human gp100 (hgp100) to

* Correspondence: jessika.cavalleri@tiho-hannover.de
[1]Clinic for Horses, University of Veterinary Medicine Hannover, Foundation, Hannover, Germany
Full list of author information is available at the end of the article

horses, and clinical study results on the anti-melanoma effect of DNA-encoded xenogenic tyrosinase and gp100 in grey horses have not been published to date.

Cytokines such as Interleukin (IL) 12 and IL18 have been applied to increase cellular immunity and reduce angiogenesis in neoplasms [18-23] and were shown to have synergistic antitumoral effects [20,24-26].

To date, all immunological melanoma treatment efforts in horses were of limited effect. A local effect was achieved with DNA encoding human [27] or either eqIL12 or eqIL18 [28]. Thus, combination of these interleukins and addition of either hgp100 or htyr, all encoded by DNA vectors, seemed to be a promising approach.

The aim of the present clinical study was to evaluate whether or not treatment with eqIL12 in combination with eqIL18 each encoded by DNA vectors has a local and systemic anti-tumoral effect on naturally occurring melanoma in grey horses, and whether or not this effect is augmented by DNA vaccination against the xenogenic melanoma differentiation antigens hgp100 and htyr, respectively.

Methods
Patients
Twenty-seven horses with one or more melanoma lesions and unaffected general condition were included in the study. Informed consent was obtained from all animal owners. Horses were not treated with any medication at least two weeks prior to immunisation.

Pre-trial evaluation included a physical examination, hematology, and blood biochemistry profile. Age, breed, gender, degree of greying and number of melanoma lesions were documented (Table 1). The diagnosis of melanoma was confirmed by examination of fine needle aspirates by board certified pathologists in 20 of 27 horses. In the remaining horses, diagnosis was made clinically with regard to typical localisation and appearance of the lesions, as the owners did not agree to aspiration biopsy. Patients were treated in the Clinic for Horses of the University of Veterinary Medicine Hannover, Foundation, from November 2009 to July 2010 in accordance with the ethical guidelines of the law of animal welfare approved by the "Lower Saxony State Office for Consumer Protection and Food Safety, LAVES" approval No. 08/1522.

Horses were assigned to three treatment groups by a stratified biphasic model to achieve equal distribution of age (<15 years or ≥ 15 years) and number of melanoma lesions (<7 or ≥ 7 melanoma lesions).

Production of MIDGE-Th1 vectors
Minimalistic immunogenically defined gene expression (MIDGE) vectors with a small peptide ("Th1") attached were produced by MOLOGEN AG (Berlin, Germany) as previously described [29] from plasmids coding for hgp 100 (pcDNA3gp100, courtesy of Dr. Robbins und Dr. Rosenberg, National Cancer Institute), htyr (pMCV1.4htyr, MOLOGEN AG), eqIL12 and eqIL18 (pUSErIRESeqIL12 and 18, courtesy of L. Nicholson, University of Glasgow, via Intervet International, Boxmeer, The Netherlands). Oligonucleotides coding for the IL-1beta receptor antagonist protein (ILRAP) (Microsynth, Balgach, Switzerland) were ligated to the IL18 gene (see Additional file 1).

Preparation of MIDGE-Th1/SAINT-18 complexes
MIDGE-Th1/SAINT-18 (1-methyl-4-(cis-9-dioleyl) methyl-pyridinium-chloride, Synvolux Therapeutics, Groningen, The Netherlands) complexes were prepared as described by Endmann et al. [30]. MIDGE-Th1/SAINT-18 complexes were formed at a ratio of 1 mg DNA dissolved in PBS to 0.75 µmol SAINT-18. The PBS concentration in the final mixture was 1× PBS.

Treatment
Three groups of 9 grey horses each were treated on days 1, 22 and 78 with MIDGE-Th1 vectors coding for eqIL12 and ILRAP-eqIL18 alone or in combination with hgp100MIDGE-Th1 or htyrMIDGE-Th1 (Table 2). Throughout the study period the test items were blinded by a color code and unblinded upon completion of data analysis only.

For each treatment, 0.5 ml (half of the vaccine dose) were injected intradermally (i.d.) peritumorally around one pre-selected, well-measureable and easily-accessible melanoma ("locally treated melanoma"). Injection was performed using a 25 G cannula and a 1 ml syringe. Another 0.5 ml (the second half of the dose) were administered intramuscularly (i.m.) into the semimembranosus muscle using a 22 G cannula and a 1 ml syringe. The identical injection sites were used for the first, second and third immunisation.

Clinical evaluation for determination of response to treatment
In each horse the locally treated melanoma and up to eight additional melanoma lesions ("non-locally treated melanoma lesions") were monitored prior to each injection and on day 120 using calipers and ultrasound (LogiQ P5, General Electrics, Connecticut, USA). The ultrasonographic measurements were performed independently by two examiners. All measurements were performed in triplicates. The length (mm, longest diameter), width (mm, perpendicular to length), and depth (mm, only by ultrasound) were documented and the tumor volume (cm^3) calculated (volume = length × width^2 × 0.5 for caliper measurements and volume = length × width × depth × 0.5 for ultrasonographic measurements).

The relative volumes were calculated in reference to the volume on day one (pre-dosing), which was defined

Table 1 Patient demographics and group assignment

Treatment (encoded genes)	Horse ID	Age (years)	Breed	Sex	Color	Number of Melanoma	FNA	Localisation
eqIL12, eqIL18	1	22	Warmblood	m	flea bitten	>7	no	vt, mu, o
	2	18	Warmblood	g	flea bitten	1	yes	vt
	7	20	Icelandic-Horse	m	white	>7	yes	pa, vt, ge
	9	12	Berber	m	white	>7	yes	pa, vt, ge, p
	12	11	Carmargue	m	dappled	>7	no	vt, pa, ge, p
	13	11	Shetland	g	dappled	3	no	pa, ge, vt
	17	17	Andalusian	m	white	>7	yes	pa, vt, ge, mu, o
	23	14	Arabian	g	flea-bitten	1	yes	p
	24	16	Warmblood	m	flea-bitten	>7	yes	pa, vt, ge
eqIL12, eqIL18, hgp100	3	18	unclassified	g	flea bitten	1	yes	pa
	5	12	Andalusian	m	dappled	>7	yes	pa, vt, mu, p, o
	6	18	Andalusian	s	white	>7	no	e, vt, ge
	8	15	Berber	s	white	>7	yes	pa, vt
	15	14	Andalusian	s	white	>7	no	pa, vt
	18	16	Warmblood	m	white	>7	yes	pa, vt, ge
	19	15	Arabian	g	flea-bitten	>7	yes	p
	22	14	Warmblood	m	flea-bitten	2	no	pa, vt
	27	22	Icelandic-Horse	m	flea-bitten	>7	yes	pa, vt, ge
eqIL12, eqIL18, htyr	4	19	Arabian	s	flea bitten	>7	yes	pa, vt
	10	15	Arabian	s	white	>7	yes	pa, vt, mu
	11	20	Carmargue	s	white	4	no	vt
	14	15	Shetland	m	white	>7	no	vt
	16	13	Warmblood	m	flea-bitten	2	yes	pa, vt
	20	22	Trakehner	g	white	>7	yes	pa, vt
	21	19	Arabian	g	white	1	yes	vt
	25	13	Arabian	m	white	>7	yes	pa, vt, ge, mu, o
	26	11	Irish horse (Hunter)	g	white	1	yes	vt

Legend:

m: mare

g: gelding

s: stallion

FNA: fine needle aspirate

vt: ventral tail

p: parotid region

ge: genitals

pa: perianal

e: eyelid

mu: muscle

o: other regions

Table 2 Treatment substances administered to horses of the three treatment groups on days 1, 22 and 78

Vaccine component	Dose per injection		
	Group eqIL12/18	Group hgp100	Group htyr
MIDGE-Th1 eqIL12	200 µg	200 µg	200 µg
MIDGE-Th1 eqILRAPIL18	200 µg	200 µg	200 µg
MIDGE-Th1 hgp100	-	500 µg	-
MIDGE-Th1 htyr	-	-	500 µg
SAINT 18	0.35 µmol	0.675 µmol	0.675 µmol

as 100%. For all recorded non–locally treated melanoma lesions of each horse, a mean value per time point was calculated to statistically evaluate the effect on these tumors, i.e. the systemic effect of the treatment. Furthermore, the change of tumor volume was calculated by subtraction of the relative volume on day 1 (100%) from the relative volume on day 120 (%), with a negative value implying tumor reduction and a positive value standing for tumor growth.

These measurements and calculations were used in previous studies investigating the effect of gene therapies against equine melanoma [28] and were found to be appropriate for this mostly slow growing tumor and for comparability with aforementioned studies.

Clinical evaluation of safety of treatment

Horses were hospitalized for 3 days after each injection. Safety and tolerability of the treatment were evaluated by clinical examination, hematologic and blood biochemistry profile: a general clinical examination was performed before injection, on each day of hospitalisation and on day 120. A hematologic examination was realized before injection, on the 3rd day after injection and on day 120, a biochemistry profile was accomplished before each injection and on day 120. The injection sites were monitored for signs of local inflammation and depigmentation. Other pigmented skin areas (eyelids, nostrils) were observed for signs of depigmentation.

Measurement of the immune response induced by vaccination

To measure specific serum antibodies against hgp100 and htyr a cell based, flow cytometric antibody assay was performed. Therefore, sera from the patients were obtained before each injection and on day 120. The sera were incubated with hgp100 and htyr plasmid transfected HEK 293 cells. Evaluation was performed by flow cytometry after staining bounded antibodies with a secondary antibody (see Appendix A, Additional file 1).

At any time post-vaccination a humoral response was considered positive when fluorescence increased ≥ 3

standard deviations over the mean value at baseline and had an absolute value > 0.1%.

The establishment of an assay to detect a potential T-cell response induced by the vaccine was not followed up after transfection rates of primary autologous dermal cells, derived from skin of patients were inconsistent and low. Thus expression of antigens was insufficient to induce T cell activation after co-culture of transfected cells and peripheral blood mononuclear cells (data not shown).

In vitro expression of transgenes eqIL12, eqIL18, htyr and hgp100 on mRNA level

Chinese hamster ovary (CHO)-K1 cells (ATCC CCL-61) were cultured in Ham`s F12 (10% FCS, 1% Penicillin/Streptomycin) medium at 37°C in 5% $CO_2$. Prior to transfection the culture medium was removed, cells were washed once with PBS, then detached with trypsin/EDTA and 0.12E + 06 cells per well suspended in 500 µL transfection medium (Ham`s F12 cell culture medium w/o additives). 100 µL of each DNA/SAINT-18 complex were prepared as follows: MIDGE-Th1 vectors were mixed with previously vortexed SAINT-18 (0.75 mM) at a ratio of 5 µl SAINT-18 per µg DNA and filled up to 100 µL with HBS. Complexes were allowed to form for 5 min. Cells were incubated with complexes containing a) MIDGE-Th1 vectors encoding eqIL12 and eqIL18 (0.5 µg per vector), b) MIDGE-Th1 vectors encoding eqIL12 (0.5 µg), eqIL18 (0.5 µg) and htyr (1.25 µg), c) MIDGE-Th1 vectors encoding eqIL12 (0.5 µg), eqIL18 (0.5 µg) and hgp100 (1.25 µg) and d) MIDGE-Th1 vectors encoding eGFP (1.25 µg) as positive control for the transfection method and CHO-K1 expression efficiency (measured by FACS). Salmon sperm DNA (Invitrogen) served as negative control item. The DNA SAINT-18 complexes were added to the cells, followed by a brief centrifugation step. After 2.5 hours of incubation, 1 mL of complete Ham`s F12 was added and cells incubated for 24 hours at 37°C in 5% $CO_2$. Cells were harvested and detached as described above, centrifuged and pellets stored on ice until RNA was extracted using the NucleoSpin RNA II Kit (Macherey & Nagel) as described in provider`s instructions.

mRNA specific Reverse Transcription quantitative PCR (RT-qPCR) was performed with 100 ng mRNA per reaction using the TaqMan® RNA-to-CT 1-Step Kit (Applied Biosystems) according to manufacturer`s instructions. Primers and probes (TIBMOLBIOL, Berlin) had specific sequences to generate and detect cDNA of eqIL12-p35 (fw 5`-AAATTGCTAACGCAGTCAGT-3`, rv 5`-GCTAGCTCCGGAGTT-3`, probe FAM-CGACTGATCACAGGGGTACC-BBQ), eqIL12-p40 (fw 5`-AAATTGCTAACGCAGTCAGT-3`, rv 5`-GACCAACCACTGGTGAC-3`, probe FAM-CGACTGATCACAGGGGTACC-BBQ), eqIL18

(fw 5`-AAATTGCTAACGCAGTCAGT-3`, rv 5`-GAGGC
CTCTGCAGATT-3`, probe FAM-CGACTGATCACAGGG
GTACC_BBQ), hgp100 (fw 5`-AAATTGCTAACGCAGTC
AGT-3`, rv 5`-AGCCAAATGAAGAAGGCATC –3`, probe
FAM-CGACTGATCACAGGGGTACC-BBQ) and htyr (fw
5`-AAATTGCTAACGCAGTCAGT-3`, rv 5`-CCACAGCA
GGCAGTAC –3`, probe FAM-CGACTGATCACAGGGGT
ACC-BBQ). Samples were measured in technical triplicates.

Statistical analysis

An Analysis of Variance (ANOVA) for repeated measurements was performed to identify statistically significant
influences on the relative tumor volume. Parameters included in the model were the individual horse, examination day (1, 22, 78, 120), treatment group (eqIL12/18,
hgp100, htyr), locally treated versus non-locally treated
melanoma lesions and examination method (caliper and
ultrasound with differentiation between the two examiners). After starting with the full model, non-significant
variables and correlations were eliminated stepwise.

For post-hoc testing a Tukey-Kramer Multiple-Comparison
Test was performed to compare the relative volumes
on the different examination days.

An ANOVA for repeated measurements was performed
to analyse changes in body temperature over time. A one-
way ANOVA was used to evaluate differences in body
temperature between the groups.

A p–value < 0.05 was considered significant for all statistical tests applied.

Statistical analyses were performed using the statistical
software JMP 8.0 (SAS Institute Inc., Cary, NC, USA)
and NCSS (NCSS, Kaysville, Utha, USA).

Results

Safety of treatment

Based on the clinical examinations of the horses the
vaccine was safe and well tolerated. The only consistent
abnormal finding was a significant increase in body
temperature on the day after injection (p < 0.00001,
Figure 1). No difference in body temperature between
the groups (p = 0.98) was observed. Hematology and
blood biochemistry profile revealed no abnormalities at
any time point. At the intradermal injection sites (3x27
injections = 81 injections in total), horses showed mild
subcutaneous swelling (81/81 injections), reddening (10/
81), exudation (7/81) and mild ulceration (2/81). These
signs of acute inflammation occurred within the first three
days after injection and resolved until the next treatment
except in horse 11 were they persisted for 21 days after
the first injection. Twentysix of 27 horses developed local
dermal depigmentation restricted to the intradermal injection sites, only. The depigmentation was first observed
after 22 days in 23 horses and after 81 days in 3 more
horses. There were no signs of depigmentation observed

in the monitored pigmented regions or melanoma lesions.
No differences of local reactions were noted between
treatment groups. No local reactions were observed at the
sites of intramuscular injections.

Caliper and ultrasonographic measurements of tumor size

In total 136 melanoma lesions (groups IL12/18: n = 42,
hgp100: n = 50, htyr: n = 44) were measured. After stepwise elimination of insignificant variables and correlations the only variable influencing the relative volume
was the examination day (p = 0.00001) and an individual
effect of the horses. Post-hoc testing showed a significant decrease of the relative melanoma-volume over
time. Mean relative volume of all measured melanoma
decreased significantly to 71.5 ± 29.73% - equalling to
28.5% of tumor volume reduction - as measured by caliper and 87.0 ± 24.42% (13% tumor volume reduction),
82.1 ± 28.02% (17.9% tumor volume reduction) as measured by ultrasonography (ultrasound examiner 1, ultrasound examiner 2) (Figure 2, Table 3). The relative
tumor volume ranged from 0 to 205% (caliper) and 0 to
194, 196% (ultrasound examiner 1, ultrasound examiner
2) at day 120.

Measurement of the humoral response induced by vaccination

No specific antibodies against htyr or hgp100 were detected in equine sera collected on days 1, 22, 78 and 120
(see Additional file 2: Figure S1).

Proof of function of DNA vectors: *In vitro* expression

The expression of all encoded genes was proven on
mRNA level after transfection of cells *in vitro*. MIDGE-
Th1 vectors were used in mixtures at weight ratios equal
to those administered to the patients and complexed with
SAINT-18. The amount of cDNA generated from mRNA
was analysed in a RT-qPCR assay using a plasmid standard, allowing for detection and estimation of the mRNA
expression levels produced from individual transgenes.
eqIL12, eqIL18, htyr and hgp100 were shown to be
expressed from all respective mixtures of MIDGE-Th1
vectors (Table 4).

Discussion

In the present clinical study, three treatments with mixtures of MIDGE-Th1 eqIL12 and ILRAP-eqIL18 alone
or in combination with MIDGE-Th1 hgp100 or MIDGE-
Th1 htyr, all complexed with the cationic transfection
agent SAINT-18, resulted in a moderate reduction of the
relative volume of examined melanoma lesions (28.5%).
The lack of differences in treatment effects between the
three groups suggests that MIDGE-Th1 hgp100 or

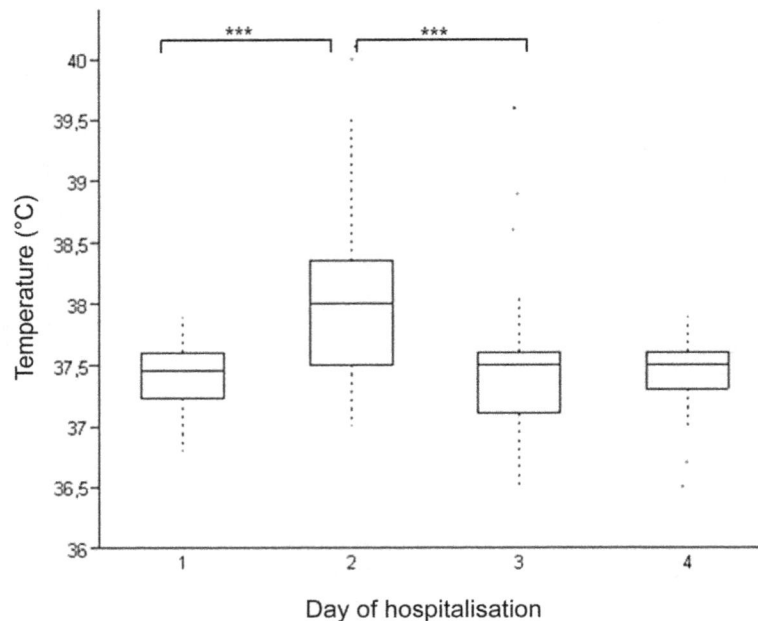

Figure 1 Daily rectal temperatures (in °C) measured in 27 horses before each injection (1) and on three consecutive days. There was a significant transient increase in the temperature on the first day after injection (Tukey-Kramer Multiple Comparison Test). The center horizontal line of the box plot marks the median of the sample. The edges of the box mark the first and third quartiles. The dotted lines define the 75th percentile plus 1.5 times the interquartile range (IQR) and the 25th percentile minus 1.5 times IQR. The singular dots represent the outside values. *** Significant difference (p ≤ 0.0001).

MIDGE-Th1 htyr did not augment the effect of the other components of the treatment.

In former studies on equine melanoma the placebo group showed progression or no change in size during the study period of 64 days [28,31]. A placebo group was not included in this study because a positive anti-tumoral effect of treatment with interleukin-12 and –18 DNA had been demonstrated in these earlier studies. Ethical considerations regarding withholding any potentially effective treatment from client-owned horses precluded inclusion of an untreated cohort. However, it is reasonable to attribute the tumor size reduction observed in this study to the treatment, as no spontaneous regression of equine melanoma lesions has been reported up to date. Importantly, the size reduction was not only seen in locally treated but also in non-locally treated melanoma lesions indicating a systemic effect of the treatment. Comparing the development of volume of peritumorally treated and distant melanoma lesions, there was no statistically significant difference observed. The systemic effect might be based on a primarily unspecific immune response that, in the presence of melanoma antigens, converted into an anti-melanoma specific immune response. However, this is a hypothesis only since such aspecific immune response has not been detected in our assays.

The present study was the first to use a combination of DNA vectors encoding eqIL12 and eqIL18 for the therapy of equine melanoma. Previously either eqIL18 or eqIL12 DNA injected intratumorally induced some size reduction in equine melanoma lesions [28] but systemic effects were not evaluated. Experimental studies in mice [24,25] have proven synergistic effects of IL12 and IL18, suppressing collateral [26] or distant tumor growth [20].

In the present study the cationic-amphiphilic transfection agent SAINT-18 was used to enhance expression *in vivo*. SAINT-18 has been reported to strengthen the immune response against antigens encoded by MIDGE-Th1 vectors [32,30]. While the complexed DNA was very well tolerated in mice and rats [30], in the horses of the study presented here it caused local inflammation at the site of intradermal injection. This could be either explained by an inflammatory reaction triggered by the two expressed cytokines eqIL12 and eqIL18 upon transfection of dermal cells, or respectively and by a higher sensitivity of horses against DNA complexed with SAINT-18. In mice, expressed cytokines were found to mediate antitumoral effects by reduction of angiogenesis [20] as well as improved cellular immunity represented by increased IFNγ production and enhanced cytotoxic T- and Natural Killer cell activities [25]. In addition to the local reaction, horses developed fever on the day post injection,

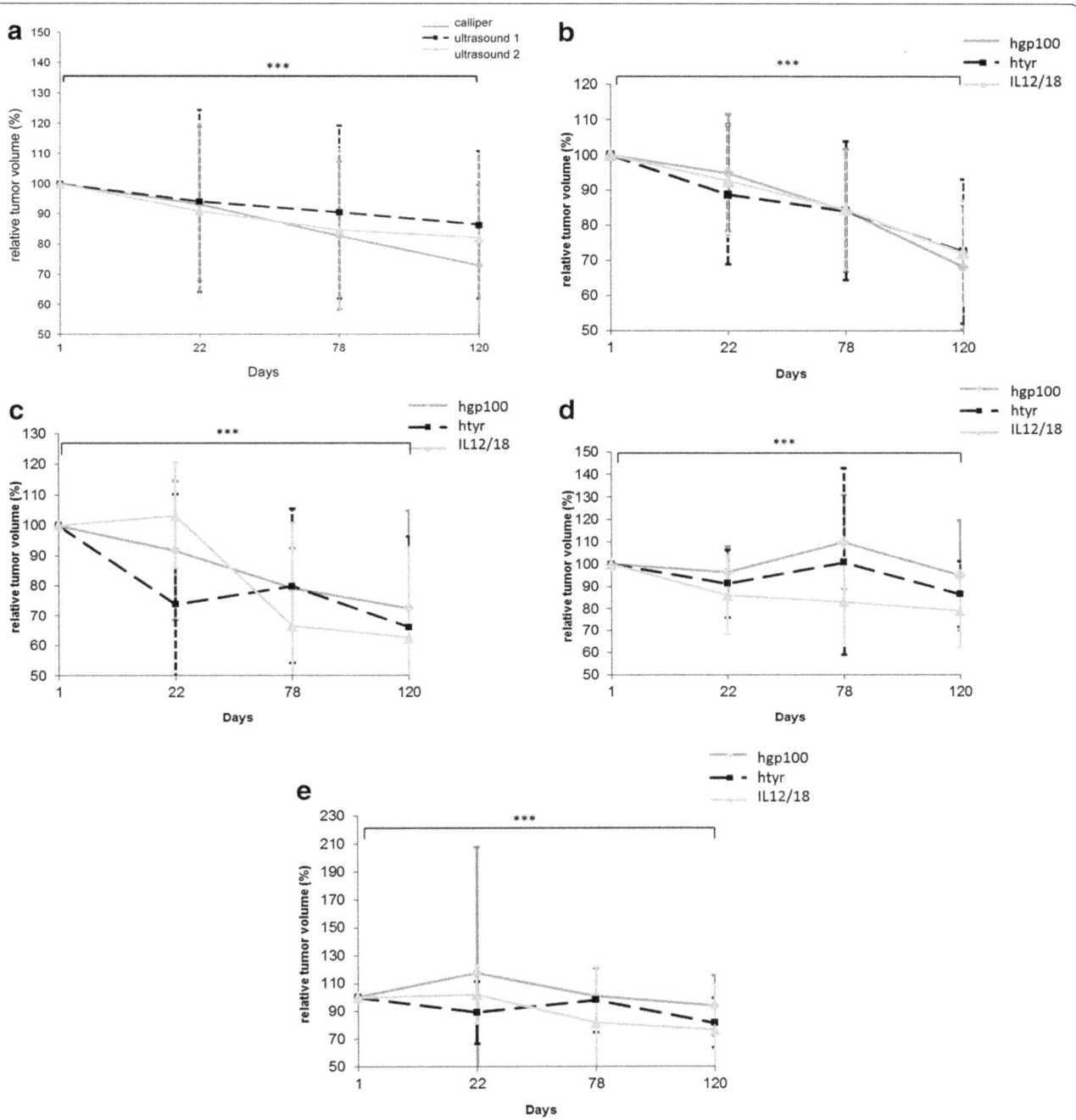

Figure 2 (See legend on next page.)

(See figure on previous page.)
Figure 2 a): Relative volumes (%) of locally and non-locally treated melanoma lesions calculated by caliper and ultrasound measurements (ultrasound examiner 1 and 2) on days 1, 22, 78 and 120. Relative volume of melanoma lesions decreased significantly from day 1 to 120 (Tukey-Kramer Multiple Comparisons Test). There were no statistically significant differences detected between the treatment groups, locally or non-locally treated melanoma lesions and measurement modality/ultrasound examiner. Dots, squares and triangles represent the median and the vertical lines the standard deviations. *** Significant difference (p ≤ 0.0001). **b)**: Relative volumes (%) of non-locally treated melanoma lesions calculated by caliper measurements on days 0, 22, 78 and 120. Relative volume of all non-locally treated melanoma lesions decreased significantly on day 120. There were no statistically significant differences detected between the treatment groups. *** Significant difference (p ≤ 0.0001). **c)**: Relative volumes (%) of locally treated melanoma lesions calculated by caliper measurements on days 0, 22, 78 and 120. Relative volume of all locally treated melanoma lesions decreased significantly on day 120. There were no statistically significant differences detected between the treatment groups. . *** Significant difference (p ≤ 0.0001). **d)**: Relative volumes (%) of non-locally treated melanoma lesions calculated by ultrasonographic measurements on days 0, 22, 78 and 120. Relative volume of all non-locally treated melanoma lesions decreased significantly on day 120. There were no statistically significant differences detected between the treatment groups. . *** Significant difference (p ≤ 0.0001). **e)**: Relative volumes (%) of locally treated melanoma lesions calculated by ultrasonographic measurements on days 0, 22, 78 and 120. Relative volume of all locally treated melanoma lesions decreased significantly on day 120. There were no statistically significant differences detected between the treatment groups. . *** Significant difference (p ≤ 0.0001).

Table 3 Relative volume of melanoma lesions measured by calipers in individual horses on Day 120, and number of new lesions by Day 120

Treatment (encoded genes)	Horse ID	% of reduction of the tumor volumes at day 120 in reference to the volume on day 1		Number of new lesions
		Peritumoral treated melanoma lesion	Distant melanoma lesions	
eqIL12, eqIL18	1	−16	−35,- 31,-30,-17, 2, 7, 10, 23	0
	2	−38	−40	0
	7	−33	−69, −7, −4	0
	9	2	−42, −24, −16	0
	12	−35	−78, −49, −46, −42, −26	0
	13	0	−39, −32	0
	17	−43	−40, −11, −8	0
	23	−47	-	0
	24	−26	−40, −21, −19, −12, −8, −4, −3, −3	0
eqIL12, eqIL18, hgp100	3	48	-	0
	5	−46	−56, −50, −36, 6	0
	6	−31	−75, −61, −40, −33, −6	0
	8	−59	−56, −49, −31, −31, −23, −15, 9, 22	0
	15	−46	−58, −43, −37, −23, −27, −21, 0, 0	0
	18	−16	−53, −41, −35, −25, −24, −23, −21, −20	0
	19	−43	−36	0
	22	−8	−47	0
	27	−45	−73, −45, −23, −15, −12, 0	0
eqIL12, eqIL18, htyr	4	−59	−79, −50, −32, −27, −24, −14, −12, 105	0
	10	−79	−65, −42, −32, −32, −22, −7, −5, 33	0
	11	−25	−58, −56, −46	0
	14	−71	−46, −32, −31	0
	16	−1	−33	0
	20	−20	−55, −46, −17, −15, −9, −5, −3, 12	0
	21	−38	-	0
	25	−18	−38, −30, −5, −15	0
	26	7	-	0

Table 4 Results of RT-qPCR to evaluate *in vitro* expression of transgenes from MIDGE-Th1 vectors encoding eqIL12, eqIL18, htyr and hgp100

MIDGE-Th1	Estimated mRNA/cDNA copy numbers per transgene (Ct values)				
Vectors [µg]	eqIL12-p35	eqIL12-p40	eqIL18	htyr	hgp100
eqIL12, eqIL18 [0.5 + 0.5]	1.14 + E03(27)	1.52 + E04(23)	3.16 + E03(25)	< LOD	< LOD
eqIL12, eqIL18, htyr [0.5 + 0.5 + 1.25]	1.01 + E03(28)	2.10 + E04(23)	5.23 + E03(25)	3.01 + E04(22)	< LOD
eqIL12, eqIL18, gp100 [0.5 + 0.5 + 1.25]	9.10 + E02(28)	9.79 + E03(24)	1.98 + E03(26)	< LOD	1.30 + E04(23)

LOD (limit of detection): = < 25 copies/reaction.

a systemic reaction to the treatment. Dow et al. [33] showed that i.v. injections of plasmid DNA complexed with lipid-protamine with non-coding DNA, resulted in local inflammation of the lung and other organs of mice. Thus, it is possible that in the present study fever and the local inflammation were in part induced by the complexes of DNA and transfection agent. In mice injection of SAINT-18 formulated DNA was tolerated well. Neither local nor systemic signs of intolerance were observed [30]. The use of SAINT-18 in pigs proved to enhance their humoral immune response to DNA vaccination. The study did not mention adverse side effects of the transfection reagent [32]. However both, the fever as well as the signs of acute inflammation were transient and are therefore considered not to be a serious drawback regarding the safety of the vaccination. As Dow et al. [33,34] showed also that lipoplexes with DNA encoding IL12 induced a more effective antitumor response than lipoplexes with non-coding plasmid DNA in mice the effect of the DNA-SAINT-18-complex might have potentially enhanced the antitumoral effect of the Interleukins.

The tumor size reduction in the present study was moderate and – according to the Response Evaluation Criteria In Solid Tumors (RECIST) [35] or immune-related Response Criteria (irRC) [36] used in human medicine - would not be considered as tumor regression but as stable disease. However, Wolchok et al. consider stable disease as a positive therapeutic outcome in cancer immunotherapy [36].

Dosages of 100, 500 and 1500 µg plasmid DNA for hgp100 in humans [8] and for htyr in dogs [12] successfully induced detectable immune responses. In the studies of Lembcke et al. [17] and Phillips et al. [37] a dosage of only 100 µg plasmid induced a measurable, though variable and relatively weak, immune response in nontumor-bearing healthy horses. Thus the doses used in our study, i.e. 500 µg per antigen encoding MIDGE-Th1 vector per application should have been appropriate to induce a detectable immune response. Moreover, MIDGE-vectors are devoid of plasmid backbone DNA and therefore have a smaller molecule size, so their effective transgene dose per microgram DNA is much higher than that of conventional plasmids [30].

Tyrosinase and gp100 were found to be (over-)expressed in equine melanoma lesions [32,38,39]. Homology between equine and human proteins is comparable to the proteins of mice compared to human for gp100 [75.5% [16]] and canine tyrosinase as well as the mouse and human equivalent [84.4% and 87.5% [12]]. Since xenogenic DNA vaccination encoding these proteins in mice and dogs induced an antitumoral immune response [10-12,14,16] it can be assumed that the proteins chosen and the difference in the amino acid sequence are adequate.

The vaccination interval used in the recent study is comparable to immunisation strategies for infectious diseases and also to a therapeutic vaccination protocol against melanoma in humans [40]. However, vaccination against tumors generally elicits a weaker immunity than vaccination against infectious diseases [41]. In other studies, in which an immunological response was successfully induced, more frequent application schemes for therapeutical antitumor vaccines [8,12,13] or cytokine gene therapy were used [42]. Lembcke et al. [17] vaccinated healthy horses four times with human tyrosinase DNA every two weeks, resulting in the successful induction of specific antibodies and IFNγ producing cells. They stated that the altered immunologic status of tumor-bearing patients (tumor tolerance) might make it more challenging to induce a specific immune response to tumor antigens than in healthy animals [17].

No specific humoral response could be observed in the present study.. In future studies additional tests to evaluate the cellular immune response [17] might give additional information about immunological mechanisms. However, in contrast to studies by Lembcke et al. [17] and Phillips et al. [37], we treated melanoma-bearing horses which might have developed an immune tolerance to gp100 and tyrosinase previously. To overcome this specific immune tolerance, higher DNA doses encoding xenogenic antigens and/or a more condensed immunisation schedule than in the present study might be necessary to induce a detectable immune response.

Conclusions

In the present study, treatment of horses with MIDGE-Th1 vectors encoding eqIL12 and ILRAP-eqIL18 alone or in combination with MIDGE-Th1 vectors encoding hgp100 or human htyr, all complexed with the transfection agent SAINT-18 resulted in a measurable systemic antitumoral effect on equine melanoma lesions. To our knowledge this is the first report on a systemic antitumoral effect against equine melanoma upon treatment with DNA vectors.

Because no specific immune response was detected, it remains to be elucidated whether this systemic antitumoral effect was caused by interleukins expressed from the DNA vectors, or an unspecific immune reaction to the combination of DNA and transfection reagent.

In future studies, a stronger anti-tumoral effect as well as a detectable specific immune response may be induced by an increased vaccine dose and/or an improved dosing schedule. Additionally, more sensitive immune assays should be applied to characterize the immune response in detail.

Additional files

> **Additional file 1: Contains supplementary text file 1.**
>
> **Additional file 2: Figure S1.** No specific antibodies were detected in serum samples from vaccinated horses on days 1, 22, 78 and 120.

Abbreviations
ANOVA: Analysis of variance; DNA: Deoxyribonucleic acid; cDNA: complementary deoxyribonucleic acid; CHO: Chinese hamster ovary; EDTA: Ethylenediaminetetraacetic acid; eGFP: enhanced green fluorescent protein; eq: equine; FACS: Fluorescence-activates cell sorting; FCS: Fetal calf serum; Gp: Glycoprotein; Hgp: Human glycoprotein; Htyr: Human tyrosinase; i.d.: intradermally; i.m.: intramuscularly; IL: Interleukin; ILRAP: IL-1beta receptor antagonist protein; irRC: immune-related Response Criteria; MIDGE: Minimalistic immunogenically defined gene expression; mRNA: messenger ribonucleic acid; PBS: Phosphate buffered saline; RECIST: Response Evaluation Criteria In Solid Tumors; RNA: Ribonucleic acid; RT-qPCR: Reverse transcription quantitative polymerase chain reaction; Tyr: Tyrosinase.

Competing interests
Christiane Juhls, Detlef Oswald and Anne Endmann are employees of Mologen AG but have no additional financial interests. Mologen AG owns a patent for MIDGE-Th1 vectors (PCT/DE02/03798P74). The other authors have no financial interest in the subject matter or materials discussed in this manuscript.

Authors' contributions
KM, HJS, KF and JMVC designed the concept of the study and the manuscript. KM and JMVC conducted the experiments of the present study. KM and MH did the ultrasonographic measurements of the tumors. CJ, AE, and DO designed the treatment constructs and determined the application details. MD performed the statistical analysis. All authors contributed to the critical revision and finalization of the manuscript. All authors read and approved the final manuscript.

Acknowledgements
We thank Silke Schöneberg and Udo Rabe from the Immunology Unit, University of Veterinary Medicine Hannover, Foundation for the support in the planning of the immunological investigations, Katrin Buettner for support in generating the expression cassettes and Nadine Gollinge of Mologen AG for mRNA analysis. The participation of the owners of the patients is gratefully appreciated.
Preliminary results were presented as an oral presentation at the 4th Vaccine and ISV Annual Global Congress, 3–5 October 2010 in Vienna, Austria and at the 5th Congress of the European College of Equine Internal Medicine, 2–4 February 2012 in Edinburgh, UK.

Author details
[1]Clinic for Horses, University of Veterinary Medicine Hannover, Foundation, Hannover, Germany. [2]Mologen AG, Berlin, Germany. [3]Immunology Unit, University of Veterinary Medicine Hannover, Foundation, Hannover, Germany. [4]Institute for Veterinary Epidemiology and Biostatistics, Free University of Berlin, Berlin, Germany.

References
1. Seltenhammer MH, Simhofer H, Scherzer S, Zechner R, Curik I, Solkner J, et al. Equine melanoma in a population of 296 grey Lipizzaner horses. Equine Vet J. 2003;35:153–7.
2. Pilsworth RC, Knottenbelt D. Melanoma. Equine vet Educ. 2006;18:228–30.
3. Montes LF, Vaughan JT, Ramer G. Equine melanoma. J Cutan Pathol. 1997;6:234–5.
4. Theon AP, Wilson WD, Magdesian KG, Pusterla N, Snyder JR, Galuppo LD. Long-term outcome associated with intratumoral chemotherapy with cisplatin for cutaneous tumors in equidae: 573 cases (1995–2004). J Am Vet Med Assoc. 2007;230:1506–13.
5. Laus F, Cerquetella M, Paggi E, Ippedico G, Argentieri M, Castellano G, et al. Evaluation of Cimetidine as a therapy for dermal melanomatosis in grey horse. Isr J Vet Med. 2010;65:48–52.
6. Hawkins WG, Gold JS, Dyall R, Wolchok JD, Hoos A, Bowne WB, et al. Immunization with DNA coding for gp100 results in CD4 T-cell independent antitumor immunity. Surgery. 2000;128:273–80.
7. Schreurs MW, de Boer AJ, Figdor CG, Adema GJ. Genetic vaccination against the melanocyte lineage-specific antigen gp100 induces cytotoxic T lymphocyte-mediated tumor protection. Cancer Res. 1998;58:2509–14.
8. Yuan J, Ku GY, Gallardo HF, Orlandi F, Manukian G, Rasalan TS, et al. Safety and immunogenicity of a human and mouse gp100 DNA vaccine in a phase I trial of patients with melanoma. Canc Immunol. 2009;9:5.
9. Zou JP, Yamamoto N, Fujii T, Takenaka H, Kobayashi M, Herrmann SH, et al. Systemic administration of rIL-12 induces complete tumor regression and protective immunity: response is correlated with a striking reversal of suppressed IFN-gamma production by anti-tumor T cells. Int Immunol. 1995;7:1135–45.
10. Bergman PJ, Camps-Palau MA, McKnight JA, Leibman NF, Craft DM, Leung C, et al. Development of a xenogeneic DNA vaccine program for canine malignant melanoma at the animal medical center. Vaccine. 2006;24:4582–5.
11. Goldberg SM, Bartido SM, Gardner JP, Guevara-Patino JA, Montgomery SC, Perales MA, et al. Comparison of two cancer vaccines targeting tyrosinase: plasmid DNA and recombinant alphavirus replicon particles. Clin Cancer Res. 2005;11:8114–21.
12. Liao JC, Gregor P, Wolchok JD, Orlandi F, Craft D, Leung C, et al. Vaccination with human tyrosinase DNA induces antibody responses in dogs with advanced melanoma. Canc Immunol. 2006;6:8.
13. Wolchok JD, Yuan J, Houghton AN, Gallardo HF, Rasalan TS, Wang J, et al. Safety and immunogenicity of tyrosinase DNA vaccines in patients with melanoma. Mol Ther. 2007;2044–2050:15.
14. Gold JS, Ferrone CR, Guevara-Patino JA, Hawkins WG, Dyall R, Engelhorn ME, et al. A single heteroclitic epitope determines cancer immunity after xenogeneic DNA immunization against a tumor differentiation antigen. J Immunol. 2003;170:5188–94.
15. Overwijk WW, Tsung A, Irvine KR, Parkhurst MR, Goletz TJ, Tsung K, et al. gp100/pmel 17 is a murine tumor rejection antigen: induction of "self"-reactive, tumoricidal T cells using high-affinity, altered peptide ligand. J Exp Med. 1998;188:277–86.
16. Zhou WZ, Kaneda Y, Huang S, Morishita R, Hoon D. Protective immunization against melanoma by gp100 DNA-HVJ-liposome vaccine. Gene Therapy. 1999;6:1768–73.
17. Lembcke LM, Kania SA, Blackford JT, Trent DJ, Grosenbaugh DA, Fraser DG, et al. Development of immunologic assays to measure response in horses vaccinated with xenogeneic plasmid DNA encoding human tyrosinase. J Equine Vet Sci. 2012;32:607–15.

18. Alton EW, Geddes DM, Gill DR, Higgins CF, Hyde SC, Innes JA, et al. Towards gene therapy for cystic fibrosis: a clinical progress report. Gene Ther. 1998;5:291–2.

19. Chow YH, Chiang BL, Lee YL, Chi WK, Lin WC, Chen YT, et al. Development of Th1 and Th2 populations and the nature of immune responses to hepatitis B virus DNA vaccines can be modulated by codelivery of various cytokine genes. J Immunol. 1998;160:1320–9.

20. Coughlin CM, Salhany KE, Wysocka M, Aruga E, Kurzawa H, Chang AE, et al. Interleukin-12 and interleukin-18 synergistically induce murine tumor regression which involves inhibition of angiogenesis. J Clin Investig. 1998;101:1441–52.

21. Gherardi MM, Ramirez JC, Esteban M. Interleukin-12 (IL-12) enhancement of the cellular immune response against human immunodeficiency virus type 1 env antigen in a DNA prime/vaccinia virus boost vaccine regimen is time and dose dependent: suppressive effects of IL-12 boost are mediated by nitric oxide. J Virol. 2000;74:6278–86.

22. Iwasaki A, Stiernholm BJ, Chan AK, Berinstein NL, Barber BH. Enhanced CTL responses mediated by plasmid DNA immunogens encoding costimulatory molecules and cytokines. J Immunol. 1997;158:4591–601.

23. Sin JI, Kim JJ, Boyer JD, Ciccarelli RB, Higgins TJ, Weiner DB. In vivo modulation of vaccine-induced immune responses toward a Th1 phenotype increases potency and vaccine effectiveness in a herpes simplex virus type 2 mouse model. J Virol. 1999;73:501–9.

24. Hara I, Nagai H, Miyake H, Yamanaka K, Hara S, Micallef MJ, et al. Effectiveness of cancer vaccine therapy using cells transduced with the interleukin-12 gene combined with systemic interleukin-18 administration. Cancer Gene Ther. 2000;7:83–90.

25. Kishida T, Asada H, Satoh E, Tanaka S, Shinya M, Hirai H, et al. In vivo electroporation-mediated transfer of interleukin-12 and interleukin-18 genes induces significant antitumor effects against melanoma in mice. Gene Ther. 2001;8:1234–40.

26. Tamura T, Nishi T, Goto T, Takeshima H, Ushio Y, Sakata T. Combination of IL-12 and IL-18 of electro-gene therapy synergistically inhibits tumor growth. Anticancer Res. 2003;23:1173–9.

27. Heinzerling L, Dummer R, Pavlovic J, Schultz J, Burg G, Moelling K. Tumor regression of human and murine melanoma after intratumoral injection of IL-12-encoding plasmid DNA in mice. Exp Dermatol. 2002;11:232–40.

28. Müller J, Feige K, Wunderlin P, Hodl A, Meli ML, Seltenhammer M, et al. Double-blind placebo-controlled study with interleukin-18 and interleukin-12-encoding plasmid DNA shows antitumor effect in metastatic melanoma in gray horses. J Immunother. 2011;34:58–64.

29. Schirmbeck R, Konig-Merediz SA, Riedl P, Kwissa M, Sack F, Schroff M, et al. Priming of immune responses to hepatitis B surface antigen with minimal DNA expression constructs modified with a nuclear localization signal peptide. J Mol Med. 2001;79:343–50.

30. Endmann A, Baden M, Weisermann E, Kapp K, Schroff M, Kleuss C, et al. Immune response induced by a linear DNA vector: influence of dose, formulation and route of injection. Vaccine. 2010;28:3642–9.

31. Heinzerling LM, Feige K, Rieder S, Akens MK, Dummer R, Stranzinger G, et al. Tumor regression induced by intratumoral injection of DNA coding for human interleukin 12 into melanoma metastases in gray horses. J Mol Med. 2001;78:692–702.

32. Endmann A, Klünder K, Kapp K, Riede O, Oswald D, Talman EG, et al. Cationic lipid-formulated DNA vaccine against hepatitis B virus: immunogenicity of MIDGE-Th1 vectors encoding small and large surface antigen in comparison to a licensed protein vaccine. PLoS One. 2014;9(7):e101715.

33. Dow SW, Elmslie RE, Fradkin LG, Liggitt DH, Heath TD, Willson AP, et al. Intravenous cytokine gene delivery by lipid-DNA complexes controls the growth of established lung metastases. Hum Gene Ther. 1999;10:2961–72.

34. Dow SW, Fradkin LG, Liggitt DH, Willson AP, Heath TD, Potter TA. Lipid-DNA complexes induce potent activation of innate immune responses and antitumor activity when administered intravenously. J Immunol. 1999;163:1552–61.

35. Therasse P, Arbuck SG, Eisenhauer EA, Wanders J, Kaplan RS, Rubinstein L, et al. New guidelines to evaluate the response to treatment in solid tumors. European organization for research and treatment of cancer, national cancer institute of the united states, national cancer institute of canada. J Natl Cancer Inst. 2000;92:205–16.

36. Wolchok JD, Hoos A, O'Day S, Weber JS, Hamid O, Lebbe C, et al. Guidelines for the evaluation of immune therapy activity in solid tumors: immune-related response criteria. Clin Cancer Res. 2009;15:7412–20.

37. Phillips JC, Blackford JT, Lembcke LM, Grosenbaugh DA, Leard T. Evaluation of needle-free injection devices for intramuscular vaccination in horses. J Equine Vet Sci. 2011;31:738–43.

38. Phillips JC, Lembcke LM, Noltenius CE, Newman SJ, Blackford JT, Grosenbaugh DA, et al. Evaluation of tyrosinase expression in canine and equine melanocytic tumors. Am J Vet Res. 2012;73:272–8.

39. Seltenhammer MH, Heere-Ress E, Brandt S, Druml T, Jansen B, Pehamberger H, et al. Comparative histopathology of grey-horse-melanoma and human malignant melanoma. Pigment Cell Res. 2004;17:674–81.

40. Livingston PO, Wong GY, Adluri S, Tao Y, Padavan M, Parente R, et al. Improved survival in stage III melanoma patients with GM2 antibodies: a randomized trial of adjuvant vaccination with GM2 ganglioside. J Clin Oncol. 1994;12:1036–44.

41. Romero P, Cerottini JC, Waanders GA. Novel methods to monitor antigen-specific cytotoxic T-cell responses in cancer immunotherapy. Mol Med Today. 1998;4:305–12.

42. Heinzerling L, Basch V, Maloy K, Johansen P, Senti G, Wuthrich B, et al. Critical role for DNA vaccination frequency in induction of antigen-specific cytotoxic responses. Vaccine. 2006;24:1389–94.

21

Evaluation of the efficacy of meloxicam for post-operative management of pain and inflammation in horses after orthopaedic surgery in a placebo controlled clinical field trial

Ulrich Walliser[1], Albrecht Fenner[2], Nicole Mohren[2], Thomas Keefe[3], Frerich deVries[2] and Chris Rundfeldt[4*]

Abstract

Background: The benefit of pre and post-operative administration of non-steroidal anti-inflammatory drugs for the relief of post-operative pain and control of inflammation in horses following orthopaedic surgery has not been previously investigated in controlled clinical field trials, and the utility of such treatment is a matter of ongoing dispute. Recently the utility of post-operative pain management was emphasized. It was therefore our aim to determine the efficacy of meloxicam in horses following partial resection of fractured splint bones. This condition was selected since the limited extent of the insult and the defined surgical intervention allowed the conduct of a randomized, double blinded, placebo-controlled, parallel group, multi-centre clinical field study in a homogenous patient population.

Results: Sixty-six client owned horses requiring unilateral partial splint bone resection were recruited in 15 centres in Germany and were allocated in a 1:1 ratio to receive meloxicam, 0.6 mg/kg for 5 days.
Lameness at trot grades prior to surgery were similar in the meloxicam and placebo treatment groups but were significantly lower in the meloxicam group on day 6 post surgery. Clinical scores for soft tissue swelling and assessment of analgesic and anti-inflammatory efficacy by the investigators at the end of the study were significantly better for the meloxicam compared to the placebo group. No treatment-related adverse reactions were observed.

Conclusion: The administration of meloxicam i.v. once prior to surgery followed by once daily oral administration for four consecutive days is efficacious for the control of post-operative pain and inflammation in horses undergoing orthopaedic surgery.

Keywords: Horse, Orthopaedic surgery, Post-operative, Pain control, Non-steroidal anti-inflammatory, Meloxicam, Splint bone fracture, Partial resection, Lameness at trot

Background

Surgical intervention on distal extremities in horses is a standard of care for many orthopaedic conditions including splint bone fractures, condylar fractures, arthroscopic joint revisions, and various other conditions [1-3]. While orthopaedic surgical procedures are well established, the medical management of pain and inflammation resulting from such intervention remains to be an under-addressed field. The benefit of pain management during and after orthopaedic surgery is a matter of controversial discussion. In the past it has been suggested that analgesics be withheld in equine patients to maintain protective reflexes and reduce the risk of injury [4], but more recently the utility of post-operative pain management was emphasized [4-6].

Nonsteroidal anti-inflammatory drugs (NSAIDs) are extensively used as analgesics in veterinary medicine, having proven efficacy in dogs and cats for post-operative pain management in orthopaedic surgery [7]. NSAIDs combine

* Correspondence: chris.rundfeldt@t-online.de
[4]Drug-Consulting Network, 01445 Coswig, Germany
Full list of author information is available at the end of the article

analgesia with anti-inflammatory activity. This pharmacology is the result of their inhibition of the cyclooxygenase pathway and prevention of the formation of pro-inflammatory prostaglandins at the site of injury [8]. Despite recommendations for the use of NSAIDs in equine orthopaedic surgery [5,9,10], evidence for efficacy from controlled clinical field studies is limited [4,11]. Meloxicam is an NSAID which is licensed and widely used for the treatment of pre- and post-operative pain and inflammation following orthopaedic and soft tissue surgery in cats and dogs [12]. It is licensed for use in horses for the alleviation of inflammation and relief of pain in both acute and chronic musculo-skeletal disorders as well as for the relief of pain associated with colic [13]. The anti-inflammatory efficacy of meloxicam in equines has been demonstrated in pharmacodynamic and pharmacokinetic studies [14,15]. But to date no data are available supporting its use in post-operative pain control in orthopaedic surgery.

The objective of this study was to examine the efficacy of meloxicam for the control of post-operative pain and inflammation in horses undergoing orthopaedic surgery in a double-blind placebo-controlled study. Partial resection of fractured splint bones is a small, well defined surgical intervention. This condition was therefore selected as a condition to demonstrate clinical efficacy of meloxicam. Both, the limited extent of pre-surgical pain and the limited and standardized surgical intervention, which involves only non-weight bearing structures and which likely does not result in severe pain, enables a placebo controlled study approach. Part of the data have been previously published in abstract form [16].

Methods

The study was designed as a randomized, double blind, placebo-controlled parallel group multi-centre clinical field study using two treatment groups with equal numbers of clinical cases per group and was conducted in compliance with good clinical practice [17]. The use of a placebo in the clinical field trial setting of the present study can be justified by the low level of post-operative pain induced by the limited surgical intervention, non-availability of a licensed veterinary medicine for peri-operative treatment, or at least a drug with proven clinical evidence for efficacy, as comparator for the clinical indication investigated. The study was approved by the local competent authority of the principle investigator Dr. Walliser, Regierungspräsidium Karlsruhe, Baden-Würtemberg, Az. 35–9182.00, and by all local authorities of all participating study centres in full compliance with German drug law, and by the local animal welfare officer of Boehringer Ingelheim Vetmedica GmbH.

Animals

Client owned horses requiring orthopaedic surgery for a closed splint bone fracture associated with marked exostosis and development of connective tissue indurations were eligible for inclusion in the study with the consent of the owner. Exclusion criteria were defined as pregnant mares, foals less than 6 weeks of age, horses with distal fractures of the splint bones with absolutely non-reactive tissue, compound fractures, proximal fractures which required internal fixation, lameness of other origin (e.g. coffin joint, fetlock joint), or clinical chemistry values indicative of hepatic, renal or hemorrhagic disease. Prior treatment with short acting corticosteroids or NSAIDs during the previous 8 days or treatment with long acting corticosteroids during the previous 8 weeks also precluded inclusion in the study.

Treatments

Premedication for surgery was performed according to the study site's usual practices (except for any treatment that might have affected or masked the clinical symptoms of post-operative pain (e.g. NSAIDs and corticosteroids). For pain control during surgery only drugs with duration of action of up to 4 hours were permitted. In most cases L-methadone and/or ketamine were administered; the use of these analgesic agents did not differ between the two treatment groups. Induction and maintenance of inhalation anaesthesia was also performed according to the study site's usual practices. To control for potential exaggerated pain after surgery during the study conduct, butorphanol was allowed as a rescue medication for the control of very strong pain but was not required or used in any case.

After an initial examination and confirmation of eligibility for inclusion in the study, the horses were allocated according to a randomization list to one of two treatments as follows: (i) a single intravenous injection of meloxicam[a] (0.6 mg/kg b.w.) immediately prior to premedication followed by (starting on the following morning) 4 once daily oral administrations of meloxicam[b] at the same dosage; or (ii) a single intravenous injection of placebo immediately prior to premedication followed (starting on the following morning) by 4 once daily equivalent volume oral administrations of placebo. The parenteral and oral investigational interventions for the two treatment groups looked identical and were identically packaged and labelled. The formulation of the placebo was identical to that of the active treatment except for the absence of the active ingredient. The administration of the interventions was carried out by the blinded investigator at each study site.

Clinical examinations

General characteristics (e.g. age, breed, and bodyweight), blood chemistry profile, affected limb, site and date of the splint bone fracture, and duration of lameness before surgery were recorded, and diagnosis was confirmed by radiographic assessment before surgery. Daily monitoring included body temperature (°C), heart rate (beats/minute), respiratory rate (breaths/minute) and food intake (scoring system: 0, unchanged (normal); 1, reduced by $\leq 1/3$; 2, by $\geq 1/3$; 3, none). Immediate post-surgery recovery was assessed in terms of the number of attempts which the horses made to stand until they actually managed to remain standing upright and the interval between the time of extubation and the time when the horse was able to remain standing upright.

The primary endpoint was prospectively defined as lameness at trot (LAMET) (prior to and at 3 and 6 days after surgery) according to the severity of lameness grading system of the American Association of Equine Practitioners (AAEP) [18]. LAMET was not assessed on day 1 post surgery due to the proximity to the surgery. To evaluate the level of pain perception at rest throughout the study, lameness at walk (LAMEW) was assessed prior to and at 1, 3 and 6 days after surgery. Assessment of soft tissue swelling, wound healing and analgesic and anti-inflammatory efficacy were additional secondary endpoints. At the surgical site, soft tissue swelling was evaluated on Days 1, 3 and 6, and local palpatory pain on Days 3 and 6, using a 4 point scoring system for both endpoints with 0, 1, 2, 3 indicating none, mild, moderate and severe, respectively. The circumference (cm) of the affected area and wound healing at the surgical site were evaluated on Days 3 and 6; wound healing was scored as either: 0, no signs of complications; 1, increased local temperature; 2, wound secretion; 3, suture dehiscence and 4, other complications such as wound infections. Dressings were changed on Days 3 and 6. At the end of the study the investigator provided a general assessment of analgesic and anti-inflammatory efficacy of the treatment for each horse using a 4 point grading system whereby 1, 2, 3 and 4 denoted excellent, good, moderate and poor, respectively.

Data analyses

Baseline characteristics for the horses in the study were summarized using descriptive statistics. Data for LAMET and LAMEW were analysed using ordinal logistic regression (OLR) analysis [19] with treatment as the main effect, first with all six AAEP categories and then for LAMET also with a reduced lameness scale, which was constructed post-hoc to focus on clinically relevant lameness at trot (CRLAT): 1, none or minimal (i.e. combination of AAEP grades 0 and 1); 2, mild (i.e. AAEP grade 2); and 3, moderate to severe (i.e. combination of AAEP grades 3, 4 and 5). To adjust for potential differences in severity of lameness prior to treatment (Day 0), the LAMET and CRLAT data on both study days 3 and 6 were also evaluated using the

OLR analysis with adjustment for the respective values at Day 0. For this purpose, the OLR model included two categorical variables, treatment (Meloxicam or placebo) as the main effect and LAMET or CRLAT, respectively, at Day 0 as a potential confounder [19,20].

Data on the categorical secondary efficacy variables (assessments of soft tissue swelling and local palpatory pain at the surgery site, wound healing and the general assessment of analgesic and anti-inflammatory efficacy) were evaluated statistically via chi-square analyses. Data on the quantitative traits, i.e. circumference of the most severely affected area, rectal temperature, heart rate, and respiratory rate, were evaluated using repeated-measures analysis of variance or covariance with treatment and day as fixed effects and, for each of the three physiological variables, with the corresponding values at Day 0 as a covariate. The analysis of each of these four variables included Tukey-Kramer mean comparisons between the meloxicam and placebo treatment groups both overall and on each study day. All statistical analyses were carried out using the SAS computer software package [20].

Results

A total of 15 investigators contributed 66 clinical cases in the study. Six of the cases enrolled (two in meloxicam and four in placebo group) were subsequently found to be in violation of the inclusion/exclusion criteria and were not further considered in the evaluation of the results for efficacy. Two cases on placebo had two fractures; one horse on placebo got a 2nd fracture on the day after surgery preventing adequate evaluation of lameness compared to pre-surgery; in three horses (one in the placebo group and two in the meloxicam group), the required pre-study procedures were not performed according to protocol or were not documented correctly, preventing the evaluation of treatment efficacy for these cases. All 6 were excluded from the primary study population.

Population characteristics of the meloxicam and placebo groups were well balanced. In particular, more than 80 % of the horses in both treatment groups were Warmbloods, and the two treatment groups were well balanced with respect to sex, age, bodyweight and duration of lameness prior to surgery (Table 1). The treatment groups were broadly similar with regard to the radiographic assessment of the affected splint bone prior to surgery and with regard to both the location of the fracture and the severity of callus formation. Fractures were most frequently presented in one of the forelimbs in both treatment groups and represented 54.8 and 69.0 % of the cases in the meloxicam and placebo groups, respectively. The distribution of fractures between left and right limbs was equal for the two groups. Mild to moderate callus formation was observed in 96.8 and 93.1 % of the cases in the meloxicam and placebo groups, respectively.

Table 1 Demographics of study population

Treatment	Number of cases [n]	Race distribution: Warmblood /Pony / Other [%]	Sex: Female /Male / Neutered male [%]	Age [years, mean ± SD]	Weight [kg, mean ± SD]	Lameness duration [days, mean ± SD]
Meloxicam	31	83.3 / 13.3 / 3.3	60 / 4 / 36	9.5 ± 4.9	537 ± 96	23.2 ± 18.4
Placebo	29	86.2 / 3.5 / 10.4	52.2 / 13 / 34.8	10.2 ± 3.7	539 ± 107	25.0 ± 24.8

Lameness at trot (LAMET) was determined on Day 0 prior to surgery and again on Day 3 and Day 6; the distribution of LAMET scores are summarised in Table 2. As determined by OLR, the lameness scores on Day 6 were significantly lower in the meloxicam group as compared to the placebo group (p = 0.007), indicating a significant clinical effect of meloxicam treatment. A similar trend towards a positive treatment effect, although not statistically significant (p = 0.067), was seen on Day 3. However, more cases with no or minimal lameness were included in the meloxicam group; 38.8 % of horses in the meloxicam group had either no or only minimal lameness at trot on Day 0 compared to 20.6 % for the placebo group (Table 1). The frequency of horses with moderate lameness (grade 3) was comparable in both groups (48.4 % and 55.2 %). While the difference in LAMET on Day 0 was not statistically significant (p = 0.162), a baseline adjustment in the evaluation of the treatment success was deemed appropriate to correct for a potential advantage

for the meloxicam group. Even with baseline adjustment, the meloxicam-treated animals had significantly less severe lameness on Day 6 (p = 0.040, Table 3). Application of the same statistical analyses to the data on the more clinically relevant lameness scale CRLAT yielded essentially similar results, however the treatment effect on Day 3 was now very close to being significant (p = 0.053, Table 3).

LAMEW scores were very low prior to, on the day after surgery, and throughout the study (Table 4). In fact, the measurements taken indicated only scores of 0 to 2 (none, minimal, or mild lameness), and the majority of measurements throughout the study reflected a score of 0, representing no lameness at all at walk. There was no difference between the placebo and the treatment group for this measure at any day, and the post-surgical grades were not significantly higher than the pre-surgical ones. There was only one animal from the placebo group which was reported on day 3 only to have a LAMEW score exceeding 2. The animal otherwise did not show any clinically relevant sign of pain at rest and therefore rescue medication was not applied.

The significant treatment effect of meloxicam as seen for the primary efficacy variable LAMET was also reflected in secondary endpoints. The treatment groups were significantly different in terms of the general assessment of analgesic efficacy at the end of the study (p = 0.029, Figure 1). Based on combining the categories "Moderate" and "Poor" to reflect treatment failure and "Excellent" and "Good" to reflect treatment success, meloxicam treatment was judged to be successful in 83.9 % of cases, compared to 51.7 % in placebo-treated animals (p = 0.008). Soft tissue swelling at the surgical site did not differ between the two treatment groups on study days 1 and 3 (p = 0.380 and p = 0.292, respectively) but was significantly less in the meloxicam group on Day 6 (p = 0.010, Figure 2). In particular, the percent of horses categorized as having moderate to severe swelling of soft tissue at the surgical site on Day 6 was only 9.7 % in the meloxicam group compared to and 34.4 % in the placebo group.

The treatment group scores for local palpatory pain at the site of surgery, circumference of the most severely affected area of the affected limb, and the scores for wound healing were similar at the various assessment time points in the study. There was no evidence for any significant difference between the two treatment groups with respect to food intake, rectal temperature or heart

Table 2 Distribution of study horses by the AAEP grade for lameness at trot (LAMET) on study days 0, 3, and 6 for the meloxicam and placebo treatment groups

Lameness at Trot		Meloxicam		Placebo	
Day	Grade	N	%	N	%
Day 0	None (0)	10	32.3	3	10.3
	Minimal (1)	2	6.5	3	10.3
	Mild (2)	3	9.7	5	17.2
	Moderate (3)	15	48.4	16	55.2
	Serious (4)	1	3.2	2	6.9
	Severe (5)	0	0.0	0	0.0
Day 3	None (0)	8	25.8	4	13.8
	Minimal (1)	3	9.7	2	6.9
	Mild (2)	8	25.8	4	13.8
	Moderate (3)	9	29.0	15	51.7
	Serious (4)	3	9.7	3	10.3
	Severe (5)	0	0.0	1	3.5
Day 6	None (0)	12	38.7	4	13.8
	Minimal (1)	11	35.5	11	37.9
	Mild (2)	5	16.1	2	6.9
	Moderate (3)	3	9.7	10	34.5
	Serious (4)	0	0.0	2	6.9
	Severe (5)	0	0.0	0	0.0
	Total	**31**	**100.0**	**29**	**100.0**

Table 3 Summary of the statistical analysis of the primary parameter lameness at trot (LAMET) and clinically relevant lameness at trot (CRLAT)

Variables	Probability value	Variables	Probability value
LAMET on Day:		**CRLAT on Day:**	
Day 0	0.162	Day 0	0.256
Day 3	0.067	Day 3	**0.053**
Day 6	**0.007**	Day 6	**0.027**
LAMET adjusted for day 0 value at Day:		**CLRAT adjusted for day 0 value at Day:**	
Day 3	0.479	Day 3	0.112
Day 6	**0.040**	Day 6	**0.043**

Results of the ordinal logistic regression (OLR) analysis of LAMET and CRLAT at Days 0, 3, and 6 and at Days 3 and 6, adjusted for the values at Day 0, based on including Day 0 in the OLR model as a categorical variable. CRLAT calculation was based on combining AEEP grades 0 and 1 and combining grades 3 to 5 to generate a 3-point scale.

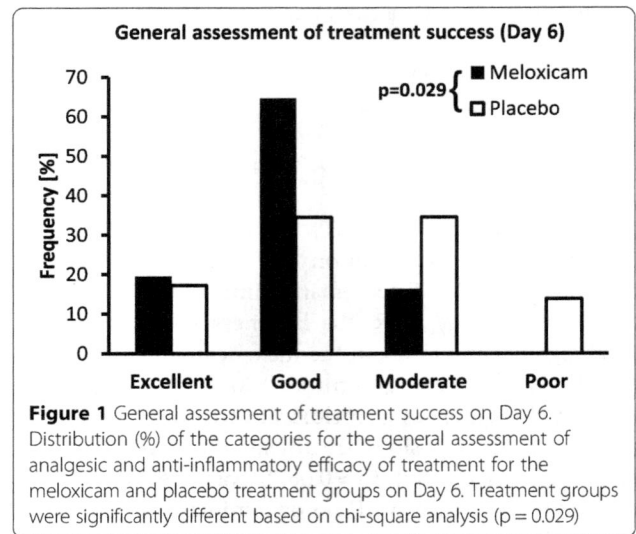

Figure 1 General assessment of treatment success on Day 6. Distribution (%) of the categories for the general assessment of analgesic and anti-inflammatory efficacy of treatment for the meloxicam and placebo treatment groups on Day 6. Treatment groups were significantly different based on chi-square analysis (p = 0.029)

Table 4 Distribution of study horses by the AAEP grade for lameness at walk (LAMEW) on study days 0, 1, 3, and 6 for the meloxicam and placebo treatment groups

Lameness at Walk Day	Grade	Meloxicam N	%	Placebo N	%
Day 0	None (0)	22	71.0	21	72.4
	Minimal (1)	1	3.2	4	13.8
	Mild (2)	8	25.8	4	13.8
	Moderate to severe (3–5)[1]	0	0.0	0	0.0
Day 1	None (0)	20	64.5	16	55.2
	Minimal (1)	2	6.5	6	20.7
	Mild (2)	9	29.0	7	24.1
	Moderate to severe (3–5)[1]	0	0.0	0	0.0
Day 3	None (0)	22	71.0	19	65.5
	Minimal (1)	7	22.6	6	20.7
	Mild (2)	2	6.5	3	10.3
	Moderate to severe (3–5)[1]	0	0.0	1	3.4
Day 6	None (0)	29	93.5	23	79.3
	Minimal (1)	2	6.5	4	13.8
	Mild (2)	0	0.0	2	6.9
	Moderate to severe (3–5)[1]	0	0.0	0	0.0
	Total	**31**	**100.0**	**29**	**100.0**

[1]Since all but one horse had LAMEW grades lower than 3, the grades 3–5 were combined.

rate at any of the assessment time points in the study. Post-surgery recovery assessments in terms of the number of attempts which the horses made to stand until they actually managed to remain standing upright and the interval between the time of extubation and the time when the horse was able to remain standing upright were similar for both groups. No abnormality was observed in the localisation of callus formation in more than 80 % of the cases in both treatment groups. No adverse events were observed in any of the horses, and all were returned to their owners at the end of the study.

Discussion

Good pain control after surgery has been recognized as important component to prevent negative outcomes including poor wound healing and prolonged recovery [21]. Exacerbations of acute pain can lead to neural sensitization and release of mediators both peripherally and centrally, contributing to delayed recovery. This phenomenon, called wind up, was found to be caused by N-Methyl D-Aspartate (NMDA) receptor activation mediated central sensitization, long-term potentiation of pain (LTP), and transcription-dependent sensitization [22]. The knowledge of these pathways has led to increased awareness on post-operative pain and has changed the attitudes towards pain management [22]. Both in human medicine and in small animal medicine, post-operative intensive pain management is now standard [21,22].

In contrast, the utility of post-operative pain management in horses undergoing orthopaedic surgery is still a matter of controversial discussion, since pain is seen as a protective mechanism resulting in reduced usage of the affected limb [4]. The fallacy, however, that pain is protective and must be allowed to avoid risk for damage after surgery should be challenged. Post-operative analgesia is directed at aching pain, whereas sharp pain associated with inappropriate movements persists [21]. While theoretical evidence is strong in support of post-operative pain management in horses undergoing orthopaedic surgery, and while post-operative pain management is used at least in a fraction of horses undergoing castration [23], clinical proof of improved outcome due to pain management is limited. In fact, only one placebo-controlled small clinical

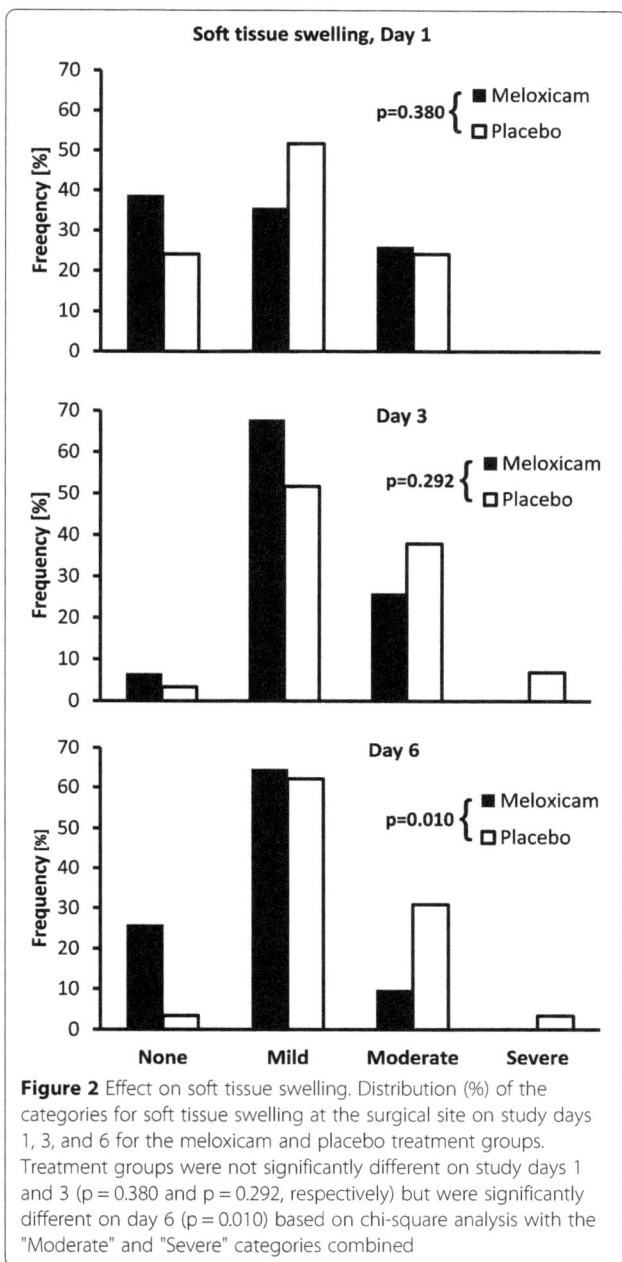

Figure 2 Effect on soft tissue swelling. Distribution (%) of the categories for soft tissue swelling at the surgical site on study days 1, 3, and 6 for the meloxicam and placebo treatment groups. Treatment groups were not significantly different on study days 1 and 3 (p = 0.380 and p = 0.292, respectively) but were significantly different on day 6 (p = 0.010) based on chi-square analysis with the "Moderate" and "Severe" categories combined

field study in horsed was identified evaluating the use of NSAIDs in post-operative pain management [11]. In that study in horses undergoing arthroscopic surgery, phenylbutazone was found to reduce the pain severity if assessed using a composite pain score, but due to the low number of cases involved (15 on phenylbutazone and 10 on placebo), the study failed to demonstrate statistically significant and clinically meaningful effects. That study also demonstrated the difficulties associated with pain assessment in horses after surgery, which is especially challenging when multiple investigators are involved, resulting in inter-rater variability [24-26].

Therefore, the current study was designed to reduce variability where possible. The surgical condition selected, i.e. unilateral closed splint bone fracture with marked exostosis and development of connective tissue induration, is a condition found in sufficient frequency to recruit a sizable clinical study in a multi-centre setting. At the same time, the condition is relatively homogenous, and the surgical procedure involved is well defined and limited in extent, thereby reducing the variability within the trial population. Since no weight bearing structures are directly involved, horses can be expected not to suffer from unacceptable postoperative pain during rest, enabling the use of placebo. In fact, while the short-acting morphine derivative butorphanol was allowed as rescue medication, no case required its use. Instead of attempting to quantify pain, we selected lameness as the primary outcome in that it reflects the pain perception of the affected horse. Lameness quantification using the AAEP scale is a routine procedure well established at all participating study sites. Two different conditions were evaluated. LAMET was selected to represent the pain perception arising from tissue movements in the surgical region induced by forcing the horses to trot. LAMEW was selected to represent the pain perception during rest and walking, and this measure was selected to best reflect the overall suffering level during the recovery. As can be expected from the medical condition, LAMEW was very low throughout the study and did not differ between the placebo and the treatment group, indicating that placebo animals were not exposed to unacceptable pain (Table 4).

We selected meloxicam as the trial drug because it is licensed for use in horses for the alleviation of inflammation and relief of pain in both acute and chronic musculoskeletal disorders, as well as for the relief of pain associated with colic [13]. Information on pharmacokinetic and pharmacodynamic relationship in orthopaedic conditions, as well as safety of single and multiple doses, is available enabling the selection of the dose and dosing interval [15,27,28]. While phenylbutazone is frequently used in horses, its use is associated with the highest rate of adverse events of NSAIDs, with a stronger effect on gastric mucosa as compared to meloxicam, and, therefore, was not considered as study medication [29,30].

Using this study design, we were able to demonstrate that preoperative and post-operative administration of meloxicam resulted in a significant reduction in lameness on the 6th day after surgery, indicating that the recovery in animals receiving pain treatment was accelerated compared to placebo-treated animals. This positive effect was also reflected by the significantly improved overall clinical assessment of treatment success, reflecting both a significant better analgesia and a significant reduction in soft tissue swelling on day 6. The reduced lameness on day 6 is clinically relevant, since it reduces the risk for development of support-limb laminitis, an unfortunate sequela that can render prior surgery needless and that often leads to the demise of the affected horse [5].

The strongest clinical effects were seen on day 6 after surgery, while immediately after surgery there was no difference as assessed by number of attempts to stand until managing to remain standing and time from extubation to time to remaining to stand upright. This indicates that early recovery from surgery may rather be related to anaesthetic procedures, which did not differ between groups, than to post-operative pain control. In fact, the pain related to the selected surgical procedure can be expected to be rather limited, having little effect on time to recovery from anaesthesia. Our data indicate that, in conditions with limited surgical intervention, early recovery cannot be improved with post-operative pain management. On day 3 after surgery, there was a trend, although not statistically significant, towards reduced lameness (Table 3). The reduced efficacy on day 3 compared to day 6 was somewhat unexpected. One reason for the delayed manifestation of clinical benefit may be the selected treatment scheme. The analgesia of an intravenous dose of 0.5-1 mg/kg meloxicam lasts in horses up to 24 hours, supporting once daily dosing [15]. In our study, an intravenous dose of 0.6 mg/kg was given immediately prior to pre-medication of anaesthesia, and the first post-surgical oral dose was administered about 24 hours later in the morning on the day following the surgery. An analgesia gap due to switching from intravenous to oral dosing could be a potential concern for inappropriate post-surgical pain relief [4,27]. In future studies, a more aggressive early treatment, potentially involving a 2nd intravenous dose, timed to bridge the gap until oral treatment reaches effective plasma levels, may result in even further improved outcome.

Our primary endpoint was based on lameness assessment using the 6-point AAEP scale for lameness at trot. Unfortunately, lameness evaluation is afflicted with low reproducibility, especially if low grades of lameness are involved, even if experienced raters are involved [18]. When the mean lameness AAEP score was lower than 1.5, the inter-rater agreement whether a respective limb was lame or not was only 61.9 %, while it was 93.1 % if the lameness score was >1.5 [18]. In view of this problem, we evaluated whether a reduction of the number of lameness scores could increase the sensitivity of this scale to treatment effects. For this purpose, the AAEP scores 0 and 1 were grouped to present the positive outcome of none or minimal lameness, while the scores 3–5 were grouped as moderate to severe lameness, leaving score 2 as well recognizable, but mild lameness. This lameness scale, revised to represent clinically relevant differences, aimed at reducing the uncertainty of evaluating low grades of lameness and also at avoiding the need for rating different grades of moderate to severe lameness. Based on application of this scale, the study result obtained was essentially similar but the difference on day 3 became almost statistically significant (p-value = 0.053, Table 3). This indicates that the reduced lameness scale may present a method which is less affected by inter-rater variability.

In carefully reviewing the data, it became evident that, despite the blinded randomization of the cases resulting in equal distribution of cases with regard to race, sex, age, weight, and lameness duration, there was a slight but statistically non-significant difference in pre-randomization lameness grade, with a tendency towards less severe lameness in the meloxicam group. While the study aimed at evaluating the drug effect on surgical pain, this slight difference could have influenced the study outcome. Therefore, the OLR analysis of lameness was repeated for day 3 and 6 with adjustment for day 0 values. This adjustment was without effect on the overall study outcome on day 6.

During the course of the study, no treatment-related adverse events were recorded, but this was expected given that meloxicam was dosed in accordance with the label and that known NSAID related toxicity, including gastric ulceration and necrosis, require longer treatment duration to develop [29,31]. In addition, NSAIDs have not been found to have a detrimental effect on wound healing [32]. In fact, we showed in this study that the scores for wound healing were similar at the various assessment time points in the study, but the treatment resulted in significantly reduced swelling of soft tissue on day 6.

Conclusions

We have demonstrated for the first time that pre and post-operative meloxicam administration has a statistically significant beneficial effect on recovery in horses undergoing orthopaedic surgery of limited degree. This positive effect could be identified and verified in a relatively small placebo-controlled field study population of 60 evaluable horses by selecting a homogenous study population and utilizing a subjective outcome measure, i.e. lameness at trot. The utilization of a clinically relevant lameness scale increased the sensitivity of the study to treatment effects. Our results for the first time support the empirical conclusion drawn by experienced clinicians that post-operative pain management using clinically safe NSAIDs, such as meloxicam, is advantageous in equine orthopaedic surgery.

Endnotes

[a]Metacam® 20 mg/ml Solution for Injection, Boehringer Ingelheim Vetmedica GmbH, Ingelheim, Germany.

[b]Metacam® 15 mg/ml Oral Suspension for Horses, Boehringer Ingelheim Vetmedica GmbH, Ingelheim, Germany.

Abbreviations
AAEP: American Association of Equine Practitioners; GCP: Good clinical practice; CRLAT: Clinically relevant lameness at trot; LAMET: Lameness at trot; LAMEW: Lameness at walk; NSAID: Non-steroidal anti-inflammatory drug.

Competing interests
The study was funded by Boehringer Ingelheim Vetmedica GmbH, 55216 Ingelheim am Rhein, Germany. Dr. Ulrich Walliser has been principal investigator of the described clinical study. Dr. Thomas J. Keefe was involved in biostatistical evaluation of the data obtained in this study and serves as scientific advisor to Boehringer Ingelheim. PD Dr. habil. Chris Rundfeldt is scientific advisor to Boehringer Ingelheim. Dr. Albrecht Fenner, Dr. Nicole Mohren and Dr. Frerich deVries are employed by Boehringer Ingelheim Vetmedica GmbH, Germany, the sponsor of this study.

Author's contribution
UW served as principal investigator and contributed to the design and conduct of the study. AF was responsible for the design and conduct of all aspects of the study including the evaluation of results. NM contributed to the design of the study, conduct of the study, collection of data, and discussion of results. TK served as statistical expert. He designed the statistical evaluation, wrote the statistical section, contributed to the data interpretation and revised the manuscript. FdV contributed to the study design, evaluated the study data, and revised the manuscript. CR served as scientific advisor, contributed to the discussion of the study results, and edited the manuscript. All authors approved the manuscript.

Acknowledgement
We thank Dr. Victor Baltus, Dr. Rüdiger Brems, Dr. Dirk Fister, Dr. Marlis Gronenberg, Dr. Josef Hollerrieder, Dr. Wigo Horstmann, Dr. Werner Jahn, Dr. Heinz Jaugstetter, Dr. Marc Koene, Dr. Kai Wigand von Salmuth, Dr. Guido Stadtbäumer, Cornelia Schnerr, Dr. Klaus Vornberger, and Dr. Bernhard Zöttl for participation in the study as clinical investigators.

Author details
[1]Clinic for Horses Kirchheim, Nuertingerstrasse 200, 73230 Kirchheim, Germany. [2]Boehringer Ingelheim Vetmedica GmbH, 55216 Ingelheim am Rhein, Germany. [3]Department of Environmental & Radiological Health Sciences, College of Veterinary Medicine & Biomedical Sciences, Colorado State University, Fort Collins, USA. [4]Drug-Consulting Network, 01445 Coswig, Germany.

References
1. Harrison LJ, May SA, Edwards GB. Surgical treatment of open splint bone fractures in 26 horses. Vet Rec. 1991;128:606–10.
2. Smith LC, Greet TR, Bathe AP. A lateral approach for screw repair in lag fashion of spiral third metacarpal and metatarsal medial condylar fractures in horses. Vet Surg. 2009;38:681–8.
3. Ljungvall K, Roneus B. Arthroscopic surgery of the middle carpal joint in trotting Standardbreds: findings and outcome. Vet Comp Orthop Traumatol. 2011;24:350–3.
4. Baller LS, Hendrickson DA. Management of equine orthopedic pain. Vet Clin North Am Equine Pract. 2002;18:117–31.
5. Goodrich LR. Strategies for reducing the complication of orthopedic pain perioperatively. Vet Clin North Am Equine Pract. 2008;24:611–20.
6. Fürst A. Postoperative pain reduction as exemplified for castration of stallions (Postoperative Schmerzreduktion am Beispiel der Kastration des Hengstes). Proceedings of the 19th conference on Horse diseases at the Equitana in Essen, 18th and 19th March 2011;19:96–100.
7. Mathews KA. Nonsteroidal anti-inflammatory analgesics: Indications and contraindications for pain management in dogs and cats. Vet Clin N Am Small Anim Pract. 2000;30:783–804.
8. Clark JO, Clark TP. Analgesia. Vet Clin North Am Equine Pract. 1999;15:705–23.
9. Matthews NS, Carroll GL. Review of equine analgesics and pain management. Proceedings of the Annual Convention of the American Association of Equine Practitioners, Orlando, Florida, Dec 01–05, 2007. American Association of Equine Practitioners, Lexington, KY, USA. 2007;53:240–4.
10. Driessen B. Peri-operative pain management in the horse: can we effectively inhibit/prevent 'wind-up'. Proceedings 14th IVECCS 2007;14:25–9.
11. Raekallio M, Taylor PM, Bennett RC. Preliminary investigations of pain and analgesia assessment in horses administered phenylbutazone or placebo after arthroscopic surgery. Vet Surg. 1997;26:150–5.
12. Perret-Gentil F, Doherr MG, Spadavecchia C, Levionnois OL. Attitudes of Swiss veterinarians towards pain and analgesia in dogs and cats. Schweiz Arch Tierheilkd. 2014;156:111–7.
13. Anonymous. Metacam 20 mg/ml solution for injection for cattle, pigs and horses. Summary of product characteristics . EMA, http://www.ema. europa.eu/docs/en_GB/document_library/EPAR_-_Product_Information/ veterinary/000033/WC500065777.pdf 2010.
14. Lees P, Sedgwick AD, Higgins AJ, Pugh KE, Busch U. Pharmacodynamics and pharmacokinetics of meloxicam in the horse. Br Vet J. 1991;147:97–108.
15. Toutain PL, Cester CC. Pharmacokinetic-pharmacodynamic relationships and dose response to meloxicam in horses with induced arthritis in the right carpal joint. Am J Vet Res. 2004;65:1533–41.
16. Walliser U, Baltus V, Brems R, Fenner A, Fister D, Gronenberg M et al. Perioperative meloxicam application- a clinical study (Perioperative Meloxicam-Applikation- eine klinische Studie). Proceedings of the 19th conference on Horse diseases at the Equitana in Essen, 18th and 19th March 2011;19:112.
17. Good clinical practice. VICH Guideline GL 9, CVMP/VICH/595/98-Final 1989. http://www.ema.europa.eu/docs/en_GB/document_library/ Scientific_guideline/2009/10/WC500004343.pdf
18. Keegan KG, Dent EV, Wilson DA, Janicek J, Kramer J, Lacarrubba A, et al. Repeatability of subjective evaluation of lameness in horses. Equine Vet J. 2010;42:92–7.
19. Hosmer Jr DW, Lemeshow S, Sturdivant RX. Logistic Regression Models for Multinomial and Ordinal Outcomes. In Applied Logistic Regression Analysis. 3rd Edition. John Wiley & Sons; Hoboken, NJ, USA. 2013; p. 269–310.
20. SAS. SAS/STAT Users guide. Release 8.2. SAS Institute, Cary, NC, USA 2001
21. Dyson DH. Perioperative pain management in veterinary patients. Vet Clin North Am Small Anim Pract. 2008;38:1309–27.
22. Vadivelu N, Mitra S, Narayan D. Recent advances in postoperative pain management. Yale J Biol Med. 2010;83:11–25.
23. Price J, Eager RA, Welsh EM, Waran NK. Current practice relating to equine castration in the UK. Res Vet Sci. 2005;78:277–80.
24. Bussieres G, Jacques C, Lainay O, Beauchamp G, Leblond A, Cadore JL, et al. Development of a composite orthopaedic pain scale in horses. Res Vet Sci. 2008;85:294–306.
25. Dalla CE, Minero M, Lebelt D, Stucke D, Canali E, Leach MC. Development of the Horse Grimace Scale (HGS) as a pain assessment tool in horses undergoing routine castration. PLoS One. 2014;19(9):e92281.
26. Vinuela-Fernandez I, Jones E, Chase-Topping ME, Price J. Comparison of subjective scoring systems used to evaluate equine laminitis. Vet J. 2011;188:171–7.
27. Vander Werf KA, Davis EG, Kukanich B. Pharmacokinetics and adverse effects of oral meloxicam tablets in healthy adult horses. J Vet Pharmacol Ther. 2013;36:376–81.
28. Noble G, Edwards S, Lievaart J, Pippia J, Boston R, Raidal SL. Pharmacokinetics and safety of single and multiple oral doses of meloxicam in adult horses. J Vet Intern Med. 2012;26:1192–201.
29. MacAllister CG, Morgan SJ, Borne AT, Pollet RA. Comparison of adverse effects of phenylbutazone, flunixin meglumine, and ketoprofen in horses. J Am Vet Med Assoc. 1993;202:71–7.
30. D'Arcy-Moskwa E, Noble GK, Weston LA, Boston R, Raidal SL. Effects of meloxicam and phenylbutazone on equine gastric mucosal permeability. J Vet Intern Med. 2012;26:1494–9.
31. Dobromyskyj P. Management of postoperative and other acute pain. In: Flecknell PA, Waterman-Pearson A, editors. Pain management in animals. Philadelphia: WB Saunders; 2000. p. 81–145.
32. McMurphy RM. Providing analgesia. In: White NA, Moore JM, editors. Current techniques in equine surgery and lameness. Philadelphia: WB Saunders; 1989. p. 2–5.

22

Reactive oxygen species generation by bovine blood neutrophils with different *CXCR1* (*IL8RA*) genotype following Interleukin-8 incubation

Joren Verbeke[1*], Xanthippe Boulougouris[2], Carolien Rogiers[2], Christian Burvenich[2], Luc Peelman[3], Bart De Spiegeleer[4] and Sarne De Vliegher[1]

Abstract

Background: Associations between polymorphisms in the bovine *CXCR1* gene, encoding the chemokine (C-X-C motif) receptor 1 (IL8RA), and neutrophil traits and mastitis have been described. In the present study, blood neutrophils were isolated from 20 early lactating heifers with different *CXCR1* genotype at position 735 or 980. The cells were incubated with different concentrations of recombinant bovine IL-8 (rbIL-8) for 2 or 6 h and stimulated with phorbol 12-myristate 13-acetate (PMA) or opsonized zymosan particles (OZP). Potential association between *CXCR1* genotype and production of reactive oxygen species (ROS) was studied.

Results: Although on single nucleotide polymorphisms (SNPs) may potentially affect CXCR1 function, SNPs c.735C > G and c.980A > G showed no association with ROS production with or without incubation of rbIL-8. Neutrophils incubated with rbIL-8 for 2 or 6 h showed higher PMA- and lower OZP-induced ROS production compared to control without rbIL-8.

Conclusions: In the present study no association could be detected between superoxide production by isolated bovine neutrophils during early lactation and *CXCR1* gene polymorphism. IL-8 showed to possess inhibitory effects on ROS generation in bovine neutrophils.

Keywords: Bovine Neutrophil, Reactive Oxygen Species Generation, *CXCR1* Polymorphism, Interleukin 8

Background

Intramammary infection induces a fast influx of blood neutrophils into the site of infection [1]. Activated neutrophils eliminate invading pathogens by phagocytosis and a diverse array of oxygen-dependent and oxygen-independent killing mechanisms. A powerful mechanism is the generation of reactive oxygen species (ROS) or superoxide [2]. It is widely accepted that neutrophils play a pivotal role in mammary gland immunity. Since 1990, an overwhelming amount of evidence has been generated of neutrophil dysfunction around parturition and early lactation with consequences on the defense of the mammary gland [3]. For example, although *E.coli* strains may influence the severity of infection, the

primary determinant of severity is the physiological state of the cow. Severity of experimentally induced *E.coli* mastitis during early lactation was tightly correlated with the pre-infection capacity of isolated blood neutrophils to generate ROS after zymosan and phorbol ester stimulation [4,5] and their chemotactic response as well [6]. Interleukin 8 (IL-8), an important chemokine in the innate immune response of the mammary gland [3], enhances ROS generation [7], causes chemotaxis [8] and delays apoptosis [9] of isolated bovine blood neutrophils *in vitro*. Interleukin 8 priming of isolated human neutrophils for higher superoxide production was mediated through CXCR1 (IL8RA) and not through CXCR2 (IL8RB) [10,11].

Many polymorphisms have been detected in the coding region of the bovine *CXCR1* gene [12,13]. Single nucleotide polymorphism (SNP) c.735C > G (dbSNP ID: rs208795699) causes an amino acid change in the third

* Correspondence: Joren.Verbeke@UGent.be
[1]M-team and Mastitis and Milk Quality Research Unit, Department of Reproduction, Obstetrics, and Herd Health, Faculty of Veterinary Medicine, Ghent University, Salisburylaan, 133 Merelbeke, Belgium
Full list of author information is available at the end of the article

intracellular loop (p.His245Glu) potentially affecting G-protein binding and signal transduction. Furthermore, c.735C > G was found to be in full linkage disequilibrium with SNPs c.37A > T (rs380621468), c.38 T > A (rs110296731) and c.68G > A (rs133273369) causing amino acid changes p.Ile13Tyr and p.Gly23Glu in the N-terminus of CXCR1 known to have an important role in the first steps of binding IL-8 [13,14]. Associations between SNP c.735C > G and neutrophil functionality have been studied: blood neutrophils with genotype c.735GG showed a higher intracellular calcium release when stimulated with IL-8 and an increased ROS generation in response to PMA compared to neutrophils with genotype c.735CC (reviewed in [15]). Single nucleotide polymorphisms c.980A > G (rs43323012) and c.995A > G (rs43323013) cause changes in the C-terminus (p.Lys327Arg and p.His332Arg) and might interfere with adaptin-2 binding and receptor internalization [12].

Previous research indicated an association between SNP c.980A > G and likelihood of intramammary infection by major pathogens in early lactating heifers [13]. In the present study we wanted to know if *CXCR1* gene polymorphism (SNPs c.735C > G and c.980A > G) could affect neutrophil functionality. Blood neutrophils, with different *CXCR1* genotype, were isolated from 20 heifers during early lactation. ROS production as detected by chemiluminescence was measured following IL-8 incubation and stimulation with either PMA or opsonized zymosan particles (OZP). Freshly calved heifers were sampled because neutrophil functionality is reduced during this period [16].

We report the results of an association study between *CXCR1* SNPs c.735C > G and c.980A > G and blood neutrophil ROS. Additionally, we discuss the unexpected effect rbIL-8 had on neutrophil ROS depending on the stimulatory agent.

Methods
Study design
The experiment has been approved by the ethical committee of the Faculty of Veterinary Medicine, Ghent University (EC2013/190). Twenty Holstein heifers with different *CXCR1* genotype were included from 5 different commercial dairy herds. Selected heifers were not siblings, had no history of diseases and all quarters were culture negative for major mastitis pathogens. Within 24 h after calving, neutrophils were isolated from blood and incubated with 0, 40 or 400 ng/ml recombinant bovine IL-8 (rbIL-8) for 2 and 6 h. Next, neutrophils were stimulated with PMA or OZP and ROS generation was measured by chemiluminescence. Finally associations between ROS generation and genotype, incubation time and rbIL-8 concentration were statistically analyzed. The sample size (n = 20) was based on previous research demonstrating significant differences in ROS generation

between 10 early and 10 mid lactating cows [16]. The incubation times were determined in a preliminary experiment in which blood neutrophils from 2 early lactating heifers were incubated for 2, 4, 6 and 18 h with 0, 40 or 400 ng/ml rbIL-8. A differential count of the isolated cells was performed to estimate the % neutrophils. Viability of neutrophils was measured after isolation and after each incubation time by trypan blue exclusion.

Bacteriological culture
As mastitis can affect functionality of blood neutrophils [17], aseptic quarter milk samples were collected at the time of blood sampling and bacteriologically cultured. Ten μL of each sample was spread on blood-esculin and MacConkey's agar and incubated aerobically for 24–48 h at 37°C. Bacteriological culture was performed according to National Mastitis Council (NMC) guidelines [18]. Four heifers were culture-positive in five quarters for major pathogens and excluded from the analysis. *Staphylococcus aureus*, esculin-positive cocci and *Escherichia coli* were isolated from 2 quarters of 1 heifers, 1 quarter of 1 heifer and 2 quarters of 2 heifers, respectively.

CXCR1 genotype
To include heifers with common and rare *CXCR1* genotypes (e.g. c.980AA), a sufficient number of heifers were genotyped before calving. A blood sample was taken from 60 Holstein heifers belonging to 5 herds and having an expected calving date between January and June 2014. Genotype at SNPs c.735C > G and c.980A > G was determined using a fluorescent multiprobe PCR assay as previously described [19]. Efforts were made to include sufficient heifers with genotype c.980AA or c.980AG. Of the 20 heifers included in the final analysis, 7, 6 and 7 had genotype c.735CC, c.735CG and c.735GG, respectively. Three, 5 and 12 had genotype c.980AA, c.980AG and c.980GG, respectively.

Reactive oxygen species assay
Seventy-five mL blood was collected from the coccygeal vein using 8 mL Vacutainer tubes (Becton Dickinson, Erembodegem, Belgium) containing 150 μL of EDTA as anticoagulant. Blood neutrophils were isolated within 1 h of collection by hypotonic lysis of red blood cells and Histopaque 1077/1119 gradient (Sigma-Aldrich, Bornem, Belgium) centrifugation according to Siemens et al. [20]. Cell concentration was measured in triplicate with a Bürker chamber.

Two hundred thousand blood neutrophils were suspended in 200 μL of 1 × Hank's balanced salt solution (HBSS; Gibco, Life technologies, Carlsbad, CA) supplemented with 0, 40 or 400 ng recombinant bovine IL-8 (rbIL-8; Kingfisher Biotech, Saint Paul, MN) per mL and incubated for 2 or 6 h at 37°C in 2 mL test tubes.

Next, blood neutrophils were pelleted by centrifugation at $1000 \times g$ for 5 min and resuspended in 120 µl $1 \times$ HBSS. Luminol (0.30 mmol/L Sigma-Aldrich) and PMA (100 ng/mL; Sigma-Aldrich) or OZP (750 µg/mL) were added to a final volume of 200 µL. Zymosan A (Sigma-Aldrich) was opsonized by washing the pellet with 60 and 30 mL $1 \times$ phosphate-buffered saline (PBS; Gibco) (centrifugation at $200 \times g$ for 10 min) followed by 1 h incubation at 37°C in 5 mL $1 \times$ PBS and 35 mL bovine serum and two additional washing steps with 30 mL $1 \times$ PBS (centrifugation at $200 \times g$ for 10 min). Bovine serum was collected from the coccygeal vein of a healthy Holstein cow using 8 mL gel and clot activator tubes (Vacutest Kima, Piove di Sacco, Italy). Reactions of blood neutrophils primed by rbIL-8 were performed in duplicate. Chemiluminescence was measured every 60 sec for 90 min with a luminometer (TriStar[2] LB 942 Multidetection Microplate Reader, Berthold Technologies, Bad Wildbad, Germany) and expressed in relative light units (RLU). Area under the curve (AUC) values (in 10^6 RLU $*$ s) were calculated to analyze the total ROS generation whereas peak values (RLUmax; in 10^3 RLU) and time of peak values (Tmax; in min) were saved in the dataset to study the kinetics of ROS generation [5].

Statistical analysis

Different linear mixed regression models (PROC MIXED, SAS 9.4, SAS Institute Inc.) were fit for AUC, RLUmax and Tmax after stimulation with PMA or OZP (6 outcome variables) and for SNP c.735C > G or c.980A > G (12 models in total). Heifer was added as random effect to correct for clustering of multiple observations (6) per heifer (RANDOM statement). The models included heifers' genotype at position of the SNP, incubation (2 or 6 h) and rbIL-8 (0, 40 or 400 ng/ml) as categorical fixed effects. All two-way interactions between fixed effects were tested but removed from the models because they were non-significant ($P > 0.05$).

Results

Preliminary experiment

A differential count demonstrated 94.3% [standard deviation (SD) 0.1%] of the isolated cells to be neutrophils. The viability of the neutrophils was 100% immediately after isolation and decreased to 96% (SD 1%), 96% (SD 2%), 98% (SD 1%) and 81% (SD 3%) after 2, 4, 6 and 18 h isolation, respectively. Differences in viability between neutrophils incubated with 0, 40 or 400 ng/mL rbIL-8 were small (data not shown). Because of the low viability and strongly diminished ROS generation after 18 h incubation, neutrophils were incubated for 2 and 6 h (Figure 1). As expected [21], chemiluminescence increased fast after PMA stimulation with a clear peak and increased more gradually after OZP stimulation (Figure 1).

Associations with ROS generation after PMA stimulation

Single nucleotide polymorphisms c.735C > G and c.980A > G were not associated with AUC, RLUmax or Tmax ($P > 0.05$) (Table 1). Incubation was associated with AUC, RLUmax and Tmax. Blood neutrophils incubated for 6 h showed higher AUC, RLUmax and Tmax values compared to blood neutrophils incubated for 2 h ($P < 0.05$). Concentration of rbIL-8 was associated with AUC and Tmax ($P < 0.01$) and not with RLUmax ($P = 0.17$). Blood neutrophils incubated with 40 or 400 ng/mL showed higher AUC and Tmax values compared to blood neutrophils incubated without rbIL-8.

Associations with ROS generation after OZP stimulation

Single nucleotide polymorphisms c.735C > G and c.980A > G were not associated with AUC, RLUmax or Tmax ($P > 0.05$) (Table 2). Incubation was associated with AUC and RLUmax and not with Tmax. Blood neutrophils incubated for 6 h showed higher AUC and RLUmax values compared to blood neutrophils incubated for 2 h ($P < 0.05$). Concentration of rbIL-8 was associated with AUC and RLUmax ($P < 0.01$) and not with Tmax ($P = 0.89$). Blood neutrophils incubated with 40 or 400 ng/ml showed lower AUC and Tmax values compared to blood neutrophils incubated without rbIL-8. Differences were mainly in neutrophils incubated with rbIL-8 at a concentration of 400 ng/mL, AUC values were smaller.

Discussion

Research on genetic polymorphisms enlarges our knowledge on mammary gland immunity and helps us to understand why certain cows are more mastitis resistant than others [15]. Because of the important function of CXCR1 in the innate immunity of the mammary gland [8,22] and a quantitative trait locus for clinical mastitis in this region of the bovine genome [23], CXCR1 polymorphisms form interesting study objects. In this study, an in vitro model was used to analyze the effect of CXCR1 SNP on neutrophil functionality in a sample population of freshly calved heifers. Associations between CXCR1 genotype and neutrophil ROS generation after rbIL-8 incubation and stimulation with PMA or OZP were studied in detail.

The association between SNP c.735C > G and PMA-induced ROS generation reported by Rambeaud et al. (2006) could not be confirmed in our model. In contrast to the previously demonstrated higher ROS generation [9], we observed numerically lower AUC values in c.735GG neutrophils compared to c.735CC neutrophils. Additionally, no significant interaction effects between c.735C > G and rbIL-8 concentration were observed. Based on previous research [13], we hypothesized a higher ROS generation and response to rbIL-8 in c.980AG

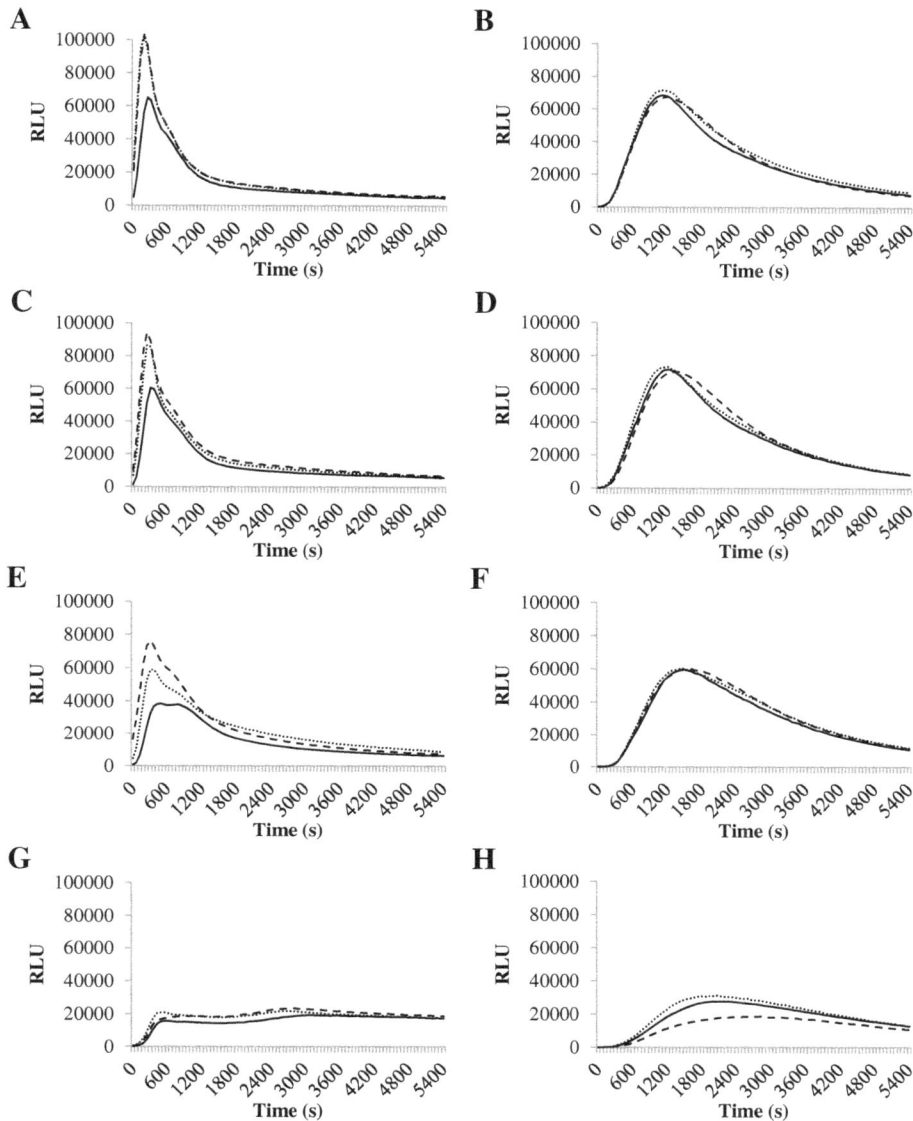

Figure 1 Effect of Interleukin-8 on reactive oxygen species generation of blood neutrophils.Preliminary experiment studying the reactive oxygen species (ROS) generation of blood neutrophils isolated from 2 early lactating dairy cows and incubated with 0 (————), 40 (••••) or 400 (– – –) ng recombinant bovine interleukin-8 (rbIL-8) per mL for 2 (**A** and **B**), 4 (**C** and **D**), 6 (**E** and **F**) or 18 (**G** and **H**) h measured using luminol chemiluminescence [expressed in relative light units (RLU)]. Prior to measurement, neutrophils were stimulated with phorbol 12-myristate 13-acetate (**A**, **C**, **E** and **G**) or opsonized zymosan particles (**B**, **D**, **F** and **H**).

compared to c.980GG neutrophils. However, neither c.980A > G nor the interaction between rbIL-8 concentration and c.980A > G were associated with AUC, RLU-max or Tmax of PMA- or OZP-induced ROS generation in our model. Despite potential effects on ligand binding, signal transduction and internalization of CXCR1 [12], no interaction between *CXCR1* SNPs and rbIL-8 incubation could be demonstrated. Human CXCR1 but not hCXCR2 was found to be important for activation of ROS [24]. Latter functional differences were partly attributed to amino acid sequence differences in the C-terminus

causing a faster receptor phosphorylation and internalization of hCXCR2 compared to hCXCR1 [25-27]. In contrast to hCXCR1 and hCXCR2, the C-terminus of both bovine IL-8R show identical amino acid sequences [28]. Hence, activation of neutrophils could be mediated by both receptors and functional effects caused by *CXCR1* SNP might be compensated by a fully functional CXCR2, explaining similar rbIL-8 responses on ROS across *CXCR1* genotypes in our study.

Several studies demonstrated a priming effect of IL-8 on ROS generation in human neutrophils [10,29,30].

Table 1 Statistical analysis of reactive oxygen species generation by blood neutrophils following phorbol 12-myristate 13-acetate stimulation

Polymorphism[1]	Fixed effect	n[2]	AUC[3]			RLUmax[4]			Tmax[5]		
			β[6]	SE[7]	P[8]	β[6]	SE[7]	P[8]	β[6]	SE[7]	P[8]
c.735C > G	Intercept		71	8		37	6		9.2	1.0	
	Genotype				0.69			0.94			0.47
	c.735CC	7	Ref.[9]	...		Ref.[9]	...		Ref.[9]	...	
	c.735CG	6	-6	11		-3	9		0.3	1.3	
	c.735GG	7	-9	11		-1	8		-1.2	1.3	
	Incubation				<0.01			<0.01			<0.05
	2 h		Ref.[9]	...		Ref.[9]	...		Ref.[9]	...	
	6 h		11	2		4	1		1.2	0.5	
	rbIL-8				<0.01			0.17			<0.01
	0 ng/ml		Ref.[9]	...		Ref.[9]	...		Ref.[9]	...	
	40 ng/ml		7	2		-3	2		3.1	0.6	
	400 ng/ml		5	2		-2	2		3.1	0.6	
c.980A > G	Intercept		66	11		29	9		8.9	1.5	
	Genotype				0.45			0.56			0.78
	c.980AA	3	Ref.[9]	...		Ref.[9]	...		Ref.[9]	...	
	c.980AG	5	10	14		12	11		0.7	1.8	
	c.980GG	12	-4	13		5	10		-0.2	1.6	
	Incubation				<0.01			<0.01			<0.05
	2 h		Ref.[9]	...		Ref.[9]	...		Ref.[9]	...	
	6 h		11	2		4	1		1.2	0.5	
	rbIL-8				<0.01			0.17			<0.01
	0 ng/ml		Ref.[9]	...		Ref.[9]	...		Ref.[9]	...	
	40 ng/ml		7	2		-3	2		3.1	0.6	
	400 ng/ml		5	2		-2	2		3.1	0.6	

[1]Linear mixed regression models describing the association between reactive oxygen species generation by blood neutrophils and *CXCR1* polymorphisms c.735C > G and c.980A > G, respectively. Neutrophils were incubated with 0, 40 or 400 ng recombinant bovine interleukin 8 per mL for 2 or 6 h and stimulated with phorbol 12-myristate 13-acetate,
[2]Number of heifers,
[3]Area under the curve values in 10^6 RLU (relative light units) * s,
[4]Peak values in 10^3 RLU.
[5]Time of peak values in min,
[6]Regression coefficient,
[7]Standard error,
[8]Overall *P*-value of the fixed effect,
[9]Reference,
All two-way interactions between the fixed effects were non-significant (P > 0.05) and removed from the model.

Enhancement of ROS generation already occurred after 5 min of IL-8 incubation [29] and was explained by intracellular calcium mobilization [30] and by activation of phospholipase D (PLD) [10], protein kinase C-ε (PKC-ε) [25] and phospholipase A_2 [29]. To the best of our knowledge, Mitchell et al. [7] were the only to study the priming effect of IL-8 on bovine neutrophils. Intracellular ROS generation was measured by 2,7-Dichloro-dihydrofluorecein diacetate (H2DCFDA) flow cytometry. Incubation with rbIL-8 for 18 h enhanced the *Mannheimia haemolytica*-induced ROS generation whereas incubation for 30 or 60 min had little effect [7]. In our study, ROS generation was measured using luminol chemiluminescence. This assay has the benefit that both intra- and extracellular ROS generation are measured and allows for measurement over time [31]. Neutrophils were exposed to the same concentrations of rbIL-8 as in the study of Mitchell et al. [7] but for only 2 or 6 h. We opted not to incubate for 18 h because our preliminary experiments showed a reduced viability and a strongly diminished ROS generation after such a long period. Associations were detected between rbIL-8 concentration and ROS generation indicating the presence of a functional IL-8 receptor on the isolated blood neutrophils. In

Table 2 Statistical analysis of reactive oxygen species generation by blood neutrophils following opsonized zymosan particles stimulation

Polymorphism[1]	Fixed effect	n[2]	AUC[3]			RLUmax[4]			Tmax[5]		
			β[6]	SE[7]	P[8]	β[6]	SE[7]	P[8]	β[6]	SE[7]	P[8]
c.735C > G	Intercept		253	32		69	10		31.7	4.0	
	Genotype				0.40			0.82			0.22
	c.735CC	7	Ref.[9]	...		Ref.[9]	...		Ref.[9]	...	
	c.735CG	6	-36	47		-6	14		-3.6	5.3	
	c.735GG	7	-63	45		-9	14		-9.2	5.1	
	Incubation				<0.01			<0.01			0.54
	2 h		Ref.[9]	...		Ref.[9]	...		Ref.[9]	...	
	6 h		20	7		5	2		1.2	1.9	
	rbIL-8				<0.01			<0.01			0.89
	0 ng/ml		Ref.[9]	...		Ref.[9]	...		Ref.[9]	...	
	40 ng/ml		-6	8		-3	2		-0.6	2.3	
	400 ng/ml		-26	8		-8	2		0.5	2.3	
c.980A > G	Intercept		248	48		63	15		32.9	6.0	
	Genotype				0.32			0.58			0.44
	c.980AA	3	Ref.[9]	...		Ref.[9]	...		Ref.[9]	...	
	c.980AG	5	13	61		12	18		-3.6	7.3	
	c.980GG	12	-51	54		-2	16		-7.8	6.4	
	Incubation				<0.01			<0.01			0.54
	2 h		Ref.[9]	...		Ref.[9]	...		Ref.[9]	...	
	6 h		20	7		5	2		1.2	1.9	
	rbIL-8				<0.01			0.17			0.89
	0 ng/ml		Ref.[9]	...		Ref.[9]	...		Ref.[9]	...	
	40 ng/ml		-6	8		-3	2		-0.6	2.3	
	400 ng/ml		-26	8		-8	2		0.5	2.3	

[1]Linear mixed regression models describing the association between reactive oxygen species generation by blood neutrophils and *CXCR1* polymorphisms c.735C > G and c.980A > G, respectively. Neutrophils were incubated with 0, 40 or 400 ng recombinant bovine interleukin 8 per mL for 2 or 6 h and stimulated with opsonized zymosan particles,
[2]Number of heifers,
[3]Area under the curve values in 10^6 RLU (relative light units) * s,
[4]Peak values in 10^3 RLU
[5]Time of peak values in min,
[6]Regression coefficient,
[7]Standard error,
[8]Overall *P*-value of the fixed effect,
[9]Reference,
All two-way interactions between the fixed effects were non-significant (P > 0.05) and removed from the model.

contrast to research on human neutrophils [29,30], IL-8 also had inhibitory effects on neutrophils ROS generation in our model. Incubation with rbIL-8 had a positive effect on the total PMA-induced ROS generation but a negative effect on the total OZP-induced ROS generation. The stimulatory agent dependent effect could be explained by differences in the pathways of ROS generation by PMA and OZP [32]. Incubation with rbIL-8 might have simultaneously activated components of the pathway induced by PMA (e.g. PKC) while inhibiting components of the pathway induced by OZP (e.g. calcium mobilization).

Conclusions

In conclusion, no differences in PMA- or OZP-induced ROS generation were detected in blood neutrophils isolated from early lactating heifers with different *CXCR1* c.735C > G and c.980A > G genotypes. The inhibitory effects of rbIL-8 on neutrophil ROS generation suggest a complex interaction between IL-8 and ROS generation in bovine neutrophils.

Abbreviations
AUC: Area under the curve; CXCR1: Chemokine (C-X-C motif) receptor 1; IL-8: Interleukin 8; IL8RA: Interleukin 8 receptor A; NMC: National mastitis council; OZP: Opsonized zymosan particles; PMA: Phorbol 12-myristate

13-acetate; rbIL-8: Recombinant bovine interleukin 8; RLU: Relative light units; RLUmax: Peak value; ROS: Reactive oxygen species; SCC: Somatic cell count; SNP: Single nucleotide polymorphism; Tmax: Time of peak value.

Competing interests
The authors declare that they have no competing interests.

Authors' contributions
JV, XB, CB, LP and SDV designed the experiment. JV, XB and CR collected milk and blood samples. JV genotyped animals. CR isolated blood neutrophils. JV, XB and CR conducted the chemiluminescence assay. JV analyzed data and drafted the manuscript. XB, CB, LP, BDS and SDV gave critical comments on the manuscript. All authors read and approved the final manuscript.

Acknowledgements
This research was financed by a PhD grant (n° 101206) by the Agency for Innovation by Science and Technology in Flanders (IWT Vlaanderen). The authors wish to thank the participating dairy producers and bovine practitioner Raf Deconinck.

Author details
[1]M-team and Mastitis and Milk Quality Research Unit, Department of Reproduction, Obstetrics, and Herd Health, Faculty of Veterinary Medicine, Ghent University, Salisburylaan, 133 Merelbeke, Belgium. [2]Department of Comparative Physiology and Biometrics, Faculty of Veterinary Medicine, Ghent University, Salisburylaan, 133 Merelbeke, Belgium. [3]Animal Genetics Laboratory, Department of Nutrition, Genetics, and Ethology, Faculty of Veterinary Medicine, Ghent University, Heidestraat, 19 Merelbeke, Belgium. [4]Laboratory of Drug Quality & Registration, Department of Pharmaceutical Analysis, Faculty of Pharmaceutical Sciences, Ghent University, Ottergemsesteenweg, 460 Ghent, Belgium.

References
1. Rainard P, Riollet C. Innate immunity of the bovine mammary gland. Vet Res. 2006;37:369–400.
2. Mehrzad J, Duchateau L, Burvenich C. Phagocytic and bactericidal activity of blood and milk-resident neutrophils against *staphylococcus aureus* in primiparous and multiparous cows during early lactation. Vet Microbiol. 2009;134:106–12.
3. Paape M, Mehrzad J, Zhao X, Detilleux J, Burvenich C. Defense of the bovine mammary gland by polymorphonuclear neutrophil leukocytes. J Mammary Gland Biol Neoplasia. 2002;7:109–21.
4. Heyneman R, Burvenich C, Vercauteren R. Interaction between the respiratory burst activity of neutrophil leukocytes and experimentally induced *Escherichia coli* mastitis in cows. J Dairy Sci. 1990;73:985–94.
5. Mehrzad J, Duchateau L, Burvenich C. High milk neutrophil chemiluminescence limits the severity of bovine coliform mastitis. Vet Res. 2005;36:101–16.
6. Kremer WD, Noordhuizen-Stassen EN, Grommers FJ, Daemen AJ, Henricks PA, Brand A, et al. Preinfection chemotactic response of blood polymorphonuclear leukocytes to predict severity of *Escherichia coli* mastitis. J Dairy Sci. 1993;76:1568–74.
7. Mitchell GB, Albright BN, Caswell JL. Effect of interleukin-8 and granulocyte colony-stimulating factor on priming and activation of bovine neutrophils. Infect Immun. 2003;71:1643–9.
8. Barber MR, Yang TJ. Chemotactic activities in nonmastitic and mastitic mammary secretions: Presence of interleukin-8 in mastitic but not nonmastitic secretions. Clin Diagn Lab Immunol. 1998;5:82–6.
9. Rambeaud M, Clift R, Pighetti GM. Association of a bovine *CXCR2* gene polymorphism with neutrophil survival and killing ability. Vet Immunol Immunopathol. 2006;111:231–8.
10. Jones SA, Wolf M, Qin SX, Mackay CR, Baggiolini M. Different functions for the interleukin 8 receptors (IL-8R) of human neutrophil leukocytes: NADPH oxidase and phospholipase D are activated through IL-8R1 but not IL-8R2. Proc Natl Acad Sci U S A. 1996;93:6682–6.
11. Jones SA, Dewald B, ClarkLewis I, Baggiolini M. Chemokine antagonists that discriminate between interleukin-8 receptors - Selective blockers of CXCR2. J Biol Chem. 1997;272:16166–9.
12. Pighetti GM, Kojima CJ, Wojakiewicz L, Rambeaud M. The bovine *CXCR1* gene is highly polymorphic. Vet Immunol Immunopathol. 2012;145:464–70.
13. Verbeke J, Piepers S, Peelman LJ, Van Poucke M, De Vliegher S. Pathogen-group specific association between *CXCR1* polymorphisms and subclinical mastitis in dairy heifers. J Dairy Res. 2012;79:341–51.
14. Liou JW, Chang FT, Chung Y, Chen WY, Fischer WB, Hsu HJ: In Silico analysis reveals sequential interactions and protein conformational changes during the binding of chemokine CXCL-8 to its receptor CXCR1. Plos One 2014, 9:e94178
15. Pighetti GM, Elliott AA. Gene polymorphisms: the keys for marker assisted selection and unraveling core regulatory pathways for mastitis resistance. J Mammary Gland Biol Neoplasia. 2011;16:421–32.
16. Mehrzad J, Dosogne H, Meyer E, Heyneman R, Burvenich C. Respiratory burst activity of blood and milk neutrophils in dairy cows during different stages of lactation. J Dairy Res. 2001;68:399–415.
17. Mehrzad J, Dosogne H, Meyer E, Burvenich C. Local and systemic effects of endotoxin mastitis on the chemiluminescence of milk and blood neutrophils in dairy cows. Vet Res. 2001;32:131–44.
18. National Mastitis Council: Laboratory Handbook on Bovine Mastitis. Madison, WI: National Mastitis Counc. Inc. Wisconsin: The National Mastitis Council; 1999.
19. Verbeke J, Van Poucke M, Peelman L, Piepers S, De Vliegher S. Associations between *CXCR1* polymorphisms and pathogen-specific clinical mastitis, test-day somatic cell count and test-day milk yield. J Dairy Sci. 2014;97:7927–39.
20. Siemens DW, Schepetkin IA, Kirpotina LN, Lei B, Quinn MT. Neutrophil isolation from nonhuman species. Methods Mol Biol. 2007;138:21–34.
21. Lieberman MM, Sachanandani DM, Pinney CA. Comparative study of neutrophil activation by chemiluminescence and flow cytometry. Clin Diagn Lab Immunol. 1996;3:654–62.
22. Caswell JL, Middleton DM, Gordon JR. Production and functional characterization of recombinant bovine interleukin-8 as a specific neutrophil activator and chemoattractant. Vet Immunol Immunopathol. 1999;67:327–40.
23. Sodeland M, Kent MP, Olsen HG, Opsal MA, Svendsen M, Sehested E, et al. Quantitative trait loci for clinical mastitis on chromosomes 2, 6, 14 and 20 in Norwegian Red cattle. Anim Genet. 2011;42:457–65.
24. Stillie R, Farooq SM, Gordon JR, Stadnyk AW. The functional significance behind expressing two IL-8 receptor types on PMN. J Leukoc Biol. 2009;86:529–43.
25. Nasser MW, Marjoram RJ, Brown SL, Richardson RM. Cross-desensitization among CXCR1, CXCR2, and CCR5: Role of protein kinase C-epsilon. J Immunol. 2005;174:6927–33.
26. Richardson RM, Marjoram RJ, Barak LS, Snyderman R. Role of the cytoplasmic tails of CXCR1 and CXCR2 in mediating leukocyte migration, activation, and regulation. J Immunol. 2003;170:2904–11.
27. Richardson RM, Pridgen BC, Haribabu B, Ali H, Snyderman R. Differential cross-regulation of the human chemokine receptors CXCR1 and CXCR2 - Evidence for time-dependent signal generation. J Biol Chem. 1998;273:23830–6.
28. Lahouassa H, Rainard P, Caraty A, Riollet C. Identification and characterization of a new interleukin-8 receptor in bovine species. Mol Immunol. 2008;45:1153–64.
29. Daniels RH, Finnen MJ, Hill ME, Lackie JM. Recombinant human monocyte Il-8 primes Nadph-oxidase and Phospholipase-A2 activation in human neutrophils. Immunology. 1992;75:157–63.
30. Wozniak A, Betts WH, Murphy GA, Rokicinski M. Interleukin-8 primes human neutrophils for enhanced superoxide anion production. Immunology. 1993;79:608–15.
31. Rinaldi M, Moroni P, Paape MJ, Bannerman DD. Evaluation of assays for the measurement of bovine neutrophil reactive oxygen species. Vet Immunol Immunopathol. 2007;115:107–25.
32. Maridonneau-Parini I, Tringale SM, Tauber AI. Identification of distinct activation pathways of the human neutrophil Nadph-oxidase. J Immunol. 1986;137:2925–9.

Permissions

List of Contributors

Hassan M Mai
Department of Production Animal Studies, Faculty of Veterinary Science, University of Pretoria, Private Bag X04, Onderstepoort 0110, South Africa
Animal Production Programme, School of Agriculture and Agricultural Technology, Abubakar Tafawa Balewa University, P. M. B. 0248, Bauchi, Nigeria

Peter C Irons
Department of Production Animal Studies, Faculty of Veterinary Science, University of Pretoria, Private Bag X04, Onderstepoort 0110, South Africa

Peter N Thompson
Department of Production Animal Studies, Faculty of Veterinary Science, University of Pretoria, Private Bag X04, Onderstepoort 0110, South Africa

Leonardo Murgiano
Institute of Genetics, Vetsuisse Faculty, University of Bern, Bremgartenstrasse 109a, CH-3001 Bern, Switzerland

Natalie Wiedemar
Institute of Genetics, Vetsuisse Faculty, University of Bern, Bremgartenstrasse 109a, CH-3001 Bern, Switzerland

Vidhya Jagannathan
Institute of Genetics, Vetsuisse Faculty, University of Bern, Bremgartenstrasse 109a, CH-3001 Bern, Switzerland

Louise K Isling
Department of Veterinary Disease Biology, Section for Veterinary Pathology, Faculty of Health and Medical Sciences, University of Copenhagen, Ridebanevej 3, DK-1870 Frederiksberg C, Denmark

Cord Drögemüller
Institute of Genetics, Vetsuisse Faculty, University of Bern, Bremgartenstrasse 109a, CH-3001 Bern, Switzerland

Jørgen S Agerholm
Department of Veterinary Disease Biology, Section for Veterinary Pathology, Faculty of Health and Medical Sciences, University of Copenhagen, Ridebanevej 3, DK-1870 Frederiksberg C, Denmark
Department of Large Animal Sciences, Section for Veterinary Reproduction and Obstetrics, Faculty of Health and Medical Sciences, University of Copenhagen, Dyrlaegevej 68, DK-1870 Frederiksberg C, Denmark

Sarah L Giles
School of Veterinary Science, University of Bristol, Langford, Bristol BS40 5DU, UK

Christine J Nicol
School of Veterinary Science, University of Bristol, Langford, Bristol BS40 5DU, UK

Sean A Rands
School of Biological Sciences, University of Bristol, Bristol Life Science Building, 24 Tyndall Avenue, Bristol BS8 1TQ, UK

Patricia A Harris
WALTHAM Centre for Pet Nutrition, Equine Studies Group, Freeby Lane, Waltham-on-the-Wolds, Leicestershire LE14 4RT, Melton Mowbray, UK

Marcio C Costa
Department of Pathobiology, Ontario Veterinary College, University of Guelph, Guelph, Canada

Henry R Stämpfli
Department of Clinical Studies, Ontario Veterinary College, University of Guelph, Guelph, Canada

Luis G Arroyo
Department of Clinical Studies, Ontario Veterinary College, University of Guelph, Guelph, Canada

Emma Allen-Vercoe
Department of Molecularand Cellular Biology, College of Biological Sciences, University of Guelph, Guelph, Canada

Roberta G Gomes
Department of Clinical Studies, "Universidade Estadual de Londrina", Londrina, Brazil

J Scott Weese
Department of Pathobiology, Ontario Veterinary College, University of Guelph, Guelph, Canada

Martin C Langenmayer
Institute of Veterinary Pathology at the Centre for Clinical Veterinary Medicine, Ludwig-Maximilians-Universitaet Muenchen, Munich, Germany

Julia C Scharr
Rammingen, Germany

Carola Sauter-Louis
Clinic for Ruminants with Ambulatory and Herd Health Services at the Centre for Clinical Veterinary Medicine, Ludwig-Maximilians-Universitaet Muenchen, Oberschleissheim, Germany

Gereon Schares
Friedrich-Loeffler-Institut, Federal Research Institute for Animal Health, Institute of Epidemiology, Greifswald-Isle of Riems, Germany

Nicole S Gollnick
Clinic for Ruminants with Ambulatory and Herd Health Services at the Centre for Clinical Veterinary Medicine, Ludwig-Maximilians-Universitaet Muenchen, Oberschleissheim, Germany

Chenchen Wu
College of Animal Veterinary Medicine, Northwest A & F University, Yangling 712100, Shaanxi, People's Republic of China

Xiaoxue Liu
College of Animal Veterinary Medicine, Northwest A & F University, Yangling 712100, Shaanxi, People's Republic of China

Feng Ma
College of Animal Veterinary Medicine, Northwest A & F University, Yangling 712100, Shaanxi, People's Republic of China

Baoyu Zhao
College of Animal Veterinary Medicine, Northwest A & F University, Yangling 712100, Shaanxi, People's Republic of China

Gillian D Alton
Department of Population Medicine, Ontario Veterinary College, University of Guelph, Guelph, ON N1G 2 W1, Canada

David L Pearl
Department of Population Medicine, Ontario Veterinary College, University of Guelph, Guelph, ON N1G 2 W1, Canada

Ken G Bateman
Department of Population Medicine, Ontario Veterinary College, University of Guelph, Guelph, ON N1G 2 W1, Canada

W Bruce McNab
Ontario Ministry of Agriculture & Food, Guelph, ON N1G 4Y2, Canada

Olaf Berke
Department of Population Medicine, Ontario Veterinary College, University of Guelph, Guelph, ON N1G 2 W1, Canada
Department of Mathematics and Statistics, University of Guelph, Guelph, ON N1G 2 W1, Canada

Jenny John
Institute of Animal Nutrition, Nutrition Diseases and Dietetics, Faculty of Veterinary Medicine, University of Leipzig, Leipzig, Germany
Present address: Tierklinik Teisendorf, Teisendorf, Germany

Kathrin Roediger
Pferdeklinik Großostheim, Großostheim, Germany

Wieland Schroedl
Institute of Bacteriology and Mycology, Faculty of Veterinary Medicine, University of Leipzig, Leipzig, Germany

Nada Aldaher
Institute of Bacteriology and Mycology, Faculty of Veterinary Medicine, University of Leipzig, Leipzig, Germany

Ingrid Vervuert
Institute of Animal Nutrition, Nutrition Diseases and Dietetics, Faculty of Veterinary Medicine, University of Leipzig, Leipzig, Germany

Xiangping Li
State Key Laboratory of Subtropical Bioresource Conservation and Utilization at Guangxi University, Nanning, Guangxi, China
Guangxi High Education Key Laboratory for Animal Reproduction and Biotechnology, Guangxi University, Nanning 530004, China

Shihai Huang
College of Life Science and Technology, Guangxi University, Nanning, Guangxi, China

Yanping Ren
State Key Laboratory of Subtropical Bioresource Conservation and Utilization at Guangxi University, Nanning, Guangxi, China
Guangxi High Education Key Laboratory for Animal Reproduction and Biotechnology, Guangxi University, Nanning 530004, China

Meng Wang
State Key Laboratory of Subtropical Bioresource Conservation and Utilization at Guangxi University, Nanning, Guangxi, China

Guangxi High Education Key Laboratory for Animal Reproduction and Biotechnology, Guangxi University, Nanning 530004, China

Chao Kang
College of Life Science and Technology, Guangxi University, Nanning, Guangxi, China

Liangliang Xie
State Key Laboratory of Subtropical Bioresource Conservation and Utilization at Guangxi University, Nanning, Guangxi, China
Guangxi High Education Key Laboratory for Animal Reproduction and Biotechnology, Guangxi University, Nanning 530004, China

Deshun Shi
State Key Laboratory of Subtropical Bioresource Conservation and Utilization at Guangxi University, Nanning, Guangxi, China
Guangxi High Education Key Laboratory for Animal Reproduction and Biotechnology, Guangxi University, Nanning 530004, China

Nicole S Gollnick
Clinic for Ruminants with Ambulatory and Herd Health Services at the Centre for Clinical Veterinary Medicine, Veterinary Faculty, Ludwig-Maximilians-Universitaet Muenchen, Sonnenstrasse 16, 85764 Oberschleissheim, Germany

Julia C Scharr
89129 Rammingen, Germany

Gereon Schares
Friedrich-Loeffler-Institut, Federal Research Institute for Animal Health, Institute of Epidemiology, Suedufer 10, 17493 Greifswald-Insel Riems, Germany

Martin C Langenmayer
Institute of Veterinary Pathology at the Centre for Clinical Veterinary Medicine, Veterinary Faculty, Ludwig-Maximilians-Universitaet Muenchen, Veterinaerstr. 13, 80539 Munich, Germany

Leandro Maia
Department of Animal Reproduction, São Paulo State University, District of Rubião Júnior, n/n, CEP: 18618970, Botucatu, São Paulo, Brazil

Fernanda da Cruz Landim- Alvarenga
Department of Animal Reproduction, São Paulo State University, District of Rubião Júnior, n/n, CEP: 18618970, Botucatu, São Paulo, Brazil

Marilda Onghero Taffarel
Department of Veterinary Medicine, Maringá State University, Av. Colombo, 5.790, CEP: 87020-900, Maringá, Paraná, Brazil

Carolina Nogueira de Moraes
Department of Animal Reproduction, São Paulo State University, District of Rubião Júnior, n/n, CEP: 18618970, Botucatu, São Paulo, Brazil

Gisele Fabrino Machado
Department of Clinic, Surgery and Animal Reproduction, São Paulo State University, Clóvis Pestano, 793, CEP: 16050-680, Araçatuba, São Paulo, Brazil

Guilherme Dias Melo
Department of Clinic, Surgery and Animal Reproduction, São Paulo State University, Clóvis Pestano, 793, CEP: 16050-680, Araçatuba, São Paulo, Brazil

Rogério Martins Amorim
Department of Veterinary Clinics, São Paulo State University, District of Rubião Júnior, n/n, CEP: 18618970, Botucatu, São Paulo, Brazil

Katia Cappelli
Department of Veterinary Medicine, University of Perugia, Via San Costanzo 4, 06126 Perugia, Italy

Chiara Brachelente
Department of Veterinary Medicine, University of Perugia, Via San Costanzo 4, 06126 Perugia, Italy

Fabrizio Passamonti
Department of Veterinary Medicine, University of Perugia, Via San Costanzo 4, 06126 Perugia, Italy

Alessandro Flati
Private Practitioner, via Roma 193, Scoppito, L'Aquila, Italy

Maurizio Silvestrelli
Department of Veterinary Medicine, University of Perugia, Via San Costanzo 4, 06126 Perugia, Italy

Stefano Capomaccio
Institute of Zootechnics, UCSC, via Emilia Parmense 84, 29122 Piacenza, Italy

Carlos E Giraldo
Grupo de Investigación Terapia Regenerativa, Departamento de Salud Animal, Universidad de Caldas, Manizales, Colombia

María E Álvarez
Grupo de Investigación Terapia Regenerativa, Departamento de Salud Animal, Universidad de Caldas, Manizales, Colombia

Jorge U Carmona
Grupo de Investigación Terapia Regenerativa, Departamento de Salud Animal, Universidad de Caldas, Manizales, Colombia

Jennifer Haupt
Department of Clinical Sciences, Cummings School of Veterinary Medicine, Tufts University, 200 Westboro Road, North Grafton, MA 01536, USA

José M García-López
Department of Clinical Sciences, Cummings School of Veterinary Medicine, Tufts University, 200 Westboro Road, North Grafton, MA 01536, USA

Kate Chope
Department of Clinical Sciences, Cummings School of Veterinary Medicine, Tufts University, 200 Westboro Road, North Grafton, MA 01536, USA

Tianle Xu
College of Veterinary Medicine, Nanjing Agricultural University, Nanjing 210095, China

Hui Tao
College of Veterinary Medicine, Nanjing Agricultural University, Nanjing 210095, China

Guangjun Chang
College of Veterinary Medicine, Nanjing Agricultural University, Nanjing 210095, China

Kai Zhang
College of Veterinary Medicine, Nanjing Agricultural University, Nanjing 210095, China

Lei Xu
College of Veterinary Medicine, Nanjing Agricultural University, Nanjing 210095, China

Xiangzhen Shen
College of Veterinary Medicine, Nanjing Agricultural University, Nanjing 210095, China

Krister Blodörn
Department of Clinical Sciences, Swedish University of Agricultural Sciences, Host Pathogen Interaction Group, Uppsala, Sweden

Sara Hägglund
Department of Clinical Sciences, Swedish University of Agricultural Sciences, Host Pathogen Interaction Group, Uppsala, Sweden

Dolores Gavier-Widen
Department of Pathology and Wildlife Diseases, National Veterinary Institute, Uppsala, Sweden
Department of Biomedical Sciences and Veterinary Public Health, Swedish University of Agricultural Sciences, Uppsala, Sweden

Jean-François Eléouët
INRA, Unité de Virologie et Immunologie Moléculaires, Jouy-en-Josas, France

Sabine Riffault
INRA, Unité de Virologie et Immunologie Moléculaires, Jouy-en-Josas, France

John Pringle
Department of Clinical Sciences, Swedish University of Agricultural Sciences, Host Pathogen Interaction Group, Uppsala, Sweden

Geraldine Taylor
The Pirbright Institute, Pirbright, Surrey, UK

Jean François Valarcher
Department of Clinical Sciences, Swedish University of Agricultural Sciences, Host Pathogen Interaction Group, Uppsala, Sweden
Department of Virology, National Veterinary Institute, Immunology, and Parasitology, Uppsala, Sweden

Shengguo Zhao
Ministry of Agriculture Laboratory of Quality & Safety Risk Assessment for Dairy Products (Beijing), Institute of Animal Science, Chinese Academy of Agricultural Sciences, No. 2 Yuanyingyuan West Road, Beijing 100193, PR China
State Key Laboratory of Animal Nutrition, Institute of Animal Science, Chinese Academy of Agricultural Sciences, No. 2 Yuanyingyuan West Road, Beijing 100193, PR China

Jiaqi Wang
Ministry of Agriculture Laboratory of Quality & Safety Risk Assessment for Dairy Products (Beijing), Institute of Animal Science, Chinese Academy of Agricultural Sciences, No. 2 Yuanyingyuan West Road, Beijing 100193, PR China
State Key Laboratory of Animal Nutrition, Institute of Animal Science, Chinese Academy of Agricultural Sciences, No. 2 Yuanyingyuan West Road, Beijing 100193, PR China

Nan Zheng
Ministry of Agriculture Laboratory of Quality & Safety Risk Assessment for Dairy Products (Beijing), Institute of Animal Science, Chinese Academy of Agricultural Sciences, No. 2 Yuanyingyuan West Road, Beijing 100193, PR China
State Key Laboratory of Animal Nutrition, Institute of Animal Science, Chinese Academy of Agricultural Sciences, No. 2 Yuanyingyuan West Road, Beijing 100193, PR China

Dengpan Bu
State Key Laboratory of Animal Nutrition, Institute of Animal Science, Chinese Academy of Agricultural Sciences, No. 2 Yuanyingyuan West Road, Beijing 100193, PR China

Peng Sun
State Key Laboratory of Animal Nutrition, Institute of Animal Science, Chinese Academy of Agricultural Sciences, No. 2 Yuanyingyuan West Road, Beijing 100193, PR China

Zhongtang Yu
Department of Animal Sciences, The Ohio State University, Columbus, OH 43210, USA

Marilda Onghero Taffarel
Veterinary Medicine Department, Universidade Estadual de Maringá, Estrada da Paca s/n, Umuarama, Brazil

Stelio Pacca Loureiro Luna
Department of Veterinary Surgery and Anesthesiology, College of Veterinary Medicine and Animal Science, UNESP – Univ Estadual Paulista, Botucatu, SP 18618970, Brazil

Flavia Augusta de Oliveira
Department of Veterinary Surgery and Anesthesiology, College of Veterinary Medicine and Animal Science, UNESP – Univ Estadual Paulista, Botucatu, SP 18618970, Brazil

Guilherme Schiess Cardoso
Department of Veterinary Surgery and Anesthesiology, College of Veterinary Medicine and Animal Science, UNESP – Univ Estadual Paulista, Botucatu, SP 18618970, Brazil

Juliana de Moura Alonso
Department of Veterinary Surgery and Anesthesiology, College of Veterinary Medicine and Animal Science, UNESP – Univ Estadual Paulista, Botucatu, SP 18618970, Brazil

Jose Carlos Pantoja
Department of Veterinary Surgery and Anesthesiology, College of Veterinary Medicine and Animal Science, UNESP – Univ Estadual Paulista, Botucatu, SP 18618970, Brazil

Juliana Tabarelli Brondani
Department of Veterinary Surgery and Anesthesiology, College of Veterinary Medicine and Animal Science, UNESP – Univ Estadual Paulista, Botucatu, SP 18618970, Brazil

Emma Love
School of Veterinary Science, Langford House, Langford, UK

Polly Taylor
Taylor Monroe, Ely, Cambridgeshire, UK

Kate White
School of Veterinary Medicine and Science, University of Nottingham, Nottingham, UK

Joanna C Murrell
School of Veterinary Science, Langford House, Langford, UK

Karol Stasiak
Department of Virology, National Veterinary Research Institute, Al. Partyzantow 57, 24-100 Pulawy, Poland

Jerzy Rola
Department of Virology, National Veterinary Research Institute, Al. Partyzantow 57, 24-100 Pulawy, Poland

Gabor Ploszay
Department of Virology, National Veterinary Research Institute, Al. Partyzantow 57, 24-100 Pulawy, Poland

Wojciech Socha
Department of Virology, National Veterinary Research Institute, Al. Partyzantow 57, 24-100 Pulawy, Poland

Jan F Zmudzinski
Department of Virology, National Veterinary Research Institute, Al. Partyzantow 57, 24-100 Pulawy, Poland

Kathrin Mählmann
Clinic for Horses, University of Veterinary Medicine Hannover, Foundation, Hannover, Germany

Karsten Feige
Clinic for Horses, University of Veterinary Medicine Hannover, Foundation, Hannover, Germany

Christiane Juhls
Mologen AG, Berlin, Germany

Anne Endmann
Mologen AG, Berlin, Germany

Hans-Joachim Schuberth
Immunology Unit, University of Veterinary Medicine Hannover, Foundation, Hannover, Germany

Detlef Oswald
Mologen AG, Berlin, Germany

Mareu Hellige
Clinic for Horses, University of Veterinary Medicine Hannover, Foundation, Hannover, Germany

Marcus Doherr
Institute for Veterinary Epidemiology and Biostatistics, Free University of Berlin, Berlin, Germany

Jessika-MV Cavalleri
Clinic for Horses, University of Veterinary Medicine Hannover, Foundation, Hannover, Germany

Ulrich Walliser
Clinic for Horses Kirchheim, Nuertingerstrasse 200, 73230 Kirchheim, Germany

Albrecht Fenner
Boehringer Ingelheim Vetmedica GmbH, 55216 Ingelheim am Rhein, Germany

Nicole Mohren
Boehringer Ingelheim Vetmedica GmbH, 55216 Ingelheim am Rhein, Germany

Thomas Keefe
Department of Environmental & Radiological Health Sciences, College of Veterinary Medicine & Biomedical Sciences, Colorado State University, Fort Collins, USA

Frerich deVries
Boehringer Ingelheim Vetmedica GmbH, 55216 Ingelheim am Rhein, Germany

Chris Rundfeldt
Drug-Consulting Network, 01445 Coswig, Germany

Joren Verbeke
M-team and Mastitis and Milk Quality Research Unit, Department of Reproduction, Obstetrics, and Herd Health, Faculty of Veterinary Medicine, Ghent University, Salisburylaan, 133 Merelbeke, Belgium

Xanthippe Boulougouris
Department of Comparative Physiology and Biometrics, Faculty of Veterinary Medicine, Ghent University, Salisburylaan, 133 Merelbeke, Belgium

Carolien Rogiers
Department of Comparative Physiology and Biometrics, Faculty of Veterinary Medicine, Ghent University, Salisburylaan, 133 Merelbeke, Belgium

Christian Burvenich
Department of Comparative Physiology and Biometrics, Faculty of Veterinary Medicine, Ghent University, Salisburylaan, 133 Merelbeke, Belgium

Luc Peelman
Animal Genetics Laboratory, Department of Nutrition, Genetics, and Ethology, Faculty of Veterinary Medicine, Ghent University, Heidestraat, 19 Merelbeke, Belgium

Bart De Spiegeleer
Laboratory of Drug Quality & Registration, Department of Pharmaceutical Analysis, Faculty of Pharmaceutical Sciences, Ghent University, Ottergemsesteenweg, 460 Ghent, Belgium

Sarne De Vliegher
M-team and Mastitis and Milk Quality Research Unit, Department of Reproduction, Obstetrics, and Herd Health, Faculty of Veterinary Medicine, Ghent University, Salisburylaan, 133 Merelbeke, Belgium